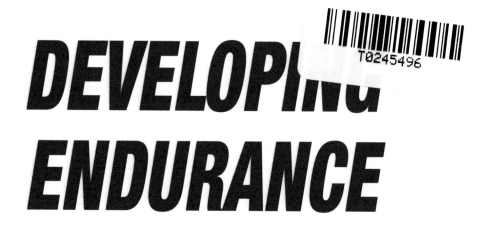

DEVELOPING ENDURANCE

SECOND EDITION

National Strength and Conditioning Association

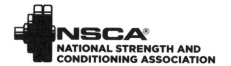

NSCA®
NATIONAL STRENGTH AND
CONDITIONING ASSOCIATION

Ben Reuter

EDITOR

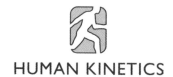

HUMAN KINETICS

Library of Congress Cataloging-in-Publication Data

Names: Reuter, Ben, editor. | National Strength & Conditioning Association
  (U.S.)
Title: Developing endurance / National Strength and Conditioning
  Association (NSCA) ; Ben Reuter, editor.
Description: Second edition. | Champaign, IL : Human Kinetics, [2025] |
  Series: Sport performance series | Previous edition published in 2012. |
  Includes bibliographical references and index.
Identifiers: LCCN 2023058696 (print) | LCCN 2023058697 (ebook) | ISBN
  9781718206960 (paperback) | ISBN 9781718206977 (epub) | ISBN
  9781718206984 (pdf)
Subjects: LCSH: Physical fitness. | Physical education and
  training--Physiological aspects. | Exercise--Physiological aspects. |
  Endurance sports. | BISAC: SPORTS & RECREATION / Training | HEALTH &
  FITNESS / Exercise / Strength Training
Classification: LCC GV481 .D47 2025 (print) | LCC GV481 (ebook) | DDC
  613.7--dc23/eng/20240212
LC record available at https://lccn.loc.gov/2023058696
LC ebook record available at https://lccn.loc.gov/2023058697

ISBN: 978-1-7182-0696-0 (print)

Copyright © 2025, 2012 by National Strength and Conditioning Association

This publication is written and published to provide accurate and authoritative information relevant to the subject matter presented. It is published and sold with the understanding that the author and publisher are not engaged in rendering legal, medical, or other professional services by reason of their authorship or publication of this work. If medical or other expert assistance is required, the services of a competent professional person should be sought.

The web addresses cited in this text were current as of November 2023, unless otherwise noted.

Senior Acquisitions Editor: Roger W. Earle; **Managing Editors:** Kevin Matz and Shawn Donnelly; **Copyeditor:** Marissa Wold Uhrina; **Indexer:** Ferreira Indexing; **Permissions Manager:** Laurel Mitchell; **Graphic Designer:** Denise Lowry; **Cover Designer:** Keri Evans; **Cover Design Specialist:** Susan Rothermel Allen; **Photographs (cover):** Nastasic/E+/Getty Images (weightlifter), Hero Images Digital Vision/Getty Images (cyclist), and .shock/fotolia.com (runner); **Photographs (interior):** © Human Kinetics, unless otherwise noted; **Photo Asset Manager:** Laura Fitch; **Photo Production Specialist:** Amy M. Rose; **Photo Production Manager:** Jason Allen; **Senior Art Manager:** Kelly Hendren; **Illustrations:** © Human Kinetics, unless otherwise noted; **Printer:** Versa Press

We thank Matthew Sandstead, NSCA-CPT,*D, Scott Caulfield, MA, CSCS,*D, TSAC-F,*D, RSCC*E, and the National Strength and Conditioning Association (NSCA) in Colorado Springs, Colorado, for overseeing (Matthew and Scott) and hosting (NSCA) the photo shoot for this book.

Human Kinetics books are available at special discounts for bulk purchase. Special editions or book excerpts can also be created to specification. For details, contact the Special Sales Manager at Human Kinetics.

Printed in the United States of America   10 9 8 7 6 5 4 3 2 1

The paper in this book is certified under a sustainable forestry program.

Human Kinetics
1607 N. Market Street
Champaign, IL 61820
USA

United States and International
Website: **US.HumanKinetics.com**
Email: info@hkusa.com
Phone: 1-800-747-4457

Canada
Website: **Canada.HumanKinetics.com**
Email: info@hkcanada.com

E8341

DEVELOPING ENDURANCE

SECOND EDITION

Contents

Introduction

There are multiple reasons people across the world train and compete in endurance sports: for recreation, as a profession, for competition, or to raise money for charity. Since the publication of the first edition of this book, endurance sport participation continues to be popular, and additional endurance events have developed. For example, the sport of cycling now has gravel racing and a growing number of Gran Fondos, a type of long-distance cycling event, for beginner cyclists through professionals. Additionally, the sport of obstacle course racing (chapter 12) has become much more common, with a variety of event distances and obstacles.

Knowledge of proper training programs and techniques for endurance training is still catching up with participation. A properly designed training program is essential for athletes to be able to enjoy endurance activities as much as possible, minimize the risk of injury, and maximize performance for those individuals who are competing.

Many endurance activities involve some amount of running. According to various research studies, as many as 75 to 80 percent of runners are injured each year; an injury is defined as something that causes the runner to miss one or more days of training. Often these injuries occur because of improperly designed training and conditioning programs. The information provided in this book can be a valuable tool to help the endurance coach or self-coached athlete develop an effective training program.

When training for endurance events, many people do not consider the importance of overall physical fitness. Physical fitness consists of three main training components: cardiorespiratory (or aerobic) training, resistance training, and flexibility training. Each component has a valuable place in a properly designed program for the endurance athlete.

Endurance sports are activities that require a high level of muscular endurance. This is achieved primarily through aerobic activities—running, cycling, swimming, and so on. The muscles are trained to contract repeatedly at a submaximal level without fatiguing. Some endurance training programs focus almost exclusively on aerobic training, using a "more is better" approach. This approach often leads to the exclusion of other aspects of fitness because athletes and coaches do not think they have time to devote to other areas. Well-trained endurance athletes do need a high level of aerobic conditioning, but long-term avoidance or minimization of the other components of overall fitness—especially resistance training—can lead to performance plateaus and chronic injuries. Most people who participate in endurance sports are recreational athletes, so overall physical fitness is an important part of maintaining a high quality of life. As a person ages, muscular strength (the ability to produce force) and power (the ability to produce force rapidly) decrease. Endurance training maximizes the ability to produce repeated submaximal muscle contractions, but it does very little to maintain or increase muscular strength or power. Thus, resistance training is a necessary component.

Endurance sports are unique. Participants have a wide range of body types, age, and experience. For example, it is not unusual for marathoners to finish in times ranging from less than 2.5 hours to over 7 hours. The age of these finishers often ranges from less than 20 years old to well over 70 years of age. Some of the participants are first-time finishers, but other participants may have previously completed numerous marathon races. No matter what the body type, age, or experience, they all complete the same event over the same terrain. Each participant needs to have adequate physical conditioning, skill, and mental fortitude to successfully complete the event.

This book is designed for endurance coaches who are looking to update or expand their expertise and also knowledgeable individuals who may be looking to improve their competition performance or be involved in an endurance activity simply for enjoyment, with no intention of ever competing in an official event or competition. Regardless of intent, the information in this book will benefit everyone from the novice who trains for health and fitness to the experienced competitor who is trying to maximize performance.

In the past, endurance coaches and athletes may not have been aware of the National Strength and Conditioning Association (NSCA) or may not have known that NSCA members could offer training knowledge relevant to endurance athletes. By the same token, many NSCA members may not have recognized that their knowledge and skills would be valuable to endurance athletes. This book takes advantage of each contributor's expertise to address all those concerns. All the contributors were selected not only for their professional knowledge but also because they practice what they preach. The About the Contributors section at the end of the book shows that the contributors are not only experts on endurance training programs but also active participants in endurance sports.

Chapter 1 provides an overview of physiology as it pertains to physical activity. It also provides information related specifically to endurance activity, which will be especially valuable for those readers without a background in endurance sports.

Chapter 2 covers testing and assessment and provides a valuable source of information that can be used to determine baseline fitness for later comparisons or whether a training program is optimally effective.

Chapter 3 provides a summary of endurance training principles with an emphasis on explaining proper program design through periodization, which is the systematic manipulation of exercise parameters (volume, intensity, and duration). Periodized training is designed to maximize healthy physiological adaptations and minimize the negative effects of too much exercise or too little recovery.

Chapter 4 has extensive information about aerobic endurance development, which is essential for many sports.

Chapter 5 is an excellent introduction to resistance training exercises specific to endurance sports. One of the highlights of this book is the detailed information on resistance training as a tool to enhance the endurance athlete's training and performance.

Chapter 6 provides explanations of resistance training programming, with practical examples of how resistance training should be incorporated into a well-designed endurance training program.

Often, warm-up methods are ignored or briefly covered when designing endurance training programs. Chapter 7 is new to the second edition. It has extensive information about the importance of warming up to increase training performance and potentially reduce risk of injury.

Chapters 8 through 12 address running, cycling, swimming, triathlon, and obstacle course racing individually with the obstacle course racing chapter being new to this edition. These chapters include sample training programs and extensive information on sport-specific program design. Of note, the triathlon chapter was largely expanded for the new edition.

Chapter 13 covers the fundamentals of recovery, defined as the process by which the body returns to resting levels after a disruption in homeostasis. The chapter also briefly touches on the subject of overtraining.

Endurance sports continue to be a growing activity worldwide, and the dissemination of knowledge to coaches and participants is essential to make the sports as safe and enjoyable as possible. This book updates and expands the information in the first edition to promote the learning of training information that is supported by science.

CHAPTER 1

Physiology of Endurance Sport Training

Randy Wilber

This chapter provides you with the basic knowledge of exercise physiology needed for coaching or participating in endurance-based sporting activities. Understanding this information is important for people who are active competitors or people who participate in endurance activities for health and recreation. A significant amount of chemical energy is expended when a person trains for and competes in endurance-based sporting events. Therefore, we begin this chapter with a discussion of energy production. Some basic questions will get us started:

- ▶ What exactly is "energy"?
- ▶ How is energy produced and used in an endurance athlete's body?

This chapter answers those questions using the basic sciences of biology and biochemistry, but for readers who are less knowledgeable about those concepts, nonscientific analogies are also provided.

ENERGETICS: THE THREE METABOLIC SYSTEMS

The basic unit of energy within the human body is adenosine triphosphate (ATP) (1, 8, 9). To make things simple, think of a molecule of ATP as an "energy dollar bill." Each of us has millions of molecules of ATP in our body, providing us with energy. We are constantly using and replenishing ATP, even when we are not exercising. Based on this money analogy, ATP usage and production can be likened to a daily scenario in which we earn and spend money to maintain our lifestyle.

The molecular structure of ATP is shown in figure 1.1. ATP is made up of three unique subunits (1, 8, 9): adenine, ribose, and the phosphate groups. Rather than memorize the structure of ATP, focus your attention on the wavy lines that connect the three phosphate groups. Each of these wavy lines represents a high-energy bond.

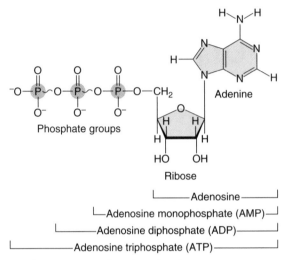

Figure 1.1 Structure of adenosine triphosphate (ATP).

Figure 1.2 shows the basic biochemical reaction whereby ATP releases energy. A single molecule of ATP is represented on the left side of the reaction. Accessing the energy from the ATP molecule requires water and the enzyme ATPase. In this reaction, one of its high-energy bonds is broken or cleaved, which releases a burst of chemical energy. This burst of chemical energy can be used for all the important physiological functions, including nerve transmission, blood circulation, tissue synthesis, glandular secretion, digestion, and skeletal muscle contraction (which we will focus on later in this chapter). When this reaction breaks a bond in ATP, it creates a molecule of adenosine diphosphate (ADP) and an inorganic phosphate molecule (P_i) (1, 8, 9).

The body has three energy systems (4, 5, 8) (see figure 1.3): the immediate (phosphagen or ATP-CP system), short-term (glycolysis), and long-term (oxidative phosphorylation) systems. The three systems differ in how quickly they replenish ATP and in the amount of ATP produced. Two of the three systems—the phosphagen and glycolytic energy systems—are anaerobic energy systems. In other words, they do not require oxygen to produce ATP (4, 5, 8). In contrast, the long-term oxidative energy system is aerobic and requires oxygen to produce ATP (4, 5, 8).

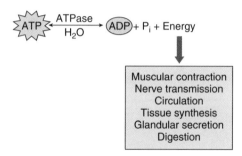

Figure 1.2 Biochemical conversion of ATP to ADP + P_i + energy.

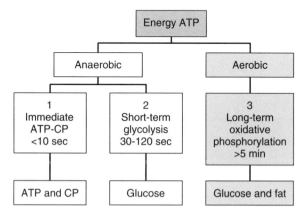

Figure 1.3 The three energy systems.

The technical name for the phosphagen energy system is the ATP-CP system (ATP stands for *adenosine triphosphate*, and CP stands for *creatine phosphate*) (4, 5, 8). The biochemical reactions involved in the phosphagen energy system are shown in figure 1.4. Notice that the first reaction is the same one that was described earlier for the conversion of ATP to chemical energy (figure 1.2). Again, one of the high-energy bonds is cleaved (broken) in that reaction. As a result, ATP, which contained three phosphate groups, is converted to adenosine diphosphate (ADP), which contains two phosphate groups, plus inorganic phosphate (P_i) and energy, and an H+ ion is released. As shown in figure 1.4, ADP is not thrown away after the initial reaction. It goes through a recycling process with CP, which has one phosphate group. The CP donates its phosphate group to ADP (two phosphate groups) to produce a new molecule of ATP (three phosphate groups), leaving a molecule of creatine (CR), which will later bond with another molecule of phosphate (4, 5, 8).

Using our money analogy, the immediate energy system is similar to the money in a person's wallet:

▶ The person can access and use the money immediately.

▶ However, the person has a very limited amount of money.

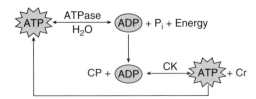

Figure 1.4 The two basic biochemical reactions of the phosphagen energy system (ATP-CP): (1) the release of energy from the breakdown of ATP to ADP and (2) the resynthesis of ATP from a "recycled" ADP and a phosphate donated from CP.

Similarly, the phosphagen energy system has the advantage of producing ATP very quickly but the disadvantage of producing a very limited supply of ATP. In terms of athletic performance, the phosphagen energy system is the dominant energy system during very high-intensity, short-duration exercise lasting approximately 10 seconds or less. Examples of athletic events in which the phosphagen energy system is dominant include the 100-meter sprint in track, a 10-meter diving event, and weightlifting events.

Like the phosphagen energy system, the glycolytic energy system is anaerobic (4, 5, 8). The glycolytic energy system gets its name in reference to the first of several biochemical reactions involved in the conversion of glycogen (stored glucose) to free glucose. A simplified version of the glycolytic energy system is shown in figure 1.5. One molecule of glucose is converted to two molecules of pyruvate; then, in the absence of oxygen, the two molecules of pyruvate are converted to two molecules of lactate. Most important, notice that two molecules of ATP are also produced (4, 5, 8).

Again using our money analogy, the glycolytic energy system is similar to the money that a person has in a checking account:

▶ The person has a larger amount of money available, compared to money in the person's wallet.

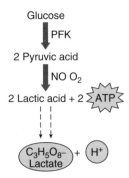

Figure 1.5 A simplified version of the biochemical reactions involving the glycolytic energy system. (PFK stands for *phosphofructokinase*.)

▸ However, accessing money from a checking account takes a little longer because the account holder must write out the check and then get it cashed at a bank.

Similarly, the glycolytic energy system has the advantage of producing more ATP than the phosphagen energy system but the disadvantage of taking a little more time to do so. Another disadvantage is that the glycolytic energy system produces lactic acid, which is quickly converted to lactate and positively charged hydrogen ions (H+) (1, 9) (refer to figure 1.5). High concentrations of H+ create the acidic burning sensation in exercising skeletal muscle and contribute along with other biochemical, neural, and biomechanical factors to premature fatigue (1). In terms of athletic performance, the glycolytic energy system is the dominant energy system during high-intensity, moderate-duration exercise lasting approximately 30 to 120 seconds. Examples include the 400-meter sprint in track, the 100-meter sprint in swimming, and the 1,000-meter track event in cycling.

The oxidative energy system is aerobic and requires oxygen to produce ATP (4, 5, 8). The technical name for this energy system is *oxidative phosphorylation*. A simplified version of this relatively complex energy system is shown in figure 1.6. Notice that the oxidative energy system starts out the same way as the glycolytic energy system—that is, a single molecule of glucose is converted to two molecules of pyruvate. However, because sufficient oxygen is available, pyruvate is not converted to lactate as in the glycolytic energy system. Rather, pyruvate enters one of many mitochondria in the cell (see figure 1.7) and is converted to acetyl coenzyme A (acetyl CoA); it then goes through a series of biochemical reactions—Krebs cycle and electron transport system (ETS)—that ultimately produces approximately 32 molecules of ATP (4, 5, 8).

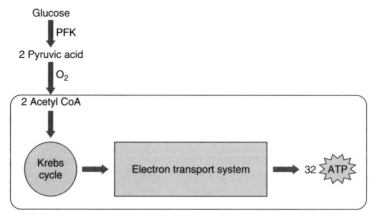

Figure 1.6 A simplified version of the biochemical reactions involved in the oxidative energy system. (PFK stands for *phosphofructokinase*.)

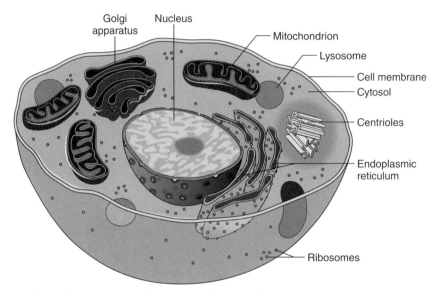

Figure 1.7 Cell structure showing several mitochondria.

Using our money analogy, the oxidative energy system is similar to the money that a person has placed in long-term investments such as mutual funds, stocks, bonds, or IRAs:

▶ The person has a significantly larger amount of money compared to the money in a checking account or the money in a wallet.

▶ However, the person must go through several more steps and must wait longer to access the funds, liquefy them, and turn them into money.

Similarly, the oxidative energy system has the advantage of producing very large amounts of ATP versus the other energy systems; however, this system has the disadvantage of taking more time than the other energy systems to produce that large amount of ATP. The oxidative energy system takes longer because it uses oxygen to produce ATP. The only place in the cell where oxygen can be used to produce ATP is in the mitochondrion, which is essentially a very large ATP factory with several stops on an assembly line. This ultimately increases the time needed for the final production of approximately 32 ATP per molecule of glucose (4, 5, 8).

In terms of athletic performance, the oxidative energy system is the dominant energy system in low- to moderate-intensity, long-duration exercise lasting longer than 5 minutes. Examples of this type of activity include the marathon, the 800-meter swim, and road events in cycling. So, the oxidative energy system is the dominant energy system used during endurance-based training and sporting events. However, athletes need to understand that the oxidative system is not the only energy system used in endurance sports, as we will discuss at the end of this chapter.

CARDIOPULMONARY PHYSIOLOGY

Because endurance-based sports rely heavily on the oxidative energy system, endurance athletes need to understand the basic concepts of cardiopulmonary physiology. The term *cardiopulmonary* refers to the heart and lungs and how those vital organs work in synchrony to ensure that the blood is carrying oxygen and nutrients to the working skeletal muscles during exercise.

Cardiopulmonary Anatomy

The primary anatomical structures of the cardiopulmonary system are the lungs, heart, and capillary beds of the skeletal muscles. We begin our anatomical tour in the lungs. Blood passes through the capillary beds of the lungs, where it unloads carbon dioxide (CO_2) and picks up oxygen (O_2). This oxygen-enriched blood travels from the lungs to the heart via the pulmonary vein. Oxygen-enriched blood initially enters the heart in the left atrium and then flows into the left ventricle. When the heart contracts, or beats, oxygen-enriched blood is ejected from the left ventricle and exits the heart via the aorta. The aorta ultimately branches into several smaller arteries that carry oxygen-enriched blood to the entire body (5, 7, 8).

Once the oxygen-enriched blood reaches, for example, the leg muscles during running, it unloads oxygen and picks up carbon dioxide. Blood exiting the exercising muscles is oxygen reduced and returns to the heart via the venous system. Oxygen-reduced blood is ultimately delivered to the heart via two large veins, the superior and inferior vena cava. The venae cavae deliver oxygen-reduced blood to the right atrium of the heart; the blood then flows into the right ventricle. When the heart contracts, oxygen-reduced blood is ejected by the right ventricle and travels via the pulmonary arteries to the lungs (5, 7, 8).

We have now arrived back at the starting point of our tour of cardiopulmonary anatomy. As the oxygen-reduced blood enters the capillary beds of the lungs, it unloads carbon dioxide and picks up oxygen and then exits the lungs as oxygen-enriched blood via the pulmonary veins (5, 7, 8). This synchrony between the lungs, heart, and tissues occurs constantly, whether the person is awake or asleep. The entire cardiopulmonary system works harder during any endurance-based sporting activity, such as a triathlon.

Oxygen Transport

As mentioned earlier, endurance-based training and sports are heavily dependent on the oxidative energy system for ATP. In the previous section, we referred to oxygen transport in very general terms: oxygen-enriched and oxygen-reduced blood. In this section, we examine oxygen transport in more detail, focusing on the gas physics and physiology of oxygen transport.

The first thing to consider when learning about oxygen transport is how oxygen is carried around in the body. Though a very small percentage of oxygen travels through the body dissolved in the plasma portion of the blood, the primary way by which oxygen is transported through the body is via the red blood cells, also called *erythrocytes*. Figure 1.8 shows the shape of a typical red blood cell. Blood within a person's body contains trillions of red blood cells. The portion of the blood containing red blood cells is referred to as the *hematocrit* (Hct) and is expressed as a percentage of volume of red blood cells relative to the total blood volume. Hematocrits for healthy individuals residing at low elevation range from 35 to 45 percent for women and 40 to 50 percent for men (5, 7, 8).

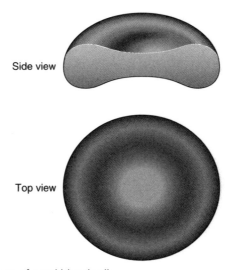

Side view

Top view

Figure 1.8 The structure of a red blood cell.

If we broke open a single red blood cell, we would find that it contains about 250 million molecules of hemoglobin (Hb). The hemoglobin molecule is what transports oxygen throughout the body. A single molecule of hemoglobin can transport 4 molecules of oxygen. Thus, a single red blood cell—and remember, each person has trillions of red blood cells—has the capacity to transport 1 billion molecules of oxygen (5, 7, 8).

Now that you understand that red blood cells—or more specifically, the hemoglobin molecules contained in red blood cells—transport oxygen throughout the body, let's look at how oxygen-reduced blood becomes oxygen-enriched blood in the lungs. The entire process of oxygen transport is regulated by changes in the partial pressure of oxygen (PO_2) that take place from the moment we inhale air through our nose and mouth until the oxygen-enriched blood reaches our body's tissues and organs. PO_2 decreases as inspired air moves from the nose and mouth to the lungs. The decrease is due to the process of diffusion whereby molecules move from an area of higher PO_2 concentration (outside the body) to an area of lower PO_2 concentration (in the lungs). Specifically, the PO_2 of inspired air at sea level is approximately 159 mm Hg (millimeters of mercury), which drops to 105 mm Hg in the lungs (5, 7, 8).

As already noted, blood entering the lungs via the pulmonary arteries contains red blood cells that are relatively low in oxygen content. The PO_2 of this oxygen-reduced blood is approximately 40 mm Hg. This pressure difference, or pressure gradient, in the lungs (PO_2 ~105 mm Hg) compared to the oxygen-reduced blood (PO_2 ~40 mm Hg) favors the diffusion of oxygen from the lungs to the oxygen-reduced blood (see figure 1.9), where it binds to hemoglobin within red blood cells. The diffusion of oxygen from the lungs to the blood takes only about 0.75 seconds and occurs across a very sheer membrane in the pulmonary capillaries that is approximately 1/10,000 the thickness of a facial tissue (5, 7, 8).

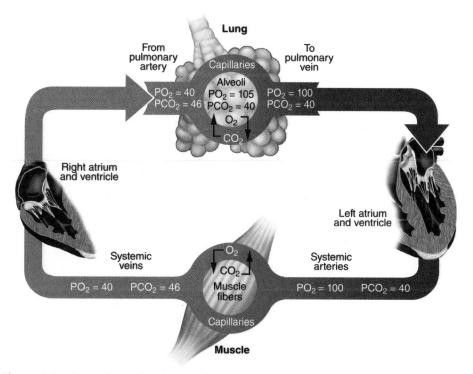

Figure 1.9 Gas exchange between air, lungs, blood, and tissue shows how partial pressures of O_2 and CO_2 drive the exchange.

As a result of the diffusion of oxygen in the lungs, oxygen-enriched blood exits the lungs with a PO_2 of 100 mm Hg. The oxygen-enriched blood is transported via the pulmonary veins to the left ventricle of the heart; the blood is then circulated throughout the body, as discussed earlier. When oxygen-enriched blood arrives at the capillary bed of a skeletal muscle, the pressure gradient favors the release of oxygen from hemoglobin to the skeletal muscle. The oxygen-enriched blood is at PO_2 ~100 mm Hg, and the muscle PO_2 is ~30 mm Hg. The oxygen that is unloaded in the skeletal muscle can now be used by the mitochondria to produce ATP via the oxidative phosphorylation energy system. Finally, the blood exits the skeletal muscle's capillary bed in an oxygen-reduced state with a PO_2 of about 40 mm Hg. The blood returns to the right ventricle of the heart to repeat the process of oxygenation in the lungs and oxygen transport throughout the body (5, 7, 8).

TRAINING EFFECTS ON THE CARDIOPULMONARY SYSTEM

The ability to transport oxygen efficiently is clearly an important factor contributing to optimal performance in endurance sport, which is heavily dependent on oxidative energy production. Of course, one question that immediately comes to mind among athletes is, "Can I improve my cardiopulmonary system and oxygen transport capabilities through training?" The answer is yes.

This section focuses on those beneficial cardiopulmonary training effects. (Chapters 8 through 12 provide specific training programs that help elicit these beneficial cardiopulmonary training effects.) Many cardiopulmonary adaptations occur because of regular endurance training. Regular endurance training is defined as a minimum of 30 to 45 minutes per training session and a minimum of 3 to 5 training sessions per week for at least 8 weeks (4). The beneficial cardiopulmonary adaptations that can occur include the following (1, 5, 8, 13):

▶ Decrease in resting and exercise submaximal heart rate

▶ Increase in cardiac output

▶ Increase in maximal oxygen uptake ($\dot{V}O_2$max)

▶ Improvement in lactate threshold

▶ Improvement in maximal exercise performance

▶ Improvement in exercise economy

▶ Improvement in endurance performance

▶ Improvement in heat tolerance

▶ Improvement in body composition

▶ Decrease in blood pressure (if moderate or high blood pressure exists)

The combined effects of the training-induced improvements in cardiac output, maximal oxygen uptake, lactate threshold, exercise economy, and maximal exercise performance clearly have a positive effect on endurance performance.

However, endurance performance will not improve significantly unless the proper training is done to bring about these cardiopulmonary training effects. The upcoming sections explore some of these benefits in greater detail (1, 5, 8, 13).

Heart Rate

Through regular endurance training, the heart becomes stronger via a progressive overload. Because the heart is stronger, it can pump out more blood with each beat. As a result, the heart does not have to work as hard, and the person's heart rate at rest and during exercise will be lower than it was before beginning an endurance training program (1, 5, 8, 13). During exercise, the person's heart rate will be lower at a specific workload. For example, let's say that the person's heart rate taken immediately after running 800 meters on the first day of training was 175 beats per minute (bpm). After 8 weeks of endurance training, the person's heart rate should be significantly lower after running 800 meters at the same pace that the person ran 800 meters on the first day of training. The exact amount is difficult to estimate because it varies from person to person.

A person's recovery heart rate will also improve because of endurance training (1, 5, 8, 13). Using the previous example, let's say that it took 3 minutes for the person's heart rate to drop from 175 bpm to 125 bpm after running 800 meters on the first day of training. After 8 weeks of endurance training, the person's

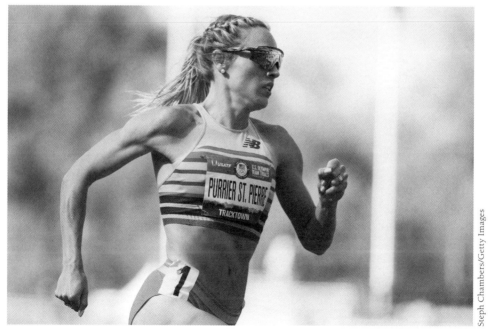

Steph Chambers/Getty Images

Well-trained endurance runners, such as professional track athletes like Elle Purrier St. Pierre, have a high cardiac output that delivers more oxygen to the working muscles.

heart rate will drop from 175 bpm to 125 bpm in less than 3 minutes. Again, the improvement in recovery heart rate will vary from person to person. Despite this individual variability, it is safe to say that after a minimum of 8 weeks of endurance training, the person can expect to see improvements in submaximal heart rate at rest (lower), heart rate during submaximal exercise at the same workload (lower), and the rate of heart rate recovery after a hard effort (less time to recover).

Cardiac Output

Endurance training also increases the level of specific hormones—renin, angiotensinogen, angiotensin, and aldosterone—that regulate the amount of blood in the body. These hormones act to increase the fluid portion of the blood, which is called *plasma*. The overall effect of this hormonal response is an increase in total blood volume. An increase in total blood volume, along with the heart being stronger and more powerful, means that the heart can pump more blood over a specific period of time at the same heart rate (1, 5, 8, 13).

This increase in the amount of blood pumped over a specific time is referred to as an increase in cardiac output. Cardiac output is measured as the amount of blood that the heart pumps through the body in a single minute. An increase in cardiac output is important because more blood is delivered to the brain, liver, kidneys, and other important organs. During endurance exercise, an increased cardiac output is important because more blood is delivered to the working skeletal muscles. As a result, more oxygen is delivered to the exercising muscles for energy, whereas carbon dioxide and other metabolic by-products are removed from the exercising muscles more rapidly (1, 5, 8, 13).

$\dot{V}O_2$max

Endurance training also improves the capacity of the lungs during exercise. This means that the person's respiratory rate (breaths per minute) and tidal volume (liters of air per breath) are improved. These improvements in lung capacity may contribute to an increase in maximal oxygen uptake ($\dot{V}O_2$max). Maximal oxygen uptake is defined as the highest volume of oxygen that a person's body can take in and use for aerobic energy production (1, 5, 8, 13). $\dot{V}O_2$max can be expressed in absolute units (liters of oxygen per minute [L/min]) or relative units (milliliters of oxygen per kilogram of body mass per minute [ml/kg/min]). $\dot{V}O_2$max is usually expressed in ml/kg/min because this relative value allows us to make comparisons between individuals and tells us who is the fittest "kilogram for kilogram" or "pound for pound."

$\dot{V}O_2$max can rise to levels of 65 to 75 ml/kg/min and 75 to 85 ml/kg/min in well-trained female and male endurance athletes, respectively (1, 5, 8, 13). By comparison, typical values for untrained females and males may range from

35 to 40 ml/kg/min and 45 to 50 ml/kg/min, respectively. An improvement in $\dot{V}O_2$max is important because it means that more oxygen is available to the exercising muscles for energy production. Research has shown that a high $\dot{V}O_2$max is one of the most important physiological factors that contribute to success in endurance sports such as distance running, cross-country skiing, and triathlon (1, 5, 8, 13).

Lactate Threshold

Scientific research has also identified a couple of additional physiological factors that are important contributors to endurance performance: lactate threshold (LT) and maximal exercise performance (1, 9). These physiological parameters are typically measured under laboratory conditions.

During a demanding endurance training session or race, the LT represents the point at which the athlete's body requires a greater contribution from the glycolytic energy system (short-term energy system) and a smaller contribution from the oxidative phosphorylation energy system (long-term energy system) (1, 9). As a result of reaching this point, lactate production exceeds lactate removal, and an exponential increase in the athlete's blood lactate level occurs. A relatively high level of lactate is accompanied by a relatively high level of hydrogen ions. As described earlier, these hydrogen ions can have a limiting effect on skeletal muscle contraction, thereby leading to premature fatigue in endurance performance. Thus, endurance athletes should devote a certain amount of their training to improve LT performance capabilities.

In evaluating LT capabilities in triathletes, swimming velocity (m/sec), cycling power output (watts per kilogram of body weight [W/kg]), and running velocity (m/min) are the measurements of interest. For example, by participating in a well-designed endurance training program, a triathlete can expect to see significant improvement in these LT parameters. The athlete will certainly see an improvement in the LT over the course of a single season. In addition, the athlete will probably see improvements in the LT from season to season depending on how many years the endurance athlete has been in training. An improvement in LT allows the maintenance of a higher intensity while still emphasizing the aerobic energy system, thus improving endurance performance.

Maximal Exercise Performance

Maximal exercise performance is simply the objective quantification of an endurance athlete's athletic capability at the point at which the athlete voluntarily stops exercising because of exhaustion (volitional exhaustion) (1, 5, 8, 13). This is determined by the time at the conclusion of a laboratory-based maximal exercise test (e.g., treadmill test). In evaluating maximal exercise performance in triathletes, for example, the same physiological measurements used for evaluating LT are of interest, but they are now measured under conditions of maximal effort instead of LT effort. Like the LT, the higher the level of maximal exercise performance, the better in terms of endurance performance (1, 5, 8, 13). By participating in a well-designed endurance training program, an athlete can expect an increase in the time to exhaustion and maximal exercise performance.

Physiological Economy

Another physiological factor that contributes to endurance performance is economy, which is purported to be a key physiological factor in discriminating between elite versus subelite endurance performance (1, 5, 8). The concept of physiological economy is similar to the concept of fuel efficiency in an automobile. We know that a more economical or efficient car uses less gas at a specific speed and gets greater miles per gallon than a less economical car. The same is true for endurance athletes.

For example, athlete A and athlete B both have a similar $\dot{V}O_2max$ value of 65 ml/kg/min. However, athlete A uses 50 ml/kg/min while running at a pace of 5 minutes per mile in the first half of a 10K race, whereas athlete B uses 53 ml/kg/min while running at the same pace in the first half of a 10K race. Thus, athlete A is more efficient and economical in terms of energy expenditure than athlete B because athlete A uses less oxygen at the 5-minute-per-mile pace. Athlete A should have a competitive advantage over athlete B in the second half of the race because of this better physiological economy. Several factors can improve physiological economy, including a well-designed endurance training program, individual running biomechanics, uphill running, bungee running, and plyometrics training (1, 5, 8).

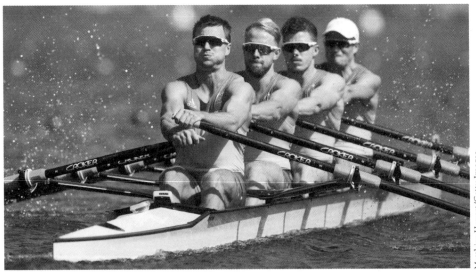

Matthias Hangst/Getty Images

In endurance competitions, having greater physiological economy is essential for success.

Endurance Performance

Research in the area of endurance training has shown that four physiological factors contribute to optimal performance in endurance performance (1, 5, 8, 13). Those factors follow:

- $\dot{V}O_2$max
- Lactate threshold
- Physiological economy
- Maximal exercise performance

Previously in this section, we have seen that a well-designed endurance training program can lead to improvements in each of these four physiological factors. It is not unusual for an athlete to improve in $\dot{V}O_2$max, LT, and maximal exercise performance simultaneously from an early-season laboratory-based testing session to a follow-up laboratory-based testing session done later in the training season (4, 6, 11). Improvement in physiological economy may require some additional specific training, and therefore improvements may not be apparent within a matter of several weeks as with $\dot{V}O_2$max, LT, and maximal exercise performance. Regardless, improvements in competitive performance are to be expected based on a logical and scientific-based endurance training program (3, 10, 13) designed to improve $\dot{V}O_2$max, LT, physiological economy, and maximal exercise performance.

Heat and Humidity Tolerance

A person's ability to work and exercise in heat and humidity is also significantly improved because of endurance training. As mentioned earlier, the body produces more plasma and increases the total blood volume when a person performs endurance training on a consistent basis. Think of total blood volume as radiator coolant in a car or truck. Endurance training leads to an increase in total blood volume, which allows a person to have more "radiator coolant" in the body. As a result, the person can produce more sweat and dissipate heat more effectively from the body, particularly when exercising in a hot and humid environment (1, 5, 8). This is a particularly beneficial effect for endurance athletes who often compete in arid or tropical environments.

Body Composition

Endurance training can lower a person's total body weight and reduce body fat (1, 5, 8). This may not be a major concern for well-trained endurance athletes, because these athletes are typically lean. However, it may become more important as athletes get older, especially when they reach a point when their lifestyle (e.g., job, family, travel) prevents them from training as they did earlier in their career.

Blood Pressure

For individuals with moderate to high blood pressure, regular endurance training can have a significant lowering effect, thereby decreasing the risk of cardiovascular disease and premature death (1, 5, 8). Again, this is probably not a major concern for most well-trained endurance athletes, because their blood pressure is typically normal. However, elevated blood pressure may become an issue as an athlete gets older and becomes less active.

SKELETAL MUSCLE CONTRACTION

The physiological process of skeletal muscle contraction is continually operating during our daily activities, even when we are not exercising. Walking up stairs, lifting a book, or even reading this sentence involves skeletal muscle contraction. Of course, the process of skeletal muscle contraction is extremely active during exercise, and it is an important training consideration for people who compete in endurance sports. As described earlier, when ATP is broken down, it provides the energy needed for several physiological functions, including muscular contraction. This section describes the process of skeletal muscle contraction, focusing on the unique anatomical structure of skeletal muscle fiber and the fascinating step-by-step process of muscular contraction.

Similar to the information presented on energy systems, the information on skeletal muscle contraction may seem very technical, but we will forgo some of the irrelevant details and stay focused on the important features of skeletal muscle contraction. Endurance athletes may gain a new appreciation for the intricacies and synchrony of this physiological process. *Note*: The terms *muscle fiber* and *muscle cell* are used interchangeably in this section.

Skeletal Muscle Anatomy

In describing the anatomy of skeletal muscle, we will move from the macrostructure to the microstructure. Having said that, a good way to think of the anatomical structure of skeletal muscle is to compare it to the cable of a suspension bridge. The cable of a suspension bridge has several internal bundles of smaller-diameter cable wrapped in an overlapping configuration that significantly enhances the strength and stability of the mother cable. The anatomical structure of skeletal muscle is similar: As we probe deeper into the muscle, the muscle fibers are progressively smaller in diameter and are bundled tightly together; the fibers are reinforced by various connective and overlapping anatomical structures that provide additional support.

Figure 1.10 shows the characteristics of skeletal muscle that are similar to the cable of a suspension bridge (5, 7, 8, 9). Notice how the muscle fibers get progressively smaller in diameter from upper right to lower left. Also notice the connective and supportive tubelike structures that surround each sequential layer of skeletal muscle. The smallest segment inside a muscle fiber, shown in figure 1.10, is the myofibril, which contains the basic functional unit of skeletal muscle contraction, the sarcomere (5, 7, 8, 9). To summarize, skeletal muscle is organized into progressively smaller subunits from the whole muscle, to bundles of muscle fibers, to the muscle fibers themselves, and then to microfilaments inside the muscle fibers that make up the myofibrils.

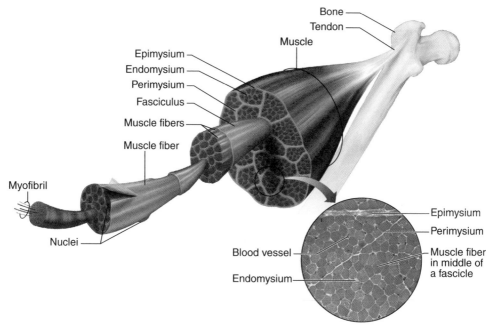

Figure 1.10 Basic structure of skeletal muscle.

A more detailed version of the myofibril and surrounding structures is shown in figure 1.11. Focus on the following important structures that surround each myofibril: transverse tubules (also known as *T-tubules*), sarcoplasmic reticulum, and terminal cisternae (5, 7, 8, 9). These structures are important because they are involved in the initial phase of skeletal muscle contraction, which is called the *excitation phase* (described in the next section). Figure 1.11 also shows the mitochondria, which you learned about earlier in this chapter in the section on the long-term energy system (i.e., oxidative phosphorylation).

Now let's take a detailed look at where the real action of skeletal muscle contraction takes place—the *sarcomere*. Briefly review the various lines, bands, and zones of the sarcomere shown in figure 1.12. The two most important structures in skeletal muscle contraction are *actin* (thin filament) and *myosin* (thick filament) (5, 7, 8, 9). The anatomical structure of myosin is shown in the blowup frame on the bottom left of figure 1.12. A myosin molecule is made up of a tail segment and two large heads (5, 7, 8, 9). An important feature of myosin is that the heads can move. To illustrate this feature, we can compare the structure

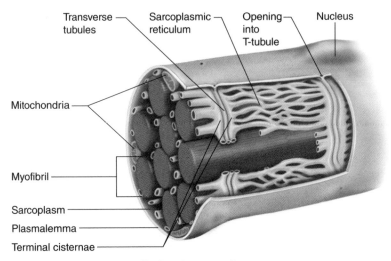

Figure 1.11 Skeletal muscle: myofibril and surrounding structures.

of myosin to the structure of a person's lower arm: forearm (myosin tail), wrist (joint between myosin tail and heads), and hand (myosin heads). Just as the hand can flex, extend, and rotate around, so do the myosin heads. This anatomical characteristic is very important in the process of skeletal muscle contraction.

The anatomical structure of actin (5, 7, 8, 9) is shown in the blowup frame on the middle left in figure 1.12. The actin filament is a double-stranded helix of globular structures like two strands of pearls wound together. A thinner protein strand called *tropomyosin* overlaps the outer surface of actin, and troponin is attached to and positioned at regular intervals on tropomyosin. The bottom half of figure 1.12 shows several actin and myosin filaments in relation to one another. Troponin and tropomyosin are regulatory proteins in a muscle cell, and actin and myosin are contractile proteins. The regulatory proteins help ensure that uncontrolled muscle contractions do not occur, and they prevent uncontrolled binding of actin and myosin.

Phases of Skeletal Muscle Contraction

Now that you are familiar with the anatomical structures involved in skeletal muscle contraction, let's look at the sequence of neural, biochemical, and physiological events that allow skeletal muscle contraction to take place. The process of skeletal muscle contraction occurs in three phases (5, 7, 8, 9), and each of these phases involves several steps:

1. Excitation phase
2. Coupling phase
3. Contraction phase

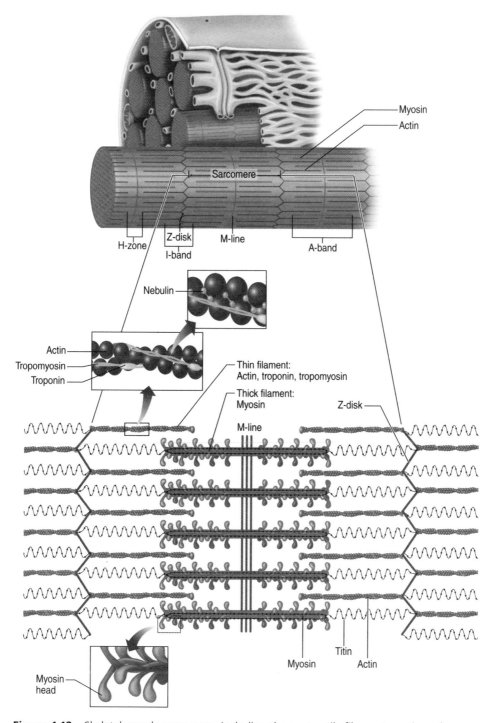

Figure 1.12 Skeletal muscle sarcomere, including the contractile filaments, actin and myosin.

The excitation phase of muscle contraction (see figure 1.13) refers to the neural impulse that serves to spark the sequence of biochemical and physiological steps that result in skeletal muscle contraction (5, 7, 8, 9). The key steps in the excitation phase are as follows (5, 7, 8, 9):

1. Motor nerves embedded in the muscle carry electrical impulses called *action potentials*. These action potentials move through the muscle fiber like electricity traveling along a power line (figure 1.13*a*).

2. The action potential moves along the sarcolemma and down the T-tubules to the sarcoplasmic reticulum (figure 1.13*b*).

3. The action potential triggers the release of calcium ($Ca2+$) from the terminal cisternae of the sarcoplasmic reticulum (figures 1.13*b* and 1.13*c*).

An interesting side note is how lactate affects this process. In the earlier discussion on energy production, associated with high-intensity exercise and anaerobic glycolysis, the rapid breakdown of ATP results in accumulation of positively charged hydrogen ions ($H+$). In addition to other physiological effects, high concentrations of $H+$ can obstruct the release of calcium from the terminal cisternae (1, 9). Essentially, high levels of $H+$ serve to gum up the process of skeletal muscle contraction, thereby contributing to premature fatigue.

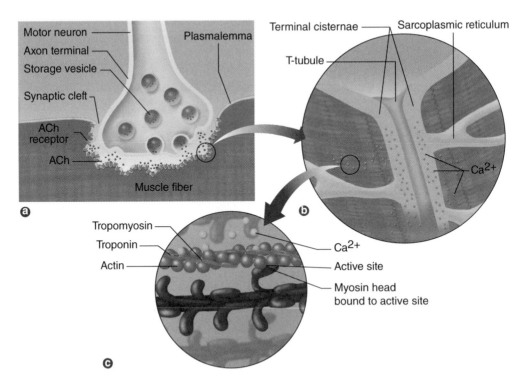

Figure 1.13 The excitation and coupling phases of skeletal muscle contraction.

The coupling phase of skeletal muscle contraction (5, 7, 8, 9) is also shown in figure 1.13c. *Coupling* refers to the interconnection of the contractile filaments, actin and myosin. Here are the key steps in the coupling phase (5, 7, 8, 9):

1. Calcium binds to the troponin complex.

2. The troponin complex changes its shape and configuration, thereby allowing tropomyosin to recede into the space between the actin strands.

3. As tropomyosin recedes from the outer surface of actin, it no longer blocks the outer surface of actin from interfacing with myosin.

4. The binding sites on actin are now fully exposed. The myosin heads quickly attach (couple) to actin at the binding sites.

The contraction phase of skeletal muscle contraction (5, 7, 8, 9) is shown in figure 1.14. *Contraction* refers to the sequence of events in which myosin

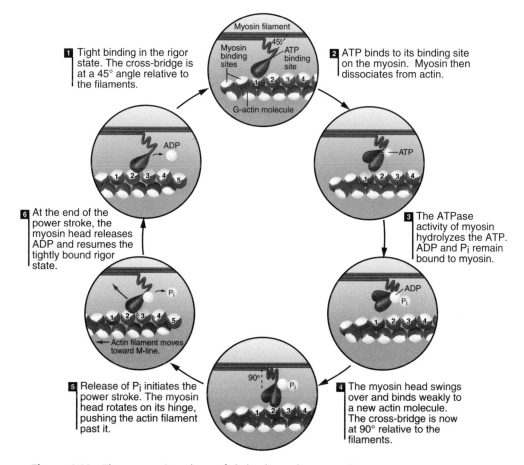

Figure 1.14 The contraction phase of skeletal muscle contraction.

Reprinted, by permission, from W.L. Kenney, J.H. Wilmore, and D.L. Costill, 2021, *Physiology of sport and exercise*, 8th ed. (Champaign, IL: Human Kinetics), 36. Adapted from SILVERTHORN, DEE UNGLAUB, HUMAN PHYSIOLOGY, 4th, © 2007. Printed and electronically reproduced by permission of Pearson Education, Inc., Upper Saddle River, New Jersey.

essentially pulls on actin, thereby drawing the two contractile filaments closer together and resulting in muscular contraction. This phase is usually referred to as the *sliding filament theory*. Remember that the contraction phase of skeletal muscle contraction will not occur unless ATP and Ca2+ are present.

After the contraction phase, the skeletal muscle will return to the relaxed, noncontractile state when the motor neuron stops carrying action potentials, which in turn shuts off the release of calcium from the terminal cisternae of the sarcoplasmic reticulum. Without calcium present, tropomyosin and the troponin complex resume their noncontractile positions—that is, they serve to block myosin from attaching to actin (5, 7, 8, 9). The process of skeletal muscle contraction is one of the most amazing aspects of human physiology.

Skeletal Muscle Fiber Types

Traditional textbooks on exercise physiology typically identify three basic types of skeletal muscle fiber in humans. However, recent research on animals and humans has provided compelling evidence of several additional pure and hybrid fiber types in skeletal muscle. This research is ongoing, and it is possible that changes in how we classify muscle fibers will occur in the future. For this chapter, we focus on the three main skeletal muscle fiber types (2, 5, 8).

▶ *Type I slow oxidative.* Type I fibers rely primarily on oxidative phosphorylation for ATP. These fibers typically have a high level of endurance, or the ability to contract repeatedly without fatigue. The soleus muscle in the lower leg is an example of a muscle with a predominance of type I muscle fibers (6).

▶ *Type IIa fast oxidative glycolytic.* Fibers of this type are often considered hybrids—that is, they have characteristics of both type I and type IIx muscle fibers. The diaphragm muscle contains many type IIa muscle fibers (6).

▶ *Type IIx fast glycolytic.* Type IIx fibers have the potential to produce a great deal of force, but they also have limited endurance because of their heavy reliance on the short-term energy system for ATP. The gastrocnemius muscle in the lower leg contains many type IIx muscle fibers (6).

Most muscles have a certain percentage of type I, type IIa, and type IIx fibers (2, 5, 8). In other words, the soleus muscle is not made up exclusively of type I fibers; rather, the soleus has predominantly type I fibers but also includes lower percentages of type IIa and type IIx fibers. Similarly, the diaphragm muscle is predominantly composed of type IIa fibers, whereas the gastrocnemius muscle is primarily made up of type IIx fibers.

Type I and type IIx fibers have very distinct metabolic features (2, 5, 8). Type I fibers are designed to facilitate oxidative phosphorylation energy production and are found in relative abundance in endurance athletes. In contrast, type IIx fibers are designed to facilitate glycolytic energy production and are found in relative abundance in sprint and power athletes. Type IIa fibers are essentially a hybrid of type I and type IIx fibers and therefore have the capability of producing ATP via oxidative phosphorylation and glycolytic metabolism.

TRAINING EFFECTS ON SKELETAL MUSCLE

Three types of training can alter the physiological and biochemical characteristics of skeletal muscle (3, 4, 6, 8, 10, 12, 13):

- ▶ Aerobic (or endurance) training
- ▶ Anaerobic (or sprint) training
- ▶ Resistance training

The following sections will examine some of the effects that each of these methods of training have on skeletal muscle.

Aerobic or Endurance Training

Endurance training stresses and challenges type I (slow oxidative) muscle fibers more than type IIx (fast glycolytic) muscle fibers. As a result, type I fibers tend to enlarge with endurance training. Although the percentage of type I and type IIx fibers does not appear to change, endurance training may cause type IIx fibers to take on more of the characteristics of type IIa (fast oxidative glycolytic) fibers if they are regularly recruited during exercise (10, 13).

The number of capillaries supplying each muscle fiber increases with endurance training (10, 13). Recall that the capillary bed is a microscopic, mesh-like structure that is embedded deep in the muscle. The capillaries serve as a transfer point through which oxygen and nutrients (e.g., glucose) are delivered to the exercising muscles via arterial blood, while carbon dioxide and metabolic by-products (e.g., lactate and positively charged hydrogen ions) are removed via venous blood. This delivery-and-pickup process is enhanced if the number of capillaries is increased, thereby allowing the exercising muscles to perform more efficiently.

Endurance training increases both the number and size of the mitochondria in skeletal muscle (10, 13). This is particularly true for type I muscle fibers. As described earlier, the mitochondria are microscopic, capsule-shaped units located in the muscle cell (see figure 1.7 on page 6) that are essential to produce ATP via the oxidative phosphorylation energy system (figure 1.6 on page 5). By increasing both the size and number of mitochondria, endurance training enhances oxidative energy production.

The activity of many oxidative enzymes is increased with endurance training (10, 13). Figure 1.6 is a simplified representation of the oxidative energy system. It shows how 2 molecules of acetyl CoA enter a mitochondrion and move into the Krebs cycle, then on to the electron transport system (ETS) to produce

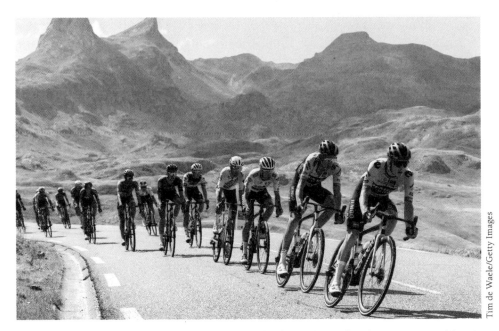

Tim de Waele/Getty Images

Endurance training leads to key physiological adaptations that increase an athlete's ability to compete.

approximately 32 molecules of ATP. The Krebs cycle is a series of biochemical reactions essential to the production of ATP, which are ultimately synthesized in the ETS. Most of the oxidative enzymes that are enhanced via endurance training are in the Krebs cycle phase of the oxidative energy system. Similar to the increase in mitochondria, an increase in the activity of oxidative enzymes serves to enhance oxidative energy production.

Finally, endurance training increases muscle myoglobin content by 75 to 80 percent (10, 13). Myoglobin is smaller than hemoglobin and has many similar structural characteristics. Like hemoglobin, myoglobin's primary physiological function is to transport oxygen. Whereas hemoglobin carries oxygen from the lungs to the exercising muscles via the bloodstream, myoglobin picks up oxygen after it has been dropped off in the capillary bed by hemoglobin. Next, myoglobin transports oxygen to the mitochondria, where the oxygen is used to produce ATP. By increasing myoglobin content, endurance training enhances oxygen delivery within the exercising muscle.

Anaerobic or Sprint Training

Anaerobic training increases ATP-CP and glycolytic enzymes in skeletal muscle (4, 8). Some of these enzymes are shown on page 4 in figures 1.4 (phosphagen energy system) and 1.5 (glycolytic energy system). Similar to the increase in the oxidative enzymes, increases in the ATP-CP and glycolytic enzymes serve to enhance the production of ATP by those two energy systems.

Another benefit of anaerobic training is that it can increase the buffering capacity of skeletal muscle (4, 7, 8). As described earlier, positively charged hydrogen ions (H+) are released via the rapid hydrolysis of ATP in activities that have a high emphasis on the glycolytic system. High concentrations of H+ slow down the release of calcium (Ca_2+) in the excitation phase of skeletal muscle contraction, thereby contributing to fatigue of the muscle. As a result of anaerobic training, the amount of bicarbonate (HCO_3–) in skeletal muscle is increased. As shown in figure 1.15 (7, 9), bicarbonate acts as a very effective buffer for reducing acidosis in the exercising muscle. Bicarbonate essentially picks up excess H+ ions and subsequently removes them from the body in the form of H_2O and CO_2.

$$C_3H_5O_8^- + H^+ + HCO_3^- \longrightarrow H_2CO_3 \longrightarrow H_2O + CO_2$$

Lactate   Bicarbonate

Figure 1.15 Biochemical reaction showing how the bicarbonate buffering system reduces acidosis in exercising muscle.

Resistance Training

Athletes may use various types of resistance training programs (e.g., heavy weight and low repetitions versus moderate weight and high repetitions), and many physiological adaptations occur because of regular resistance training (6, 12). Regular resistance training means a minimum of 3 to 5 training sessions per week for at least 8 weeks. The following are some general effects of resistance training. More detailed information regarding the effects of resistance training on the enhancement of skeletal muscle in endurance athletes is provided in chapters 5 and 6.

An increase in the actual size of the skeletal muscle fiber is known as *hypertrophy*. Most research studies have shown that regular resistance training in combination with an adequate diet will produce skeletal muscle hypertrophy (6, 12). The degree of hypertrophy will vary depending on the specific resistance training program (weight, repetitions, number of training sessions per week, and so on).

Regular resistance training also increases the number of muscle motor units that are active (6, 12). A single *muscle motor unit* is made up of several muscle fibers innervated by a single motor neuron, and stimulates them to contract in unison. To better understand how muscle motor units work, think of a group of 10 athletes pulling on a rope tied to a car. Each individual athlete can be compared to an individual muscle motor unit (in this case, the term *motor* refers to movement, not the motor of the car). If all 10 athletes are pulling hard on the rope, this represents a much stronger "muscle" than if only 5 of the 10 athletes are pulling on it because there are twice as many "active muscle motor units." The same is true in relation to resistance training. After several weeks of resistance training, the skeletal muscle has more active motor units (or people pulling on the rope) than there were before the person started the resistance training program.

Muscular strength is increased because of resistance training (4, 6, 12). *Muscular strength* is defined as the maximum force that is generated by a muscle or muscle group. Muscular strength is usually measured using a one-repetition maximum (1RM) assessment, or the maximum amount of weight that an individual can lift just once. An athlete who can bench press 300 pounds (136 kg) in a 1RM has twice the absolute muscular strength as an athlete who can bench press 150 pounds (68 kg) in a 1RM.

Resistance training also increases muscular power (4, 6, 12), which is not the same as muscular strength. Muscular power is the explosive aspect of strength and is the product of muscular strength and the speed of a specific movement. For example, athlete A and athlete B can both bench press 150 pounds (68 kg) in a 1RM. However, athlete A completes the lift in 2 seconds, whereas athlete B can complete the lift in 1 second. Although athlete B has the same muscular strength as athlete A, athlete B has twice the muscular power because he or she can lift the same weight in half the time.

Muscular endurance is another important performance characteristic for endurance athletes, and this characteristic is also enhanced via regular resistance training (4, 6, 12). *Muscular endurance* refers to the capacity to sustain repeated muscular actions, such as when running for an extended period of time. It also refers to the ability to sustain fixed or static muscular actions for an extended period of time, such as when attempting to pin an opponent in wrestling. Muscular endurance is usually measured by counting the number of repetitions an athlete can perform at a fixed percentage of the athlete's 1RM. For example, if the athlete bench presses 200 pounds (91 kg) in a 1RM, the athlete's muscular endurance can be measured by counting how many repetitions the athlete can complete at 75 percent of the 1RM (150 lb [68 kg]).

PUTTING IT ALL TOGETHER: PHYSIOLOGICAL DYNAMICS DURING ENDURANCE SPORT TRAINING AND PERFORMANCE

Now that we have learned about three critical physiological components of endurance training—energetics, cardiopulmonary function, and skeletal muscle contraction—let's look at how they come together to affect endurance performance. As described previously, ATP can be produced via three energy systems. Although we looked at each of the energy systems separately, this does not mean that only one energy system can function at a time. To understand this concept better, we use the analogy of a symphony orchestra. The orchestra includes several instrument groups, and each group plays softly, moderately, or loudly depending on the musical score.

At the beginning of the symphony, the string group may be loud, the wood-wind group may be moderate, and the percussion group may be soft. These musical emphases may be reversed by the end of the symphony to reflect soft music by the string group and loud music by the percussion group. The same is true for energy production during exercise. Each of the three energy systems is in a state of dynamic flux (4, 5, 8, 9). Like the instrument groups, each of the energy systems is operating constantly during a training session or race, but the systems operate at different levels of ATP production depending on the intensity and duration of the training session or race.

Figure 1.16a shows the symphony orchestra–type effect that takes place for the provision of energy during a cycling road race. During pack riding, the exercise intensity is moderate, and the duration is relatively long. As discussed earlier in this chapter, the dominant energy system during moderate-intensity, long-duration exercise is the oxidative energy system. Although the oxidative energy system is dominant during pack riding, it is not the only energy system that is active. The other two energy systems—phosphagen and glycolysis—are active, but they are "playing softly."

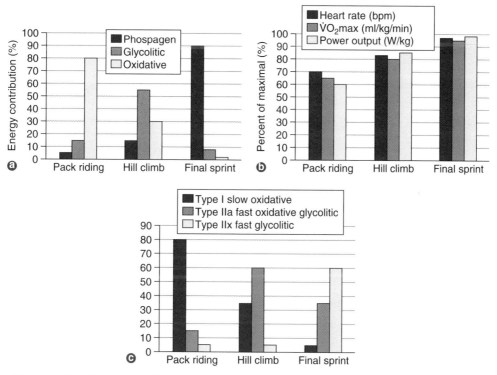

Figure 1.16 Physiological dynamics for (a) energetics, (b) cardiopulmonary function, and (c) skeletal muscle fiber recruitment during a road cycling race.

During a hill climb, the intensity picks up, but the duration is shorter compared with pack riding. This type of high-intensity, moderate-duration exercise requires the glycolytic energy system to play the loudest, the phosphagen energy system to play louder than during pack riding, and the oxidative energy system to play softer. Finally, the energy dynamics are reversed during the final sprint to the finish, which involves exercise at a very high intensity but for a short duration. In this phase, the phosphagen energy system is clearly the loudest, and the glycolytic and oxidative energy systems are relatively quiet.

The symphony orchestra analogy can also be used to describe the physiological dynamics of the cardiopulmonary system during a training session or race. As shown in figure 1.16b, heart rate (bpm), $\dot{V}O_2$max (ml/kg/min), and power output (W/kg) are all at or below 70 percent of maximal during pack riding, indicating a moderate-intensity, long-duration effort. These cardiopulmonary parameters rise during a hill climb with all reaching a level of 80 percent of maximal or greater, reflecting the increased metabolic demands and intensity. Finally, during the final sprint, heart rate, $\dot{V}O_2$max, and power output are close to maximal.

Additionally, this analogy can be used to describe the physiological dynamics of skeletal muscle recruitment during a training session or race. As shown in figure 1.16c, during pack riding, type I slow oxidative muscle fibers are recruited to a relatively high degree reflecting a moderate-intensity, long-duration effort, whereas the type IIa fast oxidative glycolytic and type IIx fast glycolytic fibers are much less recruited during pack riding. This changes during hill climbing when type IIa fibers are heavily recruited, with a decreased recruitment of type I fibers, reflecting a shift from moderate intensity to higher intensity. Finally, during the final sprint, type IIx fibers are recruited to the highest degree, followed by a moderate recruitment of type IIa fibers and minimal recruitment of type I fibers. Notice also how the patterns of energetics (figure 1.16a) and skeletal muscle recruitment (figure 1.16c) tend to be in synchrony during pack riding versus hill climbing versus the final sprint.

Finally, some physiological characteristics predict success in endurance sports. Some of these characteristics are inherent—for example, skeletal muscle fiber type (6). In other words, if you were born with the genetic profile of a sprinter with lots of type IIx fibers, it is unrealistic to think that endurance training can convert most of those type IIx fibers into type I fibers to allow someone to go out and make the Olympic team in the marathon. However, many physiological parameters are trainable and, if trained effectively, can enhance endurance performance. For example, $\dot{V}O_2$max, LT, maximal running velocity (or maximal cycling power output), and economy are responsive to training (1, 5, 8, 13). In addition, an athlete can effectively train each of the three energy systems (1, 5, 8, 13). So, although the oxidative energy system is the most important one for endurance sports, one should not focus exclusively on it in training at the expense of minimal development of the phosphagen and glycolytic energy systems. As this concluding section on the physiological dynamics and interplay of energetics, the cardiopulmonary system, and skeletal muscle contraction has shown, it is important that each "instrument section" within the "symphony orchestra" be fine-tuned via a well-designed and scientifically based training plan that considers each "instrument group" and its important impact on endurance performance (3, 10, 13). Figure 1.17 lists training emphases for energetics, cardiopulmonary function, and skeletal muscle function across five training phases of a competitive season for an endurance athlete.

TRAINING PHASE 1: FOUNDATIONAL CONDITIONING

Energetics
- Training emphasis almost exclusively on developing the oxidative energy system.

Cardiopulmonary
- Training emphasis on developing a robust level of cardiopulmonary fitness that will serve as the foundation for the entire competitive season.
- Immediate focus on enhancing physiological economy.

Skeletal muscle
- Training emphasis almost exclusively on developing the efficiency of type I slow oxidative muscle fibers.

TRAINING PHASE 2: EARLY COMPETITIVE SEASON

Energetics
- Continued training emphasis on developing the oxidative energy system.
- Minor development of the glycolytic energy system will take place via select early season races.

Cardiopulmonary
- Continued training emphasis on enhancing physiological economy.
- Added training emphasis on improvement in $\dot{V}O_2$max and LT capabilities.

Skeletal muscle
- Continued training emphasis on developing the efficiency of type I slow oxidative muscle fibers.
- Minor development of the performance capabilities of type IIa fast oxidative glycolytic muscle fibers will take place via select early-season races.

TRAINING PHASE 3: MID–COMPETITIVE SEASON

Energetics
- Continued training emphasis on developing the oxidative energy system.
- Added training emphasis on development of the glycolytic energy system.
- Minor development of the phosphagen energy system will take place via select mid-season races.

Cardiopulmonary
- Minor training emphasis on enhancing physiological economy.
- Increased training emphasis on improvement in $\dot{V}O_2$max and LT capabilities.
- Added training emphasis on enhancing maximal power output.

(continued)

Figure 1.17 Training emphases for energetics, cardiopulmonary function, and skeletal muscle function across five training phases of a competitive season for an endurance athlete.

Skeletal muscle
- Continued training emphasis on developing the efficiency of type I slow oxidative muscle fibers.
- Added training emphasis on developing the performance capabilities of type IIa fast oxidative glycolytic muscle fibers.
- Minor development of the performance capabilities of type IIx fast glycolytic muscle fibers will take place via select mid-season races.

TRAINING PHASE 4: PEAK COMPETITIVE SEASON

Energetics
- Training to maintain the efficiency of the oxidative energy system.
- Continued training emphasis on development of the short-term glycolytic energy system.
- Added training emphasis on the development of the immediate phosphagen energy system.

Cardiopulmonary
- Minor training emphasis on enhancing physiological economy.
- Increased training emphasis on improvement in $\dot{V}O_2$max and LT capabilities.
- Increased training emphasis on enhancing maximal power output.
- Ancillary training emphasis on heat and humidity acclimatization as needed.

Skeletal muscle
- Training to maintain the efficiency of type I slow oxidative muscle fibers.
- Continued training emphasis on developing the performance capabilities of type IIa fast oxidative glycolytic muscle fibers.
- Added training emphasis on developing the performance capabilities of type IIx fast glycolytic muscle fibers.

TRAINING PHASE 5: POSTSEASON REGENERATION

Energetics
- Training emphasis on maintaining the efficiency of the oxidative energy system.
- Minor training emphasis on maintaining the glycolytic energy system.

Cardiopulmonary:
- Training emphasis on maintaining approximately 65 percent level of fitness in physiological economy, $\dot{V}O_2$max, and maximal power output.

Skeletal muscle
- Training emphasis on maintaining approximately 75 percent level of efficiency of type I slow oxidative muscle fibers.

Figure 1.17 *(continued)*

Assessing Endurance Athletes

Joshua Miller
Will Kirousis

Training programs are traditionally used by competitive athletes to maximize training effectiveness and performance improvement. However, any well-designed training program can also be useful for non-competitive and recreational athletes, allowing these athletes to maximize enjoyment and minimize the risk of injury or overtraining. To measure the effectiveness of an endurance training program, regular testing should be done. The testing may be performed in a laboratory setting, but a field setting is usually more convenient for both the coach and the athletes. Ideally, testing should include measures for aerobic endurance, movement analysis, and muscle endurance. This chapter reviews some common laboratory- and field-testing protocols and the methods used to analyze the data collected during the testing sessions.

Testing for the sake of testing will not provide any guidance for a coach or athlete. For any tests conducted, the information gathered should be used to provide feedback to the athlete. The information gained in testing sessions needs to be shared with the athlete in a timely manner and then used to guide changes in training.

AEROBIC ENDURANCE MEASURES

During most endurance competitions, athletes rely heavily on energy developed through the aerobic system. For this reason, the training plans for many endurance athletes place almost exclusive focus on the development of aerobic fitness and endurance. The $\dot{V}O_2max$ test is the most effective measurement of the body's ability to deliver and use oxygen (O_2). $\dot{V}O_2max$ (also known as *maximum aerobic power*) is the highest amount of O_2 an individual can take

The authors would like to acknowledge the significant contribution of Neal Henderson and Jason Gootman to this chapter.

in, transport, and use to provide *adenosine triphosphate (ATP)* (36). ATP is the stored chemical energy that links the energy-yielding and energy-requiring functions with all cells.

This measurement is important because the more O_2 an individual can use, the more ATP can be produced by the muscles for contraction. For the athlete to move faster, more energy must be available to enable muscles to contract more rapidly, contract with more force, or some combination of these two. Therefore, the more ATP an athlete can produce through the aerobic energy system, the faster the athlete can move in endurance-based events.

Measurement of this variable requires the use of a metabolic cart, a device that measures O_2 uptake and *carbon dioxide (CO_2) production* along with a measurement of breathing volume and frequency. The metabolic cart measures the amount of $\dot{V}O_2$ used, the amount of $\dot{V}CO_2$ exhaled by the athlete, and the volume of air that the athlete is breathing in and out throughout the test. All measures are used to calculate the actual extraction of O_2 from ambient air for use by the muscles to generate usable energy.

The mathematical equation for $\dot{V}O_2$ is equal to cardiac output ($\dot{Q}$) multiplied by the difference of O_2 found in the arterial and venous blood ($a - v\ O_2$ difference) concentrations. This is expressed by the following equation (2):

$$\dot{V}O_2 = \text{cardiac output } (\dot{Q}) \times (a - v)\ O_2 \text{ difference}$$

Cardiac output is determined by the following:

$$\text{Cardiac output} = \text{heart rate (HR)} \times \text{stroke volume (SV)}$$

Therefore, $\dot{V}O_2$ can also be expressed this way:

$$\dot{V}O_2 = (\text{HR} \times \text{SV}) \times (a - v)\ O_2 \text{ difference}$$

As exercise intensity increases, $\dot{Q}$ rises and extraction of O_2 from the arterial blood by the muscles increases. This results in increasing $\dot{V}O_2$. At some point, maximal HR (and therefore, $\dot{Q}$max) is achieved, and $\dot{V}O_2$ plateaus with increasing work rate. The highest rate of O_2 consumption measured is typically defined as $\dot{V}O_2$max. (See the laboratory testing section on how to properly conduct the $\dot{V}O_2$max testing protocol.)

MOVEMENT ANALYSIS AND BIOMECHANICS

Endurance sports are typically not thought of as highly technical endeavors (unlike sports such as golf, baseball, and tennis), but efficient movement during training and competition for endurance sports can affect both performance and health. Most endurance sports movements are repeated hundreds or thousands of times during each training session. Therefore, proper mechanics are critical to an endurance athlete's ability to optimize performance and avoid injury.

Movement evaluation can be performed subjectively using a well-trained eye, or objectively using video capture, a computer, or specialized biomechanics equipment such as pressure sensors, force plates, and three-dimensional computer motion analysis programs (figure 2.1).

Every endurance athlete has a unique physical build and may have strengths, weaknesses, and asymmetries that will dictate personal movement style. However, within each sport, some movement patterns are more efficient. For example, during running, the foot should land nearly underneath the knee to

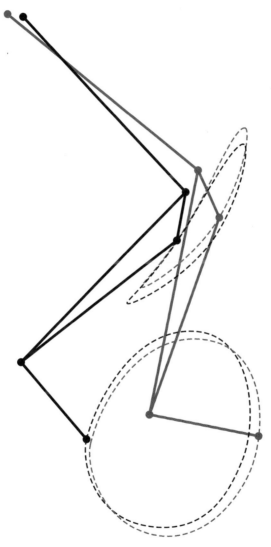

Figure 2.1 This image represents three-dimensional data of a cyclist's pedal stroke. The lower, round tracings are the trackings of the toes, and the upper, oval tracings are the paths that the kneecaps travel. The black line represents the right leg, and the gray line represents the left leg.

reduce braking movement on each stride and to reduce the stress placed on the musculoskeletal system. When cycling, the knee and foot should travel in a vertical path, overlapping one another when viewed from the front. This reduces stress on the knee joint. When swimming, proper mechanics allows the athlete to move through the water more easily by producing less drag and also reduces strain on the shoulder joint.

Coaches and athletes can learn to analyze motion by viewing performances of the proper form and mechanics within their sport. They can do this in person or by reviewing video footage. Keep in mind that the top athletes in each sport do not always use optimal biomechanics and are successful in spite of their technique. Variations from one athlete to another are normal, but coaches should be able to evaluate an athlete's biomechanics and suggest drills and corrections that will help the athlete improve. Coaches often use video to record their athletes' techniques. Video analysis can be used to slow the body movements to a speed that allows viewers to discern small details that the unaided eye might not see. Coaches should review the video with their athletes to reinforce effective movement patterns and pinpoint areas for improvement.

Athletes who do not have a personal coach can do much of this evaluation by themselves or with the help of a partner who can operate the video camera or digital camera. Free or low-cost video analysis programs often come standard on a computer. However, more technical software packages such as Dartfish technology allow for more comprehensive video analysis (including synchronizing multiple camera views, drawing angles, and adding comments or written text on videos).

More sophisticated equipment such as pressure sensors and three-dimensional imaging systems may be available at specialized sports medicine facilities, medical facilities, universities, and other research institutions. The typical thinking is that endurance athletes move the way that they naturally do and should just improve their fitness without worrying about poor mechanics. Although the differences in improved mechanics can be subtle, they are very effective in reducing injury and improving performance.

Movement analysis can also help determine the types of sport-specific and supplemental training, such as resistance training, that can improve performance. Proper analysis should include evaluation of the actual muscle groups being used (prime movers and stabilizers), the type of muscle action occurring (concentric, eccentric, isometric, or a combination of these), the velocity of contraction and movement, the range of motion of the joints, and the type of energy system used to deliver energy (immediate, short-term, or long-term energy system). All these factors should be known before prescribing training and exercises meant to improve an individual's capability and performance.

Figure 2.2 presents a worksheet that athletes can use to perform their own movement analysis. An athlete could complete this form periodically to monitor movement changes and adaptations that can occur with regular training. The best strategy might be to complete the form every 4 to 8 weeks after similar workouts. The form is subjective and can be used for any sport or activity, but it works best for those activities that are repetitive, such as running, biking, and swimming.

Figure 2.2 Movement Analysis Worksheet

Athlete's name: _____ Date: _____

Sport: _____ Location: _____

GENERAL IMPRESSION

_____

_____

_____

_____

_____

SPECIFIC OBSERVATIONS

Range of motion:

_____

_____

Symmetry and asymmetry:

_____

_____

Coordination of movement:

_____

_____

Timing and rhythm:

_____

_____

ADDITIONAL NOTES

_____

_____

_____

_____

_____

From NSCA, 2025, *Developing endurance, second edition* (Champaign, IL: Human Kinetics).

PHYSIOLOGICALLY TESTING THE ATHLETE

Evaluating an athlete's progress outside of actual competition helps determine how to adjust training loads, and it provides important feedback to the athlete during extended periods of training. In addition, some athletes do not compete in events or only compete for a limited number of times each year. For these athletes, routine testing helps ensure that the training they are performing is improving their fitness and their performance potential.

Another reason to include testing in the training schedule is to help build athletes' confidence. Evaluating the changes in performance from one training cycle to another is one of the simplest ways for athletes to gain a mental edge when they compete. Consistent testing can measure performance improvement, which helps keep motivation high. If athletes see improvement, they will be more convinced that the training program is working. Evidence of improvement can also motivate athletes who are not competing regularly. In addition, comparisons can be performed to track fitness and performance levels from season to season and from year to year. In endurance sports, it typically takes many years of dedicated training for athletes to reach their full potential. Initially, the gains are larger, but they tend to decrease over time.

Consideration of where to conduct the testing is important. The advantages of performing testing in the lab include the following:

▶ Testing is completed in a controlled condition, which allows the testing to be reliable.

▶ Submaximal and maximal data can be collected based on the selection of the test.

▶ $\dot{V}O_2$max can be determined.

▶ Threshold intensity can be established upon completion of the testing based on the thresholds determined (e.g., lactate threshold, ventilatory threshold, etc.).

▶ Economy, whether running or cycling, can be determined from serial testing.

▶ Peak power output (PPO) is measured at the end of the test.

▶ Individualized training zones can be established from the test.

The disadvantages of completed laboratory testing include the following:

▶ Performance on an ergometer may not be valid due to improper calibration.

▶ Testing is dependent on the athlete's motivation.

▶ Laboratory equipment is expensive (e.g., metabolic carts cost >$25,000).

- ▶ Testing may be very time-consuming.
- ▶ Testing cannot be performed on a regular basis.

Laboratory testing should be completed several times per year, but data should be collected in the preseason and at the end of the season. Additional testing could be completed at the beginning of the competition phase, and midway through the competition phase. Testing will help to establish goals for the season and to adjust training as necessary.

HOW TO PREPARE FOR TESTING

Prior to testing, whether in the lab or in the field, specific guidelines need to be addressed for the athlete to give their best effort on each test. Before testing, follow these criteria:

- ▶ The day prior should be a very easy training day, or take the day off completely.
- ▶ Do not eat in the 2 hours immediately before the test.
- ▶ Have a standardized nutritional intake 24 hours prior to the test (eat and drink the same foods each time). Ensure a fully hydrated and carbohydrate-loaded state prior to the test.
- ▶ Drink only water or use the same sports drink with every test.
- ▶ Avoid alcohol in the 24 hours prior to testing.
- ▶ Do not test if ill or infected in the previous 2 weeks.
- ▶ If testing outdoors, make sure the weather and road conditions will be similar each time.
- ▶ If testing in the lab on a trainer, follow the manufacturer's guidelines for calibration prior to testing.
- ▶ The data collection sheet should include the time of day and environmental factors (temperature, humidity, and barometric pressure) for comparisons for future testing.

All equipment used for testing should be maintained and calibrated according to the manufacturer's recommendations. Testing conducted with equipment that is not calibrated or is incorrectly calibrated will result in data that are not valid or reliable. If the analysis of a training program's effectiveness is based on data that are not valid or reliable, the analysis will be flawed. Table 2.1 lists different laboratory and field tests that endurance athletes can use throughout the training year to determine whether they are attaining their goals.

Table 2.1 Laboratory and Field Tests

Test	Location of test (lab or field)	Page number
Maximal Oxygen Consumption ($\dot{V}O_2$max) Testing	Laboratory	39
Threshold Tests • Lactate Threshold • D_{max} Protocol Testing • Ventilatory Threshold and Ventilatory Equivalents	Laboratory/Field Laboratory Laboratory	42 44 45
Efficiency—Cycling and Running	Laboratory	46
Critical Power and Critical Speed	Laboratory	47
Functional Threshold Power	Field	48
Lamberts and Lambert Submaximal Cycle Test	Field	49

LABORATORY TESTING

The following sections will describe both the laboratory and field testing for endurance athletes. If the athlete is unable to complete a laboratory test, the athlete should complete a field test that has the specificity of the goal that the coach is trying to obtain for the athlete. Retesting should use the same test in similar conditions to allow for comparisons to be made.

MAXIMAL OXYGEN CONSUMPTION ($\dot{V}O_2$MAX) TESTING

Traditional $\dot{V}O_2$max testing can be conducted using either a continuous or discontinuous protocol. This allows the athlete to complete the test with and without breaks during the different stages (figure 2.3).

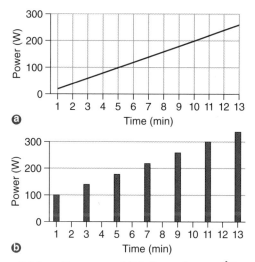

Figure 2.3 Examples of *(a)* continuous and *(b)* discontinuous $\dot{V}O_2$max testing protocols.

The protocols can include those for running, cycling, swimming, or rowing based on the athlete's sport of specialty. Traditionally, when conducting a $\dot{V}O_2$max test it may be difficult to determine if the $\dot{V}O_2$max was reached, so this test might be interpreted as the *highest achieved VO₂ (VO₂peak)*. The $\dot{V}O_2$peak can be determined when the athlete achieves fatigue without achieving the specific criteria for determination of $\dot{V}O_2$max. Depending on their specialized sport, the $\dot{V}O_2$peak may be a better test. For example, a triathlete who is a great runner but may not have a strong swimming physiology base expresses a higher $\dot{V}O_2$max when running in comparison to cycling or swimming, so using $\dot{V}O_2$peak for swimming and cycling would be a better test to use in training prescription.

The most common testing protocol is a continuous protocol in which each step lasts 1 minute. Data that are collected during the test with the use of a metabolic cart include $\dot{V}O_2$, $\dot{V}O_2CO_2$, *maximal heart rate (MHR)*, *minute ventilation (V_E)* (i.e., the maximal amount of air the person is able to breathe in and out at the end of the test), *peak power output (PPO)*, maximal power or watts (W) that can be achieved during a test, and *blood lactate (BLa⁻)* (i.e., a by-product of ATP production that is created during higher intensity exercise, if collected at the end of each stage). If the protocol is a running test, *maximal speed (mph)* will be determined. From the data that is collected, it is possible to determine different thresholds, such as ventilatory threshold (VT), *lactate threshold* (LT), *first ventilatory threshold (VT1)*, and *second ventilatory threshold (VT2)*.

(continued)

Maximal Oxygen Consumption ($\dot{V}O_2$max) Testing *(continued)*

Test Protocol

A traditional $\dot{V}O_2$max test for a running test or cycle ergometer test has similar protocols. The test is administered via an increasing workload (speed or W) when conducted on a calibrated treadmill or cycle ergometer. If the athlete participates in triathlon, consider testing both running and cycling. The reader is referred to the following reference for examples of running, sprinting, and intermittent sprint testing protocols (31).

An example for a cycling protocol is described below:

1. Calibrate the metabolic cart to the manufacturer's specifications.
2. Measure body mass and height prior to testing, and record the data on a data collection sheet.
3. Place an HR monitor on the athlete to monitor HR throughout the testing protocol.
4. Prior to beginning the test, a proper warm-up may be completed to prepare the athlete for exercise.
5. The test begins with a relatively low power output (e.g., 100 W). Power output is increased incrementally. Maintain the pedal cadence throughout the testing protocol at a comfortable range of at least 80 revolutions per minute (rpm).
6. Each stage lasts 1 minute, while power may be increased varying between 10 to 50 watts per stage.
7. At the end of each stage, collect the ratings of perceived exertion (RPE) (28).
8. The test ends when volitional fatigue occurs or the athlete can no longer maintain the starting cadence within 10 to 15 rpm.

The criteria to determine if the test is maximal or not is based on the following factors (2):

1. A respiratory exchange ratio ($\dot{V}CO_2/\dot{V}O_2$; RER) greater than or equal to 1.1
2. A heart rate of ± 10 bpm of the predicted maximal heart rate (220 − age)
3. A plateau of oxygen consumption (less than 2 mL of $\dot{V}O_2$) with an increase in workload
4. An RPE of ≥ 9 (see table 2.2)

Traditionally, an athlete should attain three out of four criteria to determine if $\dot{V}O_2$max has been achieved. Recently, verification tests have been conducted to truly determine if $\dot{V}O_2$max has been met. This test is conducted after the incremental test and a short recovery period. The test is completed as a constant speed run or power output to exhaustion. A comparison will be made between the incremental and constant run (power) tests to determine peak $\dot{V}O_2$ values.

Instructions for the Rating of Perceived Exertion

The $\dot{V}O_2$max test and any additional lab or field test allow the athlete to rate the perception of exertion (i.e., how difficult and demanding the exercise feels subjectively). The perception of exertion is mainly felt as strain and fatigue in the muscles and breathlessness. All work requires some effort, even if it is minimal. Table 2.2 describes the scale from 1 to 10.

Table 2.2   Ratings of Perceived Exertion Scale With Definitions

Rating	Description
1	Nothing at all (lying down)
2	Extremely little
3	Very easy
4	Easy (could do this all day)
5	Moderate
6	Somewhat hard (starting to feel it)
7	Hard
8	Very hard (making an effort to keep up)
9	Very, very hard
10	Maximum effort (cannot go any further)

Reprinted by permission from M. Martino and N.C. Dabbs, "Training Program Design," in *NSCA's Essentials of Personal Training*, 3rd ed., edited for the National Strength and Conditioning Association by B.J. Schoenfeld and R.L. Snarr (Champaign, IL: Human Kinetics, 2022), 432.

A typical maximal exercise test provides not only values of $\dot{V}O_2$max, but also maximal aerobic power (MAP), PPO, and MHR. Peak power output is the maximal work rate during the incremental test and is not the PPO from a sprint. It can be defined as the highest power output completed in the final stage if the entire stage is completed. If the stage is not completed, PPO can be determined using this equation:

$$PPO = Wf + [(t / D \times P)]$$

where Wf is the last completed stage (power/speed), t is the time remaining during the uncompleted stage, D is the duration of each stage in seconds, and P is the workload between each stage. The $\dot{V}O_2$max value is reported in absolute values (expressed in liters per minute [L/min] and relative expressed in liters per minute per kilogram of body weight per min [ml/kg/min]) from the highest 15-second value at the end of the test. The relative value and additional data collected allow for the comparison of other athletes ranging from sedentary to world-class athletes (table 2.3).

Table 2.3 Comparison of Metabolic Variables Collected During a $\dot{V}O_2$ Test in Different Categories of Athletes

Category	Sedentary	Trained	Well trained	Elite	World class
MAP (W)		250-400	300-450	350-500	400-600
Power:weight ratio		4.0-5.0	5.0-6.0	6.0-7.0	6.5-8.0
$\dot{V}O_2$max (L/min)	3.0-3.5	4.5-5.0	5.0-5.4	5.2-6.0	5.4-7.0
$\dot{V}O_2$max (ml/kg/min)	40-45	64-70	70-75	72-80	75-90+

Reprinted by permission from A.E. Jeukendrup and J.A. Hawley, "The Bioenergetics of World Class Cycling," *Journal of Science and Medicine in Sport* 3, no. 4 (2000): 414-433, with permission from Elsevier.

Threshold Testing

Several different thresholds have been described in the exercise physiology literature. Following is a brief explanation of some of the thresholds: the $\dot{V}O_2$ at which arterial (lactate) starts to increase is termed the *lactate threshold* (*LT*) and is also known as the *lactic acidosis threshold* (*LAT*), the *anaerobic threshold* (*AT*), and the *gas exchange threshold* (*GET*). Each threshold describes events resulting from the onset of metabolic acidosis in muscle. The distinction in terminology reflects the method of measurement (3, 4, 39).

LACTATE THRESHOLD TESTING

Lactate profile testing can be performed with or without $\dot{V}O_2$ or indirect calorimetry measurements. As previously mentioned, the method used to determine the threshold point is less important than using a consistent testing protocol. Researchers have found that valid results occur when the testing method involves using 4-minute stages; starting at a level that allows for seven to nine stages of progressive intensity; and monitoring HR, RPE, and BLa⁻ at each stage. In addition, the quality of the lactate-measuring device cannot be overlooked, and daily calibration and proper maintenance help ensure consistent results.

Test Protocol

Lactate threshold is typically performed on a treadmill or cycle ergometer in the lab; however, it can be measured in the field as well (14).

1. Calibrate blood lactate analyzer per manufacturer guidelines.
2. After an adequate warm-up period, the test begins at a low starting workload (speed or W).
3. Each stage typically lasts 4 to 5 minutes, with a small blood sample taken from the finger or earlobe during the last 30 seconds of each stage to determine blood lactate concentration.

4. The test ends when volitional fatigue occurs or the athlete can no longer maintain the starting cadence or running speed.

Figure 2.4 provides the lactate profile of a professional cyclist tested at the start of the season. All stages were 4 minutes long. The top line being plotted is HR (right vertical axis), and the bottom line is lactate level (left vertical axis). Heart rate is linear as workload increases. In other words, a direct relationship exists between HR and workload. Lactate level increases in a linear manner as workload increases until the seventh stage; at that point, a sharp upturn or increase in lactate occurs, indicating LT. The goal of training is to move the upturn to the right on the graph—that is, the goal is for the LT to occur at a higher workload.

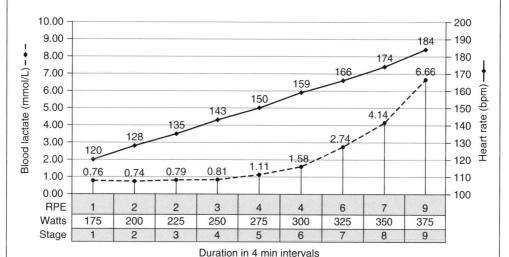

Duration in 4 min intervals

Threshold data		Prescribed training zones					
		By power output (watts)		By perceived effort (RPE)		By heart rate (bpm)	
Power output (watts):	325	Zone 1	<175	Zone 1	<1	Zone 1	<120
Heart rate at LT:	166	Zone 2	175-250	Zone 2	1-3	Zone 2	120-143
Percent of peak heart rate (194)	86%	Zone 3	250-320	Zone 3	3-5	Zone 3	143-164
Mass (kg):	67.3	Zone 4	325-370	Zone 4	6-8	Zone 4	166-180
Power/weight ratio (watts/kg):	4.83	Zone 5	>375	Zone 5	>8	Zone 5	>180

Normal blood lactate resting range: 0.7-2.1 mmol/L

Figure 2.4   Lactate profile of a professional cyclist.

D_{MAX} PROTOCOL TESTING

Upon completion of the LT test, determination of the LT may be difficult to determine using the traditional method described in the previous section. Cheng and colleagues proposed the D_{max} method to overcome the disadvantages of visual, subjective determination of thresholds (7).

The D_{max} is calculated as the maximal perpendicular distance from a curve representing work and lactate variables to the line drawn from the lowest to highest blood lactate points collected during the test (5) (figure 2.5).

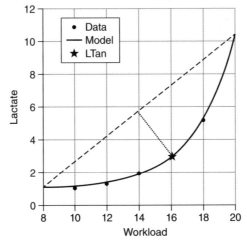

Figure 2.5 Example of D_{max} method for determining LT.

VENTILATORY THRESHOLD AND VENTILATORY EQUIVALENTS

The ventilatory threshold (VT) is the point where the rectilinear rise in V_E breaks from linearity during an incremental test to the maximum. The slope of the line may have two points of rise from linearity (40, 41). These breakpoints from linearity have different names but in the literature have been called the *ventilatory thresholds* (figure 2.6).

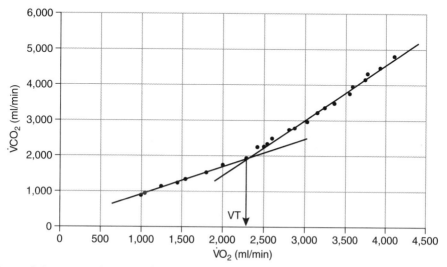

Figure 2.6   Determination of the ventilatory threshold.

The data collected during the $\dot{V}O_2$max test can be used to determine additional thresholds called the *ventilatory equivalent method* using VT1 (estimation of the LT) and VT2 (also called the *respiratory compensation point*). The ventilatory equivalents of oxygen ($V_E/\dot{V}O_2$) and ventilatory equivalents of carbon dioxide ($V_E/\dot{V}CO_2$) are simply the amount of air that moves into and out of the lungs to move 1 ml of O_2 and CO_2, respectively. Plotting these values versus time allows for the determination of VT1 and VT2 (figure 2.7).

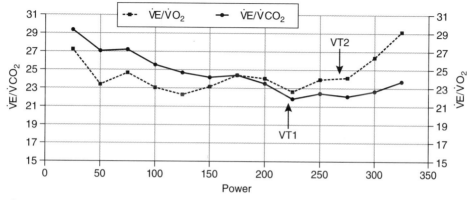

Figure 2.7   Determination of VT$_1$ and VT$_2$ using ventilatory equivalents method.

(continued)

Ventilatory Threshold and Ventilatory Equivalents *(continued)*

Test Protocol

Throughout the $\dot{V}O_2$max testing protocol, V_E, $\dot{V}O_2$, and VCO_2 are collected and can be plotted at the end of the test to correctly define the VT (V_E vs. power output). Graphing V_E will show a disproportionate increase in V_E; this point typically occurs between 55% and 70% of $\dot{V}O_2$max.

Similar data are collected to determine the ventilatory equivalents for O_2 and CO_2. When reviewing the graph of V_E/VO_2 and V_E/VCO_2, the lowest point on the plot of V_E/VO_2 without an accompanying increase in V_E/VCO_2 is determined to be VT1. The second VT or respiratory compensation point is determined at the point prior to an increase in V_E/VCO_2 values.

Normative Data

Table 2.4 Normative Data for LT and VT in Sedentary Individuals and Athletes

Threshold type	Sedentary or untrained	Trained or athlete
Lactate	40-60% of $\dot{V}O_2$max	75-90% of $\dot{V}O_2$max
Ventilatory	40-60% of $\dot{V}O_2$max	70-85% of $\dot{V}O_2$max

CYCLING AND RUNNING EFFICIENCY

Efficiency is a submaximal variable that is measured routinely and relates to the amount of energy required to perform that work. Higher efficiency will decrease the percentage of $\dot{V}O_2$max required to sustain a given amount of mechanical work. This indicates that an athlete is becoming better at the specificity of their sport. Efficiency is the ratio of work generated to the total metabolic energy cost, or delta efficiency, and is expressed as a percentage ratio of the change in work performed per minute to the change in energy expended per minute.

Test Protocol

1. This test requires the direct assessment of $\dot{V}O_2$ during exercise.
2. The athlete completes several (3-4) different running speeds or constant power output during cycling lasting 6 minutes.
3. At the last minute of each stage, O_2 is collected for analysis. At the end of each stage, a brief rest period is taken. All stages must be below the LT.
4. Using the same speeds or power allows for successive comparisons over time to determine any changes occurring due to training.

CRITICAL POWER (CP) AND CRITICAL SPEED (CS)

Critical power (CP) or critical speed (CS) testing provides a form (i.e., power output or running speed) that is more relevant across most physiological systems (anaerobic and aerobic energy systems) (15, 37). The CP and CS models describe power output or speed as a function of time. It is based on how long an athlete can complete a set power output or running speed. Three separate stages can be completed while timing until failure occurs. The models indicate the relationship of the athlete's power to speed or time. This relationship is depicted as a curve (figure 2.8) and can be used to directly establish weaknesses and allow for training to work in these areas.

The equation of the power to speed or time curve follows:

$$P = W' / t + CP$$

The equation demonstrates the sustainable power output (P) and is dependent on anaerobic capacity (W') divided by time (t), added to critical power (CP). Critical power is, in theory, the highest power output that can be sustained for an extended period without fatigue. The reader is referred to Hill (12), Jones and Vanhatalo (19), and Pettitt (32) to read more on CP and CS and how to use it for training.

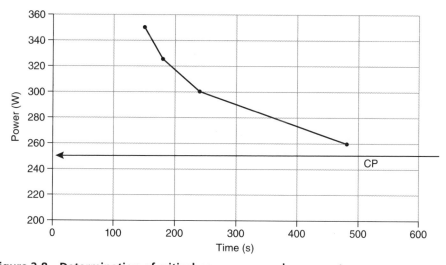

Figure 2.8 **Determination of critical power on a cycle ergometer.**

Test Protocol

For this test, a bicycle with a trainer or treadmill and a stopwatch are needed. Multiple maximal efforts will be necessary for the completion of the test. Three to five trials are usually recommended to allow for a better fit for the test. Recovery between stages can range between 30 minutes to 48 hours depending on the effort.

1. Prior to the test begins a proper warm-up should be completed.

2. The goal is to select three to five different workloads that can be completed in at least 1 to 10 minutes but may last longer, so workloads should not too easy.

3. Upon completion of the test, a proper cooldown should be completed. Heart rate and RPE can be collected for inclusion of data (20).

FIELD TESTING

Tools such as wireless HR monitors and GPS units allow athletes to track speed and HR and then download these data for further analysis after the performance. Using a portable power meter on a bicycle is an effective way to evaluate the power sustained during field tests. A chief advantage of using these tools is that they provide excellent information that can be compared season after season.

FUNCTIONAL THRESHOLD POWER (FTP)

Functional threshold power (FTP) is defined as the power a rider can maintain in a steady state without fatiguing for at least 60 minutes (1). Allen, Coggan, and McGregor stated the FTP test can be conducted in the field satisfactorily and can be used to create objective training metrics for cyclists (1). From a physiological standpoint, FTP is the demarcation point for the power or effort that an athlete can maintain where blood lactate production and combustion are equal with no increase in blood lactate. Once the FTP is exceeded, the amount of time that the intensity can be maintained is reduced. Several research studies have demonstrated that completion of a 20-minute protocol is just as good as performing a 1-hour time trial (21, 26, 30). Functional threshold power can be determined by either running or cycling.

Test Protocol

Similar to any laboratory test, FTP is conducted after a warm-up to make sure the athlete is ready to perform the test. See table 2.5 below on how to perform a cycling FTP test.

Table 2.5   Functional Threshold Testing Protocol

	Time	Description	% of FTP	% of FTHR
Warm-up	20 minutes	Endurance pace	65	70
	3 × 1 minute fast pedaling with 1 minute recovery between	Fast pedaling (100 rpm)	N/A	N/A
	5 minutes	Easy riding	65	<70
Main set	5 minutes	All-out effort	Max	>106
	10 minutes	Easy riding	65	<70
	20 minutes	Time trial	Max	99-105
Cooldown	10-15 minutes	Easy riding	65	<70

FTP = functional threshold power; FTHR = functional threshold heart rate; N/A = nonapplicable (adapted from 1).

Reprinted by permission from H. Allen, A. Coggan, and S. McGregor, *Training and Racing with a Power Meter*, 3rd ed. (Boulder, CO: VeloPress, 2019), 31.

After completing the test, download the data and average the watts for the 20-minute time trial. Use the average value and subtract 5% from it. The resulting value is your FTP.

- For example, your average power during the 20 minutes is 350 watts. You would calculate 350 × 0.05 = 17.5 watts, and 350 − 17.5 = 332.5 watts or 333 watts. Thus, your FTP is 333 watts.
- The reason for subtracting 5% from the average value during the 20-minute time trial is that the shorter test includes the athlete's anaerobic capacity, which skews the data.
- If an athlete has a higher anaerobic capacity, consider subtracting 7% or more, and athletes who are purely aerobic will need to subtract about 2% to 3%.

LAMBERTS AND LAMBERT SUBMAXIMAL CYCLE TEST (LSCT)

The Lamberts and Lambert Submaximal Cycle Test (LSCT) is a short, structured test protocol that is used to assess the fatigue state and training readiness of cyclists and triathletes, where the tests help to make more informed decisions on

- how fatigued a cyclist is,
- whether a particular planned session or current week's training plan is too hard,
- when an athlete is ready to return to inducing training stress within a recovery-focused week, and
- to what extent key physiological markers (i.e., HR, power output, speed) are improving because of the training program (25).

The LSCT is typically a 16- to 17-minute-long test, which can be used as a warm-up or as a stand-alone session when training stress is intended to be kept low. The goal of the LSCT test is to predict performance increases and determine training and fatigue status in the athlete, and is helpful when specifically looking for signals of potential overtraining in the athlete. Previous research has demonstrated that it is highly reliable (22, 23, 24) and able to demonstrate change in training and nonfunctional overtraining in athletes (23).

Test Protocol

Cyclists performing the test are required to ride at intensities that elicit certain percentages of their maximum HR values. The athlete can be tested on their bicycle attached to a trainer. An HR monitor is worn and can be recorded to a device during the test. Throughout the test, power output, HR, cadence, and RPE are recorded. It is also worth noting that pretest dietary patterns, particularly the consumption of caffeine (which can increase HR) are controlled; it is advised that no caffeine is consumed within 3 hours prior to the test. The test itself is split into four distinct blocks of riding (figure 2.10):

1. The cyclist rides at an intensity that elicits 60% of maximum HR for 6 minutes, and data are recorded and averaged during minutes 1 to 6. The goal is to maintain HR within ± 2 beats during the stage.

(continued)

Lamberts and Lambert Submaximal Cycle Test (LSCT) *(continued)*

2. The cyclist rides at an intensity that elicits 80% of maximum HR for 6 minutes, and data are recorded and averaged during minutes 7:30 to 12:30. The goal is to maintain HR within ± 1 beat during the stage.

3. The cyclist rides at an intensity that elicits 90% of maximum HR for 3 minutes, and data are recorded and averaged during minutes 13:30 to 15:30. The goal is to maintain HR within ± 1 beat during the stage.

4. Stop pedaling after the final stage, and allow HR to drop, where heart rate recovery (HRR) is measured during minutes 15:30 to 17:00.

In numbers 1, 2, and 3, the performance data analysis is conducted from 1 minute into each stage, setting aside this initial 60 seconds where the power output is higher than typically would be associated with the target HR to raise the HR to the desired level quickly. RPE is recorded for the final minute of steps 1, 2, and 3 (figure 2.9).

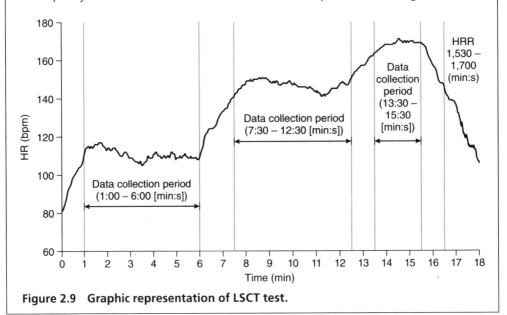

Figure 2.9 **Graphic representation of LSCT test.**

IMPLICATIONS OF ENDURANCE TEST RESULTS

For coaches and athletes a primary goal of purposeful training is to see the athlete's ability to perform in sport improve. Often this is viewed solely through finish times and podium positions. In fact, to train with purpose, coaches and athletes need to understand as well as possible the abilities, skills, and readiness an athlete has in order to prescribe, perform, and modify training centered on the athlete.

From a broader view of the sport's season and the athlete's career, performance testing can help the athlete team direct training toward the athlete's key performance indicators relative to their sport and ability. On the workout execution level, field and lab testing can help organize which intensity domain an athlete needs to target for specific performance purposes, while readiness tests can help the athlete team better understand how to adjust prescribed training based on the athlete's ability to perform and absorb training at a given point in time, reducing the risk of nonfunctional overreaching or underrecovery.

Taken together, test data from the lab and field help the athlete team plan and then adjust the athlete's preparation over the course of the year such that workouts consistently fit where that individual is at each point in time as they progress into and through their season (table 2.6).

Table 2.6 Relationship Between Domains, Zones, Paces, and Expected Adaptations

	Zones	Percentages	Key concepts	Specific adaptations
Moderate domain Lactate threshold	Zone II Endurance	• %HR @ CP/CS 69%-83% • %CS swim pace 107%-103% • %CS run pace 124%-115% • %$\dot{V}O_2$max run pace 134%-125% • %CP 56%-75%	• Training of slow-twitch muscle fibers • Fatigue resistance	• Increased muscle capillarization (9, 38) • Increased mitochondrial enzymes in slow-twitch muscle fibers (33)
Heavy domain	Zone III Tempo	• %HR @ CP/CS 84%-95% • %CS swim pace 103%-101% • %CS run pace 104%-95% • %$\dot{V}O_2$max run pace 114%-95% • %CP 76%-90%	• Training of slow- and fast-twitch muscle fibers (8) • Maximize metabolic fitness	• Improved LT (35) • Improved glycogen storage and use (10) • Reduction in $\dot{V}O_2$slow component (6) • Improved economy (6) • Improved V$\dot{V}O_2$max (10) • Increased critical power • Increased size of types I and II fibers (10) • Convert fast-twitch muscle fibers from type IIx to type IIa • Increased capillarization (35)

Reprinted by permission from P.F. Skiba, *Scientific Training for Endurance Athletes* (New Jersey, NJ: PhysFarm Training Systems, L.L.C., 2021), 80-81.

(continued)

Table 2.6 Relationship Between Domains, Zones, Paces, and Expected Adaptations *(continued)*

	Zones	Percentages	Key concepts	Specific adaptations
Heavy domain Critical power Severe domain $\dot{V}O_2$max	Zone IV Threshold	• %HR @ CP/CS 95%-105% • %CS swim pace 101%-98% • %CS run pace 104%-95% • %$\dot{V}O_2$max run pace 114%-95% • %CP 91%-105%	• Maximal training of fast-twitch (type IIa) muscle fibers • Some training of fast-twitch (type IIx) muscle fibers (protocol dependent) • Increased cardiac output	• Improved glycogen storage and use (10) • Improved $\dot{V}O_2$max • Improved critical power (34) • Increased size of muscle fibers (types I and II) (10)
	Zone V $\dot{V}O_2$max	• %HR @ CP/CS 106%-120% • %CS swim pace 98%-92% • %CS run pace 94%-84% • %$\dot{V}O_2$max run pace 104%-95% • %CP 106%-120%	• Maximal training of fast-twitch (type IIx) muscle fibers • Moderate training of slow- and fast-twitch (types I and IIa) muscle fibers	• Improved $\dot{V}O_2$max (34) • Improved CP (34) • Improved glycogen usage (10) • Hypertrophy of muscle fibers (types I and II) (10) • Increased capillarization of types I and II fibers (13, 17) • Increased oxidative enzymes (27) • Increased mitochondria (27)

Zones	Percentages	Key concepts	Specific adaptations
Extreme domain Zone VI Anaerobic	• %HR @ CP/CS N/A • %CS swim pace <92% • %CS run pace <84% • %$\dot{V}O_2$max run pace <95% • %CP >120%	• Anaerobic training of type IIx muscle fibers • Improvement in neuromuscular system • Improved sprint ability • Some improvement in aerobic system (seen in untrained individuals)	• Minimal improvement in $\dot{V}O_2$max (protocol dependent) (11, 29) • Fiber shift from type I to type IIx muscle fibers (8) • Increased capillarization of types I and II fibers (17, 27) • Increased W' (16) • Increased PPO (35, 38) • Improved muscle (enzyme) oxidative capacity (35, 38) • Improved fatigue resistance (38) • Improved glycogen storage (35, 38) • Improved muscle creatine phosphate (35)

Test data can be helpful for clarifying athletes' current fitness levels and customizing their training accordingly. In turn, this can help athletes and coaches determine training ranges, which can help target work during training sessions. There are many systems of organizing training intensity ranges in use today, including those of many national governing bodies, individual coaches or coaching groups, or online training platforms.

CONCLUSION

Data collection is important when organizing training programs based on the time of the season and goals that have been discussed by the coach and athlete. Fitness tests can be conducted in a laboratory or the field, and have specific pros and cons for each athlete, sport, and situation. Testing gives valuable information, which helps to understand the athletes' training status and can help athletes organize their training approach. With a sound testing strategy in place throughout the year, athletes and coaches can make evidence-based decisions that support continued growth over the long term.

CHAPTER 3

Endurance Training Principles and Considerations

Ben Reuter
Bob Seebohar*

One of the primary goals of a well-designed endurance training program is to help the athlete achieve positive physiological adaptations through proper training and recovery so that the athlete can peak optimally for competition (22). A well-designed program may also reduce the chance of injury and illness while promoting systematic recovery throughout the training plan. When an athlete experiences a high training load, the body is placed under a great deal of physiological stress. The body does not begin to adapt positively to that stress until proper recovery takes place (8, 34). A common error is believing that more is always better when it comes to endurance training. However, training without adequate recovery leads to overtraining, illness, and burnout (8). In contrast, too much recovery without training can lead to a deconditioned state or lack of preparation. The amount and timing of both training and recovery are important when designing a training program for endurance athletes.

This chapter provides an overview of periodization, which is the main principle for endurance training programming. The chapter on resistance training programming for endurance sports as well as the chapters on individual sports expand on the overview of periodization with sport-specific information and sample programming. No matter the sport, the periodization is individualized for the athlete. Level of competition, training experience, past and current injuries, and training and racing environmental conditions are all considered when the coach develops the training plan for the athlete. The plan should always be

---

*Ben Reuter was contracted to author this chapter; Bob Seebohar's name was added to acknowledge his significant contribution partially retained from the previous edition.

considered fluid, with changes to it made as required to ensure the athlete is able to work toward improved performance.

PROGRAM DESIGN

Recovery-based training should be a primary focus of program design. Without adequate recovery, athletes will not progress optimally and reach their full potential (8, 34). Recovery takes many forms, including rest, skill and technique practice, good sleep, aerobic cross-training, and proper nutrition (34). All are important when implementing recovery within a training program. Designing a training program for endurance athletes requires four steps:

1. Gather information.
2. Focus on initial planning components.
3. Examine the training program in more detail.
4. Plan the periodization of each cycle.

Step 1, information gathering, includes determining the athlete's short- and long-term goals, overall focus for the competitive season, and race priorities and objectives (18, 27, 34). The coach needs to determine the athlete's current training program and whether the athlete prefers group or individual training. The coach also should identify the current equipment available and any new equipment that will be needed throughout the training program. In addition, the coach should determine what type of terrain (geographical location) is available as well as the environment and climate in that area.

This step also involves determining the athlete's sport background, competitive history, sport-specific strengths and weaknesses, injury history, muscular imbalances, physiological variables (based on lactate threshold, metabolic, and body composition testing), biochemical variables (based on blood work analysis), and biomechanical variables (body movement efficiency patterns). Most important, the coach and athlete need to determine the amount of time that the athlete realistically can devote to training daily. This should include identifying the athlete's life commitments (e.g., family, social, and career) and details on the athlete's daily commute (mode and time to and from work). Many new endurance athletes are overzealous and take on more than they can handle. Athletes must differentiate between realistic and idealistic time goals so that they can achieve a proper balance between sport and life.

Step 2 involves focusing on the initial planning components. These components include the type and frequency of high-quality training sessions, the time between training sessions, the type and frequency of recovery sessions, and the proper build-to-recover ratio of the periodization program (and when this may fluctuate throughout the training year) (14). In this step, the coach and athlete also should determine the mental training and nutritional strategies that will be used. In addition, they should identify the method of communication and type of feedback that will be used between the athlete and coach.

Step 3 begins the process of planning the training program in more detail. This includes determining the specific training techniques that will be used at specific times of the year. An additional part of the program design is ensuring that the athlete is able to work on tactical skills in relation to race-specific scenarios. The coach and athlete should work together to determine when and where specific training sessions should be placed throughout each training plan and identify the associated goals and outcomes, including specific physical, mental, and nutritional goals for each training session. Additionally, recovery opportunities should be emphasized, and the structure of recovery sessions throughout the training program should be planned in this step.

The last step includes planning each periodization cycle (11, 34). The goal of the training program is to systematically improve fitness to allow the athlete's maximal performance in competitions.

Here are some additional things that coaches and athletes need to consider when determining the structure and timing of training throughout the year:

▶ When and how resistance training fits into the program

▶ When to implement drills that require fine movements and a high amount of focus

▶ How many high-quality training sessions should be implemented during each training cycle

▶ Whether two high-quality training sessions should be completed in one day (referred to as *combo workouts* or *bricks* for multisport athletes; referred to as *doubles* for single-sport athletes)

PERIODIZATION

Periodized training uses groups of training sessions. These sessions are typically combined into microcycles, mesocycles, and macrocycles (11, 14, 34). A *microcycle* is a cycle of training sessions lasting a few days or weeks. A *mesocycle* is a group of microcycles that is generally around 4 weeks in length. A *macrocycle* is a period of training time often 12 to 16 weeks in duration, but may be as long as a year. A macrocycle is made up of a group of mesocycles (34).

For endurance athletes, the normal progression of fitness begins by developing a good aerobic base (see figure 3.1). Overdistance (OV) and endurance (EN) training are used to build the base of the aerobic system. This is followed by more high-aerobic and tempo work (moving up the pyramid). Then lactate threshold and maximal effort sessions (top of the pyramid) are added when the body has built up a strong foundation of aerobic fitness and strength (22, 27, 34).

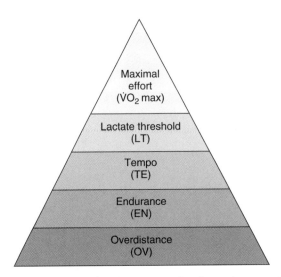

Figure 3.1 Sample traditional periodization progression for endurance athletes.

An example of a normal distribution outlining the volume, intensity, and percentage of each type of training during each macrocycle can be seen in table 3.1. Throughout the cycles, most training is devoted to overdistance and endurance training. As the competition season approaches, the athlete gradually increases higher intensity training and reduces training volume.

Table 3.1 Distribution of Training Load for Each Type of Training

Cycle	Volume	Intensity	Overdistance	Endurance	Tempo	Lactate threshold	$\dot{V}O_2$max
Preparatory (off-season or base)	Moderate to high	Low	60%	30%	5%	5%	0%
Precompetition (preseason)	Moderate	Moderate to high	55%	25%	5%-10%	10%-15%	0%-10%
Competition (race or in-season)	Low to moderate	High	55%	20%	5%-10%	5%-10%	0%-5%
Tapering and peak	Low to moderate	Moderate to high	55%	25%	5%-10%	10%-15%	2%-5%
Transition (active rest or postseason)	Low	Low	85%	5%-10%	0%-5%	0%	0%

The information in table 3.1 can be used as a guide for planning the volume, intensity, and relative contributions of each cycle shown in figure 3.1.

Two types of periodization are commonly used by endurance athletes: traditional and reverse (11, 15). In *traditional periodization with standard progression*, the athlete progresses through the typical cycles of preparatory (off-season or base), precompetition (preseason), competition (race or in-season), and transition (postseason or active rest). For athletes who compete in multiple events, a short tapering cycle is generally used before key competitions.

Figure 3.2 presents an example of the traditional periodization with standard progression of building volume and intensity. The example depicts a 3-week build followed by 1 week of recovery. The athlete can slowly build volume and intensity over 3 weeks. The standard 3:1 build-to-recover progression is merely an example of the many ways to periodize a training program. This method can lead to high fatigue during the third week if the athlete is not ready for the load or if the athlete has many outside stressors that influence recovery.

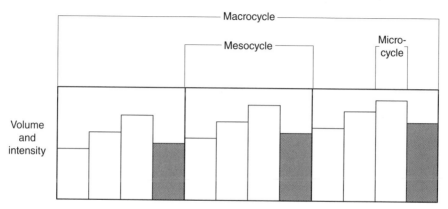

Figure 3.2   Sample traditional periodization with a standard method of progression.

Traditional periodization with a reverse of progression (figure 3.3) begins with a higher load and gradually decreases through the cycle (15). Because the training load is highest in the first week of training, this strategy is more demanding and should only be used by athletes who are capable of withstanding high training loads.

A periodization mesocycle can be planned in many ways. The traditional 3:1 week build-to-recover cycle is probably the most popular for endurance athletes. For novice athletes a 2:1 week build-to-recover model is a good option because it ensures sufficient recovery. Remember that any single approach to training may not work throughout the entire season. For an athlete to continue progressing toward optimal performance, various training methods may need to be used throughout the athlete's training year. Once the athlete's body begins to develop and the athlete's performance begins to level off, it may be time to change the periodization method or look at the recovery program in more detail.

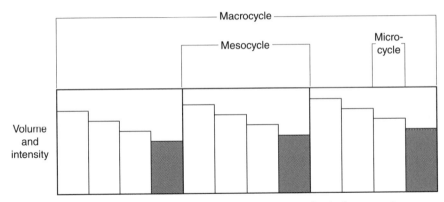

Figure 3.3 Sample traditional periodization with a reverse method of progression.

Preparatory (Off-Season or Base)

In a traditional periodization plan, the *preparatory* period (sometimes termed *off-season* or *base*) enables the athlete to build the aerobic foundation, strength, and flexibility needed to progress to the next cycle, which is more physically, mentally, and nutritionally challenging. This base period can last 12 to 16 weeks (34).

Precompetition (Preseason)

The *precompetition* period (sometimes termed *preseason* or *build*) is the next cycle in the program. During this cycle the goals are to improve speed, economy, power, and race-specific strength (29). Like the preparatory phase of training, this period can last 12 to 16 weeks (34). Generally, volume during the precompetition period is lower than during the preparatory period, with a concomitant increase in training intensity (22).

Competition (Race or In-season)

The *competition* season (sometimes termed *race* or *in-season*) commonly lasts 12 to 16 weeks (29, 34). Some experienced athletes may have longer competition seasons. For example, triathletes may race shorter distances during the early competition season and schedule longer ultradistance races later in the cycle. During the race season volume is lower than during preparatory or precompetition cycles.

The goal of the competition season is racing or performance. Many coaches break up the competition cycle into blocks of 1- to 4-week cycles if competitions will take place each week (29). This allows the body to recover. In addition, because most athletes can only achieve two or three formal peaks in the competition season, top-priority competitions are often separated into two or three separate blocks throughout the season.

Tapering and Peaking

Part of successful competition and a well-designed competition period is using tapering to allow peaking for key races (34). The challenge often lies in planning the taper so that the athlete peaks at the right time. Many athletes miss their peak because of an inappropriately timed taper. A *taper* is a progressive reduction in training load. This reduction in the training load is meant to reduce the physical and psychological stressors incurred on a daily basis in order to enhance the body's adaptation to training—and thus optimize performance—to reach a peak (17, 19, 21). Many physical and psychological factors are improved with a properly implemented taper. Two main training variables are usually adjusted for a taper: volume and intensity. Both must be balanced carefully to reap the positive effects. A properly designed taper can result in performance improvement as much as 6% (18).

Tapers generally last 1 to 4 weeks (19). Training volume is reduced, but intensity is maintained. The specific length of the taper is based on a variety of factors, including athlete experience, length of the event being trained for, and the importance of the competition. Novice athletes or coaches may want to discuss these factors with a more experienced mentor or friend. There is often no rhyme or reason in an athlete's decision on the duration of the taper; however, athletes who compete over shorter distances usually use a shorter taper, and athletes who compete over longer distances usually use a longer taper.

Transition (Active Rest or Postseason)

A transition between competitions or intense training blocks can be included to implement short recovery bouts, which usually last 1 or 2 weeks. Additionally, a full transition cycle (postseason) of 4 to 8 weeks can be scheduled at the end of the competition season (29). This gives the athlete a full block of recovery. During this transition cycle, the athlete's goals are to exercise without structure, cross-train, have fun, and take a mental and physical reprieve.

TYPES OF TRAINING

During the periodization cycles athletes train at different intensities and durations for individual sessions. Generally, for a given session the higher the intensity, the lower the duration of the activity. Most training programs for endurance sports rely heavily on low-intensity training for most of the training volume (29, 34). The emphasis on the type of training depends on the training cycle. Table 3.2 provides general guidelines for each type of training.

Table 3.2 General Guidelines for Types of Training

Type of training	Duration	Intensity	Frequency
Overdistance	Longer than race time or distance	Below lactate threshold	1-2 times/week
Endurance	30 minutes to race distance or time	Below lactate threshold	1-2 times/week
Tempo (to include lactate threshold training)	20-30+ min specific to race distances; lactate threshold training should be 20-30 min total	At or slightly below race intensity; lactate threshold training is at lactate threshold	1-2 times/week
$\dot{V}O_2$max	Interval duration of a few seconds to a few minutes	Close to $\dot{V}O_2$max	1 time/week

Adapted by permission from B.H. Reuter and J.J. Dawes, "Program Design and Technique for Aerobic Endurance Training," in *Essentials of Strength Training and Conditioning*, edited for the National Strength and Conditioning Association by G. Haff and N.T. Triplett (Champaign, IL: Human Kinetics, 2016), 567.

Overdistance and Endurance

Overdistance and endurance training is sometimes called *long slow distance* (LSD) (22). The intensity of this training is below the lactate threshold. *Overdistance training* is typically longer and at a lower intensity than *endurance training*. Both overdistance and endurance training sessions are at an intensity below lactate threshold (22). Overdistance training sessions may be longer than race times, and endurance training sessions may be as short as half an hour (22). During the base or preseason overdistance and endurance training is over 70% of the training volume (27, 29). The main goal of training at these intensities is to increase aerobic capacity (22). For longer race distances the overdistance training can also help the athlete prepare for the mental stress of competing for a long period of time.

Tempo and Lactate Threshold

Tempo and lactate threshold are a small part of the preparatory and base cycles. *Tempo training* (sometimes called *pace training*) is training at an intensity that is at or slightly below racing intensity (22). The longer the duration of competition, the lower the pace for tempo training. *Lactate threshold training* is a specific form of tempo training that is performed at lactate threshold. Tempo training is performed either as one continuous session at a tempo intensity or as a series of time periods or intervals at tempo intensity. When intervals are used athletes recover between intervals with lower-intensity activity (22). Tempo training is used to allow the athlete to become familiar with race intensity. Tempo training also increases the athlete's ability to use lactate as a fuel as well as trains the anaerobic glycolytic energy system (22). As the athlete progresses closer to competition, tempo training is increasingly used to better prepare the athlete to perform.

$\dot{V}O_2max$

$\dot{V}O_2max$ is a smaller but very important component of training. Intensity of this training is close to $\dot{V}O_2max$ (6). Training sessions are generally used during the precompetition and competition cycles, as well as part of tapering. The sessions are typically interval sessions of a few seconds to a few minutes (5, 6). These sessions are quite intense, and it is important to allow adequate recovery between intervals. The goals of these sessions are to stimulate the anaerobic energy systems as well as to familiarize athletes with higher intensities that may be needed during the final part of a competition (22).

Planning an athlete's endurance training program takes knowledge of the various components that make up the program; however, the many variables in the athlete's life and training are also important when fine-tuning the program to meet the athlete's needs. Once the planning stage is complete, the athlete's progress should be monitored continually to assess positive physiological adaptations. A training program that is effective in bringing about positive physiological adaptations will not necessarily result in optimal adaptations year after year. For the athlete to achieve optimal performance year after year, different goals and strategies must be implemented.

Training Intensity and Training Zones

Individual endurance sport workouts are often programmed using heart rate training zones to delineate workout intensities. The zones are based on percentage of maximum heart rate (MHR), or estimated maximum heart rate. A heart rate monitor is reasonably priced, and many models record data for review after a workout. This makes heart rate zone training a convenient way to provide programming without requiring extensive equipment for other intensity measures such as blood lactate levels and power measurement. A key to using training zones is to understand the training zone categorization used by the coach. Commonly a five-zone training system is used, but depending on the sport and the background of a coach, the five zones may be further divided. In some programming a six- or seven-zone categorization is used. The sport-specific chapters and chapter 2 provide detailed information on the different training zone categorizations. These sections of the book also discuss the relationship between percentage of MHR and other intensity measures such as rating of perceived exertion (RPE) and power production.

ENVIRONMENTAL CONDITIONS

Environmental conditions can influence the performance of even well-trained and prepared athletes. The environment can dramatically increase the physiological stresses encountered during endurance activity. Extremes in temperature and humidity can result in less-than-optimal performance from even elite athletes. In all environmental conditions, athletes should strive to maintain core temperature, fluid balance, and blood glucose levels while maximizing performance. The combination of exercise stresses and environmental stresses does not allow maintenance of homeostasis, but ideally, the athlete's body can maintain a steady state, or a constant internal environment. Environmental extremes, especially for athletes traveling to unfamiliar environments, make it difficult to maintain a steady state. In response to the heat produced by exercise and the environmental temperature, an athlete's body works to maintain a constant internal environment by attempting to regulate body temperature.

Heat Transfer

The human body can gain or lose heat in four ways: conduction, convection, radiation, and evaporation (2). *Conduction* is heat transfer from contact between two surfaces (9). For example, when a person sits on a cold metal bench, heat is conducted from the body to the cooler bench.

Convection is a specific type of conduction that occurs via the transfer of heat between a person and air or fluid (9). When an athlete is immersed in water (e.g., a triathlete or distance swimmer), the conductive and convective heat exchange that occurs between the athlete and the water is much greater than heat exchange created by other conditions. Figure 3.4 shows an estimate of survival times with water immersion without a wetsuit. Wetsuits are allowed for many triathlons. The wetsuit traps a layer of water between the skin and the suit, and it reduces the rate of convective heat loss. Most triathlon swims will not occur in extremely cold water that will be life threatening; however, endurance swimming events in northern parts of the world could take place in temperatures cold enough to be a concern. Unlike triathlons, many open-water swim events do not allow wetsuits, regardless of the water temperature.

Another example of convection in the triathlon occurs during the bike and run. Because of the greater speed of the bike compared to the run, the convective heat exchange is much greater. In fact, during a race, triathletes on the bike and cyclists may not be aware of extreme heat conditions until the start of the run.

Radiation is heat gain or heat loss by way of electromagnetic waves (9). An extreme example of radiative heat exchange for endurance athletes is the environmental stress experienced by Ironman athletes competing on the lava fields of Kona, Hawaii. The athletes absorb heat from the environment, both from the sun and from the heated lava fields.

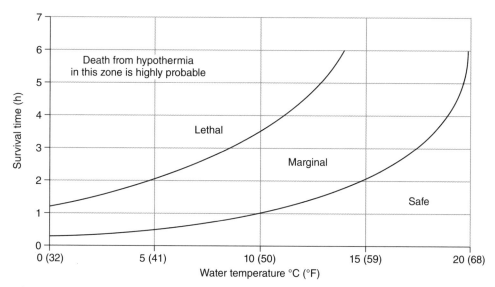

Figure 3.4 Estimated survival time during immersion of lightly clothed, non-exercising humans in cold water. The boundaries (solid lines) would be shifted upward by wearing survival gear or a wetsuit.

Adapted by permission from L. Armstrong, *Performing in Extreme Environments* (Champaign, IL: Human Kinetics, 2000), 96. Previously adapted from M.M. Toner and W.D. McArdle, "Physiological Adjustments of Man to Cold," in *Human Performance Physiology and Environmental Medicine at Terrestrial Extremes*, edited by K.B. Pandolf, M.N. Sawka, and R.R. Gonzalez (Indianapolis: Brown & Benchmark, 1988), 361-400.

Evaporation is the conversion of water-to-water vapor (9). Athletes lose a lot of heat through the evaporation of sweat. The body loses 580 kilocalories (kcal) of heat for each liter of evaporated sweat (20). However, if the sweat does not evaporate and soaks clothing or drops to the ground, no evaporative cooling can occur. The environmental humidity has the greatest effect on the rate of sweat evaporation. The more humid the environment, the lower the level of sweat evaporation. The cooling effect of sweat only occurs when the sweat evaporates. Higher air humidity reduces sweat evaporation (9).

When exercising in a cold environment, athletes need to be concerned about maintaining core temperature above 95 °F (35 °C) to avoid developing *hypothermia* (10). In cooler environments, heat loss from the body often occurs in windy conditions or when the athlete's clothing becomes wet, such as when a novice competitor wears clothing that does not wick sweat (e.g., a cotton T-shirt). Minimizing skin exposure to the wind and protecting the extremities from the cold can go a long way toward ensuring safe exercise (10). By taking these precautions, athletes can minimize the occurrence of frostnip (cold damage to the epidermis of the skin) and the more severe frostbite (fluid freezing in and between the skin cells) (2). Many of the effects of cold exposure can be controlled by making well-planned clothing choices. Dressing in layers, using clothing that wicks moisture, and wearing an outer layer that protects against the wind help to minimize the development of cold-related problems (10).

Acclimatization

Proper acclimatization will help an athlete minimize the potential for heat-related problems. A proper acclimatization program takes 10 to 14 days and involves gradually increasing the exercise intensity and duration (4). A variety of physiological changes occur during the acclimatization process, including increased sweat rate, increased plasma volume, decreased salt content of the sweat, lower heart rate and core temperature at a given exercise intensity, and increased blood flow to the skin (25).

An athlete who is unable to be at a race site long enough to acclimate can mimic race conditions by dressing in layers, which acts to create a microenvironment. For a coach who primarily works with athletes in a hot and humid environment, a useful tool to gauge environmental conditions is a sling psychrometer. The psychrometer is used to measure *wet bulb global temperature (WBGT)*. Although coaches and athletes cannot control the environmental conditions, having knowledge of extreme conditions will enable them to modify daily training or race goals. The WBGT is a popular heat stress index. The following equation is used to determine the WBGT*:

$$WBGT = (0.7 \times T_{wb}) + (0.2 \times T_g) + (0.1 \times T_{db})$$

T_{wb} is the wet bulb temperature, T_g is black globe temperature is , and T_{db} is dry bulb temperature (temperature in the shade). The WBGT equation is a more accurate measure of heat stress than ambient temperature. The WBGT takes into account the radiant heat from the sun (T_g) as well as the relationship of environmental humidity (T_{wb}) on heat stress (2). The greatest influence on heat illness risk is the humidity (T_{wb}) because the main way the body cools itself is via sweat evaporation. As already discussed, the greater the environmental humidity, the more difficult it is for sweat to evaporate.

A sling psychrometer typically comes with a chart or table to show the relationship of environmental temperature (T_g), environmental humidity (T_{wb}), and radiant heat (T_{db}) on the risk for heat-related problems during exercise.

Heat Illness

Even with acclimatization, athletes and coaches need to be aware of the three forms of heat illness: heat cramps, heat exhaustion, and heatstroke. *Heat cramps* may affect a single muscle, or in more extreme cases, an athlete may experience whole-body cramping. Athletes who develop *heat exhaustion* will have a heavy

---

*WBGT equation reprinted from L. E. Armstrong, 2000, *Performing in extreme environments* (Champaign, IL: Human Kinetics), 310.

sweat rate, may look pale, and may complain of gastrointestinal distress or not feeling well in general (3).

The most serious heat-related problem is *heatstroke* (9). The major sign of heatstroke is a lack of sweating (hot and dry skin) in a hot environment (9). This is a life-threatening condition because sweat evaporation is the major method of heat loss in a hot environment. Keep in mind that heat-related problems—cramps, exhaustion, and stroke—are not sequential; an athlete can develop heatstroke without first having heat cramps or heat exhaustion.

Terrain

Most amateur endurance athletes are not able to travel to a race destination until a few days before the competition. As previously mentioned, this is potentially problematic when athletes need to acclimate to hot and humid environments. Similarly, most athletes do not have the luxury of always training on terrain that is like race terrain, especially if the race is held in a hilly or mountainous part of the world. Unfortunately, athletes who live in areas without significant elevation changes will have a difficult time training for the terrain extremes seen at some race venues. However, with some ingenuity, athletes can create a training situation that partially mimics race conditions. Highway on-ramps, stadium ramps, a bicycle trainer with the front wheel elevated on blocks, and a treadmill with an incline all can help athletes arrive at a race with at least some training that simulates the race terrain.

Altitude

Some endurance competitions are held at altitude. Many athletes competing in these events live at sea level. Effective program design recognizes that training modifications may be necessary as part of preparation for altitude events. Aerobic performance decreases as altitude reaches 3,281 feet (1,000 m) above sea level (33). A variety of physiological changes occur at altitude, which result in decreased performance. The main reason is a decrease in oxygen use by the athlete. The percent of oxygen in the air is the same at sea level and at higher altitudes. However, *partial pressure of oxygen (PO$_2$)* decreases as altitude increases. The decreased PO$_2$ reduces the saturation of oxygen in the blood. As a result, aerobic performance decreases (33). For most athletes competing at altitude the best plan is to arrive within 48 hours of the competition. This minimizes the physiological effects of altitude, which take time to become evident. Athletes with more flexibility in their lives may want to arrive up to 3 months prior to competition to allow acclimatization (33). Athletes who live at altitude may travel to lower elevations for some or all of their training. This is commonly termed *live high, train low*. The lower elevation allows the athlete to train at a higher intensity than is possible when training at altitude (32). A third option is to make use of a hypoxia chamber for sleeping. This can simulate the popular live high, train low practice of athletes who live at altitude (7).

Air Pollution

Endurance athletes spend significant time training and competing outdoors. To minimize health risks, athletes and coaches should be aware of air pollution and air quality levels. Many weather apps and websites include air quality values, and release air quality alerts when the pollution is at a dangerous level. Air pollution can cause acute and chronic respiratory and cardiovascular problems with both short-term and long-term exposure (24, 31). Exposure to pollution may also reduce oxygen uptake (31), which will directly affect athletic performance. Athletes with preexisting cardiovascular and respiratory conditions, such as asthma, are at greater risk for problems than athletes without these conditions (31). Athletes can minimize exposure by avoiding training in high-traffic or industrial areas. Avoiding training during morning or afternoon rush-hour traffic also can help reduce exposure to pollution.

INJURY PREVENTION

Injuries are a common part of endurance training. The optimal race performance or fitness level is achieved by pushing to maximize conditioning without overtraining or injury (27). A breakthrough performance occurs when the athlete and coach are able to maximize the training load without going too far. Experienced coaches often talk about training their athletes on "the knife-edge"—pushing them to maximize adaptations without pushing them over the edge to overtraining or injury.

The rate and severity of injuries can be reduced by using periodization and a well-designed resistance program as part of the training. Coaches and athletes need to recognize that stress occurs not just from training and inadequate rest, but also from other areas of life. Poor work conditions, family problems, and trying to do too much all create stress that requires recovery (13). If athletes try to do too much training, fit too much into their life, or skimp on recovery and rest, they will eventually be unable to recover from the stresses of training. As a result, injuries will occur. It is better for an athlete to be on the starting line slightly undertrained than to be overtrained or injured.

If an injury occurs, the coach and athlete need to identify it before it becomes too severe. Especially at high training volumes, small irritations can become big problems if they are not recognized and dealt with. Coaches and athletes must understand the difference between muscle soreness from training and muscle pain from the beginning of an overuse injury. This is something that is difficult to teach, but it is a valuable skill for to develop.

Athletes can take steps to minimize the loss of training time due to injury. These steps include following a proper training program, allowing adequate recovery from training, and developing a network of medical professionals to go to if injury does occur (13, 27). A short course of physical therapy, combined with modifications in training, can often reduce the loss of training time from an acute injury—or prevent a slight problem from developing into a chronic injury.

COMMON INJURIES

Injuries can be placed into two etiologies or methods of injury: acute and chronic. Acute injuries are those that have an immediate and identifiable onset. Examples of this include inverting (turning) an ankle while running on a trail or finishing a swim session and noticing shoulder pain. Chronic injuries have a more gradual onset. The athlete may notice pain or discomfort (for part of a workout or after a workout) that subsides after a short period of time. As training progresses, the pain or discomfort may become more severe or may be noticeable for a longer period. Chronic injuries are generally more common than acute injuries for endurance athletes (16).

Some of the more common types of acute injuries are muscle strains, ligament sprains, and fractures. Common chronic injuries for endurance athletes are stress fractures and tendinopathies. Table 3.3 shows common areas of the body where each of these injuries occur (1, 12, 23, 26). Unless an athlete sustains a specific injury, most endurance athlete injuries are those from overuse. Too much training, too little recovery, and inadequate nutrition are all related to an increased risk of injury (34).

Table 3.3 Common Injuries in Endurance Sports

Injury	Common body areas
Strain	Hamstring, quadriceps, lumbar back muscles, hip flexors, gastrocnemius-soleus complex
Sprain	Ankle, foot
Fracture	Tibia, fibula, bones of the foot
Stress fracture	Femur, tibia, fibula, bones of the foot, femur
Tendinopathy	Achilles, patella, iliotibial band, shoulder

Basic treatment of these chronic conditions and a general timeline for these conditions to subside is beyond the scope of this chapter. Readers are encouraged to consult references 1, 12, 23, and 30.

A muscle *strain* or pulled muscle is a tearing of a muscle (1). A strain commonly occurs when a muscle is lengthened too far or it contracts with a force greater than the tissue can withstand. For example, a common mechanism for a hamstring strain occurs during sprinting when the athlete overstrides.

Ligaments attach bone to bone, and they provide strength and structure to joints. A ligament *sprain* is a stretching, tearing, or rupture of a ligament (1). For example, an inversion ankle sprain occurs when the foot is inverted to a degree that is not able to be controlled by the muscles crossing the ankle joint.

A *fracture* is the cracking or complete breaking of a bone. A compound or open fracture occurs when the fracture is visible through the skin. A closed or simple fracture is when the fracture is not visible. X-rays are used to identify the extent of a closed fracture (1). Fractures are less common than muscle strains and ligament sprains (1, 23, 26). However, they are seen more commonly in older athletes (26).

A *stress fracture* is an overuse injury and is microtrauma to the bone. It is caused by repetitive stress without adequate recovery (12). For example, an increase in running milage or intensity with a concomitant onset of foot pain that does not dissipate may be an indication of a stress fracture. Often x-rays do not show stress fractures, and diagnosis requires use of other radiography methods such as a bone scan or MRI (12).

Tendons connect muscles to bone. In the past a tendon overuse injury was called *tendonitis*. Currently, the term used for a tendon overuse injury is *tendinopathy*. Tendinopathy occurs more commonly in older athletes. Tendinopathy usually develops because of a training program error (30). Tendinopathy most commonly occurs when the tendon is loaded with a stress greater than it can adapt to. For example, a sudden change in running milage, intensity, or training surface could predispose an athlete to the development of Achilles tendinopathy or tendinopathies of tendons in the foot.

CHAPTER 4

Aerobic Endurance Development

Will Kirousis

Improving aerobic endurance has come a long way since Flavius Philostratus (170-245 CE) organized what may have been the first structured training plans for physical performance millennia ago (2). Many training strategies have been used since then. By the mid-20th century, the growth of sport science led to training plans focused on structured interval strategies, with coaches like Mihály Iglói and even the first sub-4-minute miler, Sir Roger Bannister, using structured bouts of work and rest to build higher performance (7). This period formed the start of a seesaw between higher-intensity intervals and long steady distance (LSD) training for the ensuing decades (8). Over time, this evolution of training approaches led to the methods of aerobic endurance development most used today.

A key component regarding the development of training methods is that they tend to be coach- and athlete-driven and have expanded via the sport science community. Coaches and athletes typically drive progress in training strategies. At the same time, sport science explores what is occurring, allowing coaches and athletes to understand their processes, which leads to more evidence-informed training decisions.

THE CHALLENGE

Humans are an amalgamation of overlapping systems. Coaches, athletes, and scientists often look at performance with a heavy focus on specific physiological markers that can be measured. For example, almost every training discussion will work toward measurable factors such as $\dot{V}O_2max$, lactate threshold, aerobic threshold, maximal lactate steady state, and so on. Athletes are complex systems, and that complexity needs to be recognized openly to help them develop best. This means acknowledging factors such as the status of the mental, emotional, and neuromuscular systems and their constant flux. Why? Because the body's systems work together to yield movement through and over the constantly changing environment (6). For example, athletes must climb hills or work through winds, currents, and changing temperatures. The athletes' perception of these factors changes based on their readiness to tackle them and on the impact of non-sport factors they are encountering throughout their daily life (e.g., final exams for a student-athlete, the death of a loved one, or an upsetting discussion with a spouse). Throughout this chapter, concepts will be reviewed related to the development of aerobic endurance and examples of workouts will be shown that can be used to develop this ability.

In his writing about coaching endurance athletes, Andrew Kirkland presents a key question for all coaches and athletes (6): Why do we do what we do when we participate in a training program?

▶ To improve (enhance one's ability to move over the earth, minimally affected by fatigue from challenges encountered along the way, including environmental, topographical, competitive, equipment, mental, etc.)

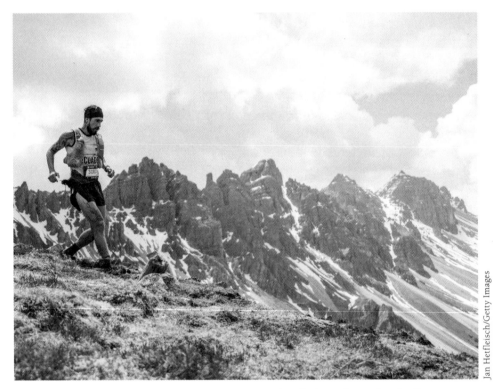

Jan Hetfleisch/Getty Images

One reason endurance athletes train is to minimize fatigue from the challenges encountered along the way.

▶ To enjoy (regardless of professional status or age group, if the athlete does not broadly enjoy the process of preparing for sport, odds of burnout rise and any potential for improvement fades)

▶ To be durable (both reducing injury odds and reducing the rate of fatigue as the duration of a training session or competition expands)

These points blend, helping form a developmental belief system by recognizing that athletes are training to compete and should approach workouts to improve their understanding of how to use the complex system (body and mind) they direct.

MEETING THE CHALLENGE: ADAPTIVE LOADING

For the training process to work best, the coach and athlete need to consider the athlete's desire for self-determination. The athlete needs a stake in the process versus simply following what the coach or plan says; the athlete should feel competence grow from training and being a part of a team, group, or something bigger than him- or herself during the pursuit of the training adventure. This does not mean every training session is done with peers. It means that an athlete's training process is not just checking boxes but intentionally exploring different concepts and methods based on current health and performance status and identified performance targets. When performing endurance workouts, an area where this process is often overlooked is the use of training intensity zones. Intensity zones tend to be based on physiological parameters and help orient athletes' efforts during specific workouts. Here is an overly simplistic example of this point: An athlete needs to improve the capacity for aerobic work, so he or she focuses on moderate-intensity domain work within zones 1 and 2 (in most systems) during a specific phase of the training year. A challenge that has emerged using zone-based training is an assumption that there are strict boundaries between different zones, leading to vastly different physiological responses to the training session. While this mindset is well intended, it misses the reality that no one can constantly train within such tight parameters, that adaptation to training occurs across a range of physiological systems regardless of training intensity zone, and that attempting to teach within such tight parameters increases the odds of burnout over time. Given humans' complex systems, athletes need to remember that many factors interact to guide them toward improved performance. While intensity zones can help target, they need to be used with different approaches to lead to improved performance. The following should be considered:

1. Over time, athletes will recognize relationships between physiology and perception or mindset (e.g., heart rate, pace or power, rating of perceived exertion) when fresh, fatigued, less or more fit, cold, hot, and so on, which they can use to adjust their training strategy.

2. Athletes should use those observations to help manage and adjust training within workouts and over longer training blocks to help build competence within their sport.

3. Athletes should be willing to modify and adjust their training based on the variation in day-to-day experience in sports and life to help them grow more adaptable and sustain a sense of autonomy.

Hearing and applying these messages help athletes look for ways to expand rather than constrain their approach, which empowers them to make decisions, take reasonable risks, gain experiences, and learn. This open approach to training incorporates intensity zones to help broadly orient or calibrate workouts to specific performance goals without removing vitally important decision-making skills from the training process.

The adaptable approach acknowledges that the individual changes slightly daily. These changes mean work performed at one rate one day may elicit a slightly different response than the same work rate another day. To account for this, athletes must take an adaptable approach to training, incorporating all intensity tools they have—power, pace, heart rate (HR), ratings of perceived exertion (RPE)—to understand and modify training each day. This allows targeting a specific training intensity zone while staying ready to adjust the approach by triangulating decisions via multiple sources of information. Adaptable approaches to training reduce the odds of pushing too hard when tired, leading to underrecovery and nonfunctional overreaching, both of which will stop athletes from having the best experience they can in sports and will reduce physical performance. For example, when athletes are triangulating metrics over time, then notice that their HR seems low and their RPE is high relative to their pace or power, the odds are good that fatigue is affecting them and therefore they should shift the workout to focus on low-intensity work for a similar duration as the planned session. If the same thing is repeated multiple days in a row, additional days off training may make more sense than the planned training. The goal of adjusting the training approach day over day like this is to:

▶ Increase the sense of autonomy an athlete has in their training process

▶ Improve athlete freshness and ability to recover from training over the long haul

▶ Improve athlete satisfaction and enjoyment

- ▶ Shift higher load training days to fit the athletes' freshness, thus handling high loads best
- ▶ Help athletes learn to read their body's signals well, which is an essential skill for performing training and racing as well as possible

Figure 4.1. describes the broad connection between an athlete's decision to perform work, the resulting changes in their physiology, their perception, and, potentially, alterations to their current workout or future workouts. Table 4.1 provides a few of the most common things athletes experience during training and actions they can take to adjust.

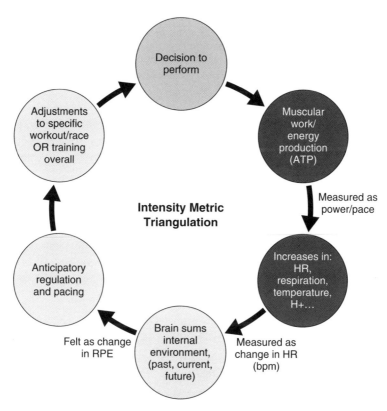

Figure 4.1 This figure illustrates intensity metric triangulation: how athletes blend incoming information (pace or power, HR) with perception (RPE) to generate changes in pacing and to alter a workout in progress or future training.

A deeper discussion of this adaptable training approach is beyond this chapter's scope. The next section covers the physical goals of aerobic development training followed by details regarding the specifics of workouts.

Table 4.1 Commonly Encountered Signals for Athletes to Adapt to During Training

Symptom	Action based on common causes
RPE increases beyond normal at a given power or pace.	Fatigue is likely, so it is best to reduce the intensity to the moderate domain, or zones 1-2, for the remainder of the workout. If this persists the following day, a 1- to 2-day period of rest makes sense. This may relate to low glycogen or low available energy during a workout as well. Increasing fueling may help, but more important is ensuring adequate energy in the athlete's daily diet—in particular, carbohydrates—to help restore glycogen rapidly after training.
Over a workout, HR increases relative to pace or power and RPE.	The temperature may be high, making cooling challenging, or the athlete may be getting dehydrated. Increase fluid consumption and consider cooling strategies if possible (e.g., ice pack on the back of the neck or head or held in hand, drink cold fluids, pour water on the head and upper body). This may require reducing the intensity
A change in HR coupled with decreasing pace or power	Fatigue is likely, so it is best to reduce the intensity to the moderate domain, or zones 1-2, for the remainder of the workout. If this persists the following day, a 1- to 2-day period of rest makes sense.

INTENSITY DOMAINS AND TRAINING INTENSITY ZONES

Training for endurance athletes presents many challenges. One key challenge is the variety of terms used to describe how intensely one should train for a specific purpose. Much of this discussion is focused on using a system of zones roughly related to specific physiologic areas that represent the increasing use of slow (type I), fast oxidative (type IIa), and fast glycolytic (type IIx) muscle fibers, working together to create the athlete's desired intensity of movement (see chapter 1 for more detail). This is great for helping athletes avoid overwork and targeting specific adaptations—for example, using lower-intensity work to help increase the density of capillary beds, which support muscular work (11).

Broadly, these zones are oriented around exercise *intensity domains*. These domains begin with the *moderate domain*, which covers very light activity to the *lactate threshold* (LT) (5, 11). Broadly, the LT can be considered the highest intensity that can be maintained before lactate levels begin to rise above the exercise baseline. There are many methods used for determining the LT, as noted in chapter 2. Within the moderate domain, oxygen uptake rises and levels off into a steady state quickly, resulting in a relatively stable physiologic state (5, 10). The *heavy domain* is from the LT to the area of *critical power* (CP) or *critical speed* (CS) (5, 11). CP or CS roughly represents the highest power or speed that can be sustained without continuously increasing oxygen uptake, which would lead to rapid fatigue. Within the heavy domain, oxygen uptake rises quickly and then gradually stabilizes around the area of CP or CS (5, 11). Beyond the heavy domain lies the *severe domain*. When working in the severe domain, oxygen uptake continues rising despite roughly constant power or pace levels (5, 11). At this rate, the athlete perceives this work as unsustainable and challenging. The extreme domain occurs during concise and aggressive efforts, and exercise fatigue occurs quickly (5, 11).

While coaches are increasingly using these intensity domains to describe training intensity targets for athletes, the decades-long history of using numbered zones remains the more common way for coaches to prescribe intensity targets during workouts. Training systems may use three to more than nine zones, though using five to six zones is the most common. Generally, the moderate domain contains zone 1 (used for recovery or very long, low-intensity, training) and zone 2 (focuses on steady, moderate to very long duration workouts). The heavy domain generally is broken into zones 3 and 4, representing increasing use of fast oxidative (type IIa) and fast glycolytic (type IIx) muscle fibers and the resulting higher rates of glycolytic metabolism needed to meet the energy needs of high pace, power, or effort exercise. In some systems, the severe domain includes the high end of zone 4 and zone 5. Finally, the extreme domain is home to zone 6 and any zone beyond that. Refer to table 4.2 to see the relationship between RPE, intensity domains, and intensity zones.

Early in the training year or the athlete's career, using zones with physiologic grounding as described previously is helpful. It can prevent overwork and help target weak areas that athletes and coaches have identified. However, one key aim of training for sports is performance. Performance is tied to many components, not just physiology. Athletes receive feedback through their sensory system during workouts; this helps calibrate how hard they feel they are working, which is constantly referenced against the known variables they are encountering on the course relative to their current level of fatigue and readiness (14). As a result, it can be helpful to incorporate maximal session effort (10) or pace-oriented training as the athlete gets closer to racing. This approach enables the athlete to aim to perform at the highest pace for a specific distance or set of intervals within a workout (highest average pace or power for the total duration of an interval set or period of a workout) or use intensities at or slightly over goal race intensity. This work style forces the athlete to face pacing questions they must work through and solve to complete the workout well. In this situation, the distance or duration of the work performed, the athlete's pacing decisions, and the environment experienced drive what physiologic systems must contribute while simultaneously forcing the athlete to think, orienting their output to the situation at hand. This can be challenging work and lead to premature fatigue as the athlete learns, but that is okay. Those experiences help the athlete take the foundational, capacity-oriented work they perform early in the season and help sharpen that so they can use greater levels of race readiness as peak events approach.

Table 4.2 Example Relationship of Perceived Exertion, Intensity Domains, and Intensity Zones

RPE	RPE description	Intensity domain	Intensity zone	Description
1	Nothing at all (lying down)	Moderate	Zone 1	Lying down, relaxing
2	Extremely little		Zones 1 and 2	Very comfortable; walking effort to very relaxed all day effort. Very controlled breathing and no burning in the limbs. Breathing is noticeable, but solid sentences can be spoken and nasal breathing is doable. No burning in the limbs. Confident this could be sustained for many hours.
3	Very easy			
4	Easy (could do this all day)			
5	Moderate			
6	Somewhat hard (starting to feel it)	Heavy	Zone 3 and low end of zone 4	Breathing rate nudges up. Short sentences or phrases can be spoken, and nasal breathing is no longer doable. Burning in the limbs gradually increases the higher into this range one works. Not confident this could be sustained for more than 1-2 hours.
7	Hard			
8	Very hard (making an effort to keep it up)	Severe	High end of zone 4 and zone 5	Breathing is very noticeable, and speaking beyond 1-3 words between breaths is unlikely. Significant burning in the limbs and a sense that this is not sustainable for more than around 10-30 min at most.
9	Very, very hard	Extreme	High end of zone 5 to zone 6 or above	Hyperventilating, speaking unlikely, heavy burning, and a strong sense that this will not be sustainable more than a few minutes at a time.
10	Maximum effort (cannot go any further)			

Adapted from M. Martino and N.C. Dabbs, "Aerobic Training Program Design," in *NSCA's Essentials of Personal Training*, 3rd ed., edited for the National Strength and Conditioning Association by B.J. Schoenfeld and R.L Snarr (Champaign, IL: Human Kinetics, 2022), 432.

CAPACITY AND UTILIZATION

Developing aerobic endurance involves using several training methods and ideas limited only by the sport and the coach and athlete's ingenuity. Because of this, different people use a range of terms to describe similar training strategies, even within a given sport. While coaches and athletes use training intensity zones to target workouts around specific levels or intensity, it is helpful to have a broad concept in mind for orienting the use of those intensity zones to develop fitness. In particular, the two areas of training most specific to aerobic endurance are the capacity to handle the distance and the ability to cover the needed distance as fast as possible without fatigue. As swim coach Bob Bowman describes, an athlete's capacity is the foundation of performance and forms the size of the cup or barrel the athlete has built (1). Ideally, *capacity*-focused work makes the athlete's cup as big as it can be created. On the other hand, *utilization*-focused work is about filling the cup (1). Another example of this breakdown is presented by House and colleagues, who describe capacity development as analogous to building a giant vacuum cleaner to draw up and use pyruvate or lactate for fuel, while utilization training is about growing the lactate shuttle and making a more powerful vacuum (4). While a small handheld vacuum may work well, it is limited in what it can do. Put in too big a motor, and it would vibrate apart or overheat. But if that vacuum is enlarged using durable parts, it has the infrastructure (capacity) to handle much more power (utilization) and thus perform much more work per unit of time. The foundation of performance is built when the athlete has the most significant capacity that can be created. That foundation is maintained with consistent capacity work throughout the athlete's career.

As House and colleagues described, capacity-focused training increases the ability of slow (type I) fibers to take up pyruvate or lactate to produce energy (4). These adaptations delay the onset of LT or CP and extend endurance. Using traditional zone-based training systems, capacity training focuses on zones 1 and 2; this is low-intensity, long-duration work. Capacity-oriented work is long term and can range from generalized to more specific in nature. Endurance athletes often cross-train in the off-season to help build capacity; for example, cross-country skiers use hiking or cycling in the off-season. The training of Nils van der Poel (15), outlined in his manifesto after setting a world record during his gold medal performance in the 10K speed skate at the 2022 Winter Olympics, outlines massive volumes of low-intensity work on the bike as the foundation of his capacity for specific work on the ice. Capacity is the work that ensures an endurance athlete can cover the distance and do the higher-intensity work ultimately needed for success.

Utilization training is focused on work within or above the heavy intensity domain, or intensity zone 3 or above. This work is focused on improving the athlete's ability to produce more work per unit of time. Physiologically, this includes work at greater-than-LT intensities or from the lower border of the heavy-intensity domain up. A key outcome of utilization work is that it helps increase the function of the glycolytic system and improves how well the athlete's lactate shuttle performs, thus allowing higher work rates to be sustained over time. Utilization training also changes an athlete's relationship with RPE: Doing intense work leads to lower-intensity work feeling easier.

APPLYING WORK ORIENTED TO CAPACITY OR UTILIZATION

Capacity training primarily consists of continuous training in the moderate-intensity domain below the LT, within intensity zones 1-2. Long slow distance or duration training (LSD) is the classic example of capacity development. Greater than 75% of the training done by endurance athletes (3, 10) should be focused on capacity development. Capacity training offers athletes a chance to practice fueling for races, builds the ability to continue without fatigue, and improves recovery from higher-intensity training or racing. Increasingly, high volumes of capacity-oriented moderate domain training have been associated with increased aerobic durability—that is, the ability to produce and sustain the highest percentage of the athletes' fresh output after having performed 1,500 to 3,500 or more kilojoules of work within a single exercise bout, a critical factor in competitive success (12). A note of caution for those working with or competing at high levels: High fitness leads to a greater risk of fatigue from capacity training. A national-caliber cyclist, for example, could be performing near 300 watts while within the moderate-intensity domain or zone 2. Despite this being highly oxidative and not acutely fatiguing, the energy demand to sustain work rates at such high levels can lead to significant fatigue. Figure 4.2 shows an example of how challenging a long capacity session can be. A good rule of thumb for long-duration capacity training is that the higher the performance level of the athlete, the better it is to anchor training toward the lower end of zone 2—and even within zone 1 in some cases—to manage the athlete's energy balance best.

Utilization training focuses on intensities that are above the moderate- to heavy-intensity domain transition or zones 3 or above within most modern training intensity zone systems. These workouts include work at or above the LT via intensity progressions, fartlek-style training, time trial efforts, interval workouts, and even shorter duration races. Utilization training helps athletes learn how they fatigue during higher-intensity training or racing, helps tune race pacing strategies, and improves athlete decision making regarding how to distribute work over a given duration or distance. Many training systems

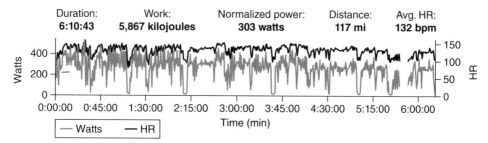

Figure 4.2 The energy demand challenge of extensive low-intensity training. This figure shows a workout performed by a national-caliber gravel and endurance mountain bike racer, which was performed at just over 300 watts, yet still within zone 2 (moderate domain). A workout like this required several days for recovery, despite the relatively low intensity at which it is performed, due to the huge energy demand (5,867 kilojoules [1,402 kcals]) it placed on the athlete.

attempt to plan variation (periodization) of these higher-intensity utilization workouts. Regardless of the training system employed, a good rule of thumb for this work style is to start with a comfortable duration at the targeted intensity and extend the time at that intensity before increasing to higher work rates. Figure 4.3 describes one strategy for growing time at intensity before increasing intensity as the athlete progresses. This approach allows athletes to explore high-intensity work, gain competence, and expand their readiness to tackle higher work rates over similar durations. Specifically, figure 4.3 provides an example of utilization workouts (zone 3 and above; heavy domain) that are progressed via extending duration before intensifying. The top workout incorporates 5 × 5-minute intervals at zone 4 with 2 minutes at zone 1 rest intervals. The total time at intensity is 25 minutes (5 intervals × 5 minutes = 25 minutes at intensity). The second workout is 4 × 7 minutes at zone 4 with 2 minutes at zone 1 rest intervals. Total time at intensity has extended to 28 minutes during this workout. The last workout is 4 × 8 minutes at zone 4, for a time at intensity of 32 minutes. These workouts could be repeated for 2 to 3 weeks each before adjusting. Note that time at intensity can be increased via more intervals or longer intervals at the same intensity. Once the goal duration at intensity has been reached, slightly intensifying with shorter intervals restarts the process. The intervals performed at a given point in the year are based on coach- and athlete-determined needs, goals, and training outline for the season.

Ultimately, the ideal approach for building aerobic endurance uses a foundation of primarily capacity-oriented work throughout the athletes' career, augmented by utilization-oriented work that goes from less to more race-like the closer to key races an athlete is. Repeated over many years, this progression helps ensure athletes race with competence and confidence.

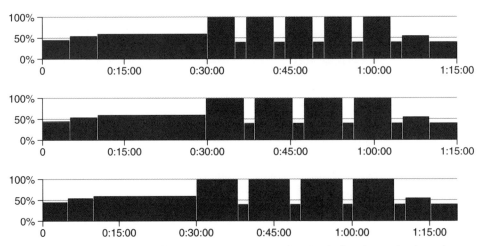

Figure 4.3 The progression of workouts via increasing duration before increasing intensity.

DISTRIBUTION OVER YEAR/WEEK

While debate persists over whether there is an ideal distribution of aerobic development work over the training year, a few broad points are repeatedly borne out in practice and research: athletes should do most (75%-90%) of their training in the moderate-intensity domain and a smaller but no less critical portion of their training (10%-20%) in the heavy-intensity domain or above (11, 13). This is commonly described as polarized or pyramidal training intensity distribution (TID) (3). Within polarized TID, most training is done at lower intensities within the moderate domain; the next most used intensity is at or above the heavy and severe intensity domain border; and finally, work within the heavy domain is least used. Within a pyramidal TID, most work is again performed within the moderate-intensity domain. However, more training is conducted in the heavy domain than at or over the heavy and severe domain border. Most coaches and athletes tend to blend these over the course of the year to fit a critical need of athletes: to become more specifically fit as they approach their target races. Note that both intensity distribution patterns relate to completed workouts and not training minutes (11).

These approaches mean an endurance athlete's training consists mainly of capacity-oriented work. It is augmented with different utilization-themed workouts based on proximity to critical races and athlete need. The key point is that an athlete should use all intensity levels to varying degrees throughout the training year. For example, early in an athlete's training year, the focus may be on a polarized approach with a heavy emphasis on capacity training at low intensities. During this time, the athlete touches on small doses of utilization training in or above the heavy-intensity domain to build those skills more generally toward their specific performance goals and reduce the detraining of abilities built during previous training periods. This distribution would change as the athlete approaches key races, with more work near race intensity—a pyramidal TID. As legendary running coach Renato Canova said, "You lose what you don't use, hence why it is important to train across as many paces as possible to keep improving."

If athletes train at similar load levels day over day, week over week, the regular monotony of training can increase the risk of burnout and under-recovery. It takes time to recover from higher-intensity workouts, very long workouts, or workouts combining duration and intensity. Training weeks should follow a hard–easy pattern, with days or short blocks of days with higher load training coupled with slightly more extended periods of lower load training (see figure 4.4).

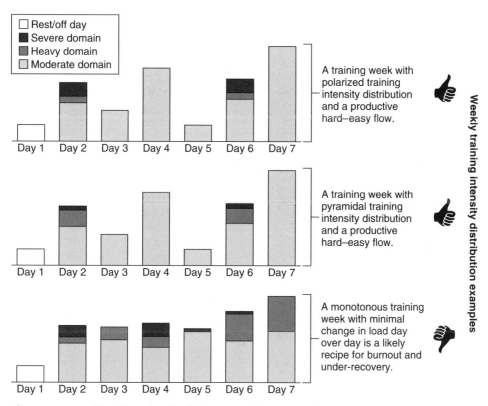

Figure 4.4 Training intensity distribution over the week.

WORKOUT TYPES

The following segments of this chapter generally describe workouts for capacity and utilization. While there are some specific examples, initially, the approach provides concepts and ideas that the reader can use to create training formats that work within their context. For example, within the capacity-focused phase of the year, overdistance and endurance training sessions are a focus. Capacity workouts like these are focused on zones 1 and 2. During the utilization training phase of the year, a nearly limitless number of interval workouts could be performed that challenge the athlete via work in zone 3 and above. This includes workouts broadly focused on tempo, LT, $\dot{V}O_2$max, and anaerobic power via repeated sprint training; micro-interval sets; fast-start intervals; fast-finishing intervals; hill repeats; short, medium, and long intervals; variably paced intervals (going over and under a target intensity area); descending and ascending interval sets; fartlek; and so on. Each group can have many subgroups or variations as well. When selecting what sessions to use when, keep as a guiding principle the concept of becoming increasingly race-like while getting closer to target events.

While determining how much volume or intensity is enough within a workout or extended training period, always remember that consistency is the keystone of peak performance. If a workout or training period is designed with the highest load an athlete can tolerate, the risk is high that the athlete could end up breaking down. Instead, aim to target a workload that often leaves the athlete wanting a little more. This approach focuses on stimulating adaptation while allowing reasonably quick recovery, thus, the greatest consistency of training over the long haul.

WORKOUTS FOR CAPACITY

Capacity-oriented workouts focus on the ability to cover the distance required and resist fatigue.

LSD (Overdistance)

▶ *Warm-up:* This is sport specific; the aim is to build to workout intensity, potentially including form drills before reaching the target intensity. Use a consistent warm-up so it can become a tool to assess readiness for training over time by determining how metrics such as RPE, HR, and pace or power relate.

▶ *Workout:* 60 minutes to 6 or more hours depending on the sport. Target the workout to the low end of the zone 2 intensity range. On hills or headwinds, allow drifting toward the high end of the zone before settling back to the lower end of the range once the challenge is lower. Maintain intensity discipline during this workout, resisting the urge to drift up in effort over the session.

▶ *Cooldown:* Reduce to walking intensity during the sport to ease out of the session over the last 5 to 10 minutes, potentially followed by light stretching or relaxing visualization before moving on with the day.

Steady Distance or Duration

▶ *Warm-up:* This is sport specific; the aim is to build to workout intensity, potentially including form drills before reaching the target intensity. Use a consistent warm-up so it can become a tool to assess readiness for training over time by determining how metrics such as RPE, HR, and pace or power relate.

▶ *Workout:* Aim for 45 to 120 minutes, depending on the sport. Target the workout to the low end of the zone 2 intensity range. On hills or headwinds, allow drifting toward the high end of the zone before settling back to the lower end of the range once the workout is completed. Maintain intensity discipline during this workout, resisting the urge to drift up in effort over the session. Within this workout, the athlete can include three to six bouts of short (<10 min) higher speed movement to maintain speed skill. Examples include a cyclist rapidly spinning up to the highest cadence they can sustain without bouncing on the bike's saddle, or a runner, skater, skier, or paddler performing pickups or strides, which are evenly distributed over the entire duration of the workout.

▶ *Cooldown:* Reduce to walking intensity during the sport to ease out of the session over the last 5 to 10 minutes, potentially followed by light stretching or relaxing visualization before moving on with the day.

Active Recovery

▶ *Warm-up:* This is sport specific; the aim is to build to workout intensity, potentially including form drills before reaching the target intensity. Use a consistent warm-up so it can become a tool to assess readiness for training over time by determining how metrics such as RPE, HR, and pace or power relate.

▶ *Workout:* Aim for 20 to 90 minutes, depending on the sport (longer for higher performing athletes and non-weight-bearing sports; shorter for lower performing athletes and weight-bearing sports) at zone 1 intensity. These sessions should feel easy to the athlete.

▶ *Cooldown:* Reduce to walking intensity during the sport to ease out of the session over the last 5 to 10 minutes, potentially followed by light stretching or relaxing visualization before moving on with the day.

WORKOUTS FOR UTILIZATION

Utilization training aims to increase the work rate that can be sustained during racing and can improve the ability to repeat high work rate bouts during extended activity.

Progressions

▶ *Warm-up:* This is sport specific; the aim is to build to workout intensity, potentially including form drills before reaching the target intensity. Use a consistent warm-up so it can become a tool to assess readiness for training over time by determining how metrics such as RPE, HR, and pace or power relate.

▶ *Workout:* The duration is sport specific, possibly lasting up to several hours. Start the workout anchored to the base of zone 2; once a targeted point of the workout is reached, the intensity begins to build up to a specific area. This area could range from just below the target race pace to 10% over that pace, or it could be performed such that intensity abruptly steps up to the target race pace or up to 10% over the target race pace, depending on the duration of the workout.

▶ *Cooldown:* Reduce to walking intensity during the sport to ease out of the session over the last 5 to 10 minutes, potentially followed by light stretching or relaxing visualization before moving on with the day.

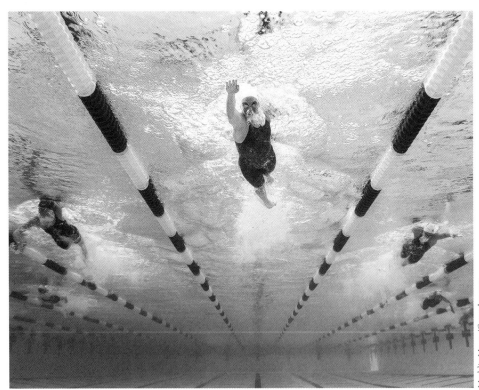

Maddie Meyer/Getty Images

Utilization training aims to increase the sustainable work rate and the ability to do repeated bouts at a high work rate.

Intervals

▶ *Warm-up:* This is sport specific; the aim is to build to workout intensity, potentially including form drills before reaching the target intensity. Use a consistent warm-up so it can become a tool to assess readiness for training over time by determining how metrics such as RPE, HR, and pace or power relate.

▶ *Workout:* Start the workout at the low end of zone 2 intensity. Use this as the base intensity for the workout. During the workout, perform 20 to 90 minutes of total time at or over the moderate- to heavy-intensity domain border: zone 3 and above.

  • *Short example:* Perform 8 to 12 intervals of a maximal yet repeatable effort of 30 seconds (likely at zone 5 or above; i.e., the highest intensity that can be maintained or slightly increased throughout the workout), with 2- to 4-minute easy recovery intervals in zone 1 (a walking level of effort).

  • *Moderate example:* Perform 4 to 6 intervals of 3 minutes at zone 4 or above, with 2- to 3-minute recovery intervals in zone 1.

  • *Moderately long example:* Perform 4 intervals of 8 minutes in zone 4 or above, with 2-minute recovery intervals in zone 1.

  • *Long example 1:* Perform 2 to 4 intervals of 12 minutes in zone 4, with 2-minute recovery intervals in zone 1.

  • *Long example 2:* 1 Perform 2 to 4 intervals of 16 minutes in zone 3 building to zone 4, with 2-minute recovery intervals in zone 1.

  • *Long example 3:* Perform 2 to 4 intervals of 20 minutes in zone 4, with 5-minute recovery intervals in zone 1.

  • *Fast starts:* Perform 4 to 6 intervals of 5 minutes paced such that the first 1 to 2 minutes per interval are targeting zone 5 or above and the next 2 to 5 minutes per interval are in zones 3 or 4, with 2-minute recovery intervals in zone 1.

  • *Micro-intervals:* Perform 2 or 3 sets of 20- to 60-second intervals in zone 5 or above, with equal duration rest intervals (i.e., 20 to 60 seconds, between the 20- to 60-second efforts) in zone 1. Allow 2-5 minutes in zone 1 between sets.

▶ *Cooldown:* Reduce to walking intensity during the sport to ease out of the session over the last 5 to 10 minutes, potentially followed by light stretching or relaxing visualization before moving on with the day.

Hill Repeats

▶ *Warm-up:* This is sport specific; the aim is to build to workout intensity, potentially including form drills before reaching the target intensity. Use a consistent warm-up so it can become a tool to assess readiness for training over time by determining how metrics such as RPE, HR, and pace or power relate.

▶ *Workout:* Start the workout at the low end of zone 2 intensity. Use this as the base intensity for the workout. During the workout, perform 1 to 15 minutes at or over the upper end of the heavy-intensity domain (zone 4 and above). For example:

- 10-12 intervals × 10-second maximum repeatable effort (zone 5 or above), with 2- to 3-minute recovery intervals in zone 1
- 8-12 intervals × 30-second maximum repeatable effort (zone 5 or above), with 2- to 3-minute recovery intervals in zone 1
- 4-8 intervals × 90-second maximum repeatable effort (zone 5 or above), with 2- to 3-minute recovery intervals in zone 1

▶ *Cooldown:* Reduce to walking intensity during the sport to ease out of the session over the last 5 to 10 minutes, potentially followed by light stretching or relaxing visualization before moving on with the day.

Fartlek Training

▶ *Warm-up:* This is sport specific; the aim is to build to workout intensity, potentially including form drills before reaching the target intensity. Use a consistent warm-up so it can become a tool to assess readiness for training over time by determining how metrics such as RPE, HR, and pace or power relate.

▶ *Workout:* Start the workout at the low end of zone 2 intensity. Use this as the base intensity for the activity. During the workout, perform 10 to 90 minutes at or over the heavy-intensity domain (zone 3 and above). Accumulate this time with fun- or terrain-oriented intervals. For example, cyclists could choose to ride all the hills they feel are short and steep at a fast and robust pace over the final half of a ride, recovering to a zone 1 level after each effort. Runners could select various distances or durations and run those segments fast, recovering to zone 1 after each effort.

▶ *Cooldown:* Reduce to walking intensity during the sport to ease out of the session over the last 5 to 10 minutes, potentially followed by light stretching or relaxing visualization before moving on with the day.

WORKOUTS FOR SPECIAL SITUATIONS

These workouts apply to race simulation, benchmarks, specific environments (e.g., hills, heat, cold), and taper.

Race Intensity Intervals

▶ *Warm-up:* This is sport specific; the aim is to build to workout intensity, potentially including form drills before reaching the target intensity. Use a consistent warm-up so it can become a tool to assess readiness for training over time by determining how metrics such as RPE, HR, and pace or power relate.

▶ *Workout:* Start the workout at the low end of zone 2 intensity. Use this as the base intensity for the workout. During the workout, perform 10 minutes or 2 hours or more at or up to 10% over the goal pace for the athlete's target race. The specific duration is based on the athlete's ability and the duration of the race. For example, an elite athlete could safely handle more volume at this intensity than a recreational athlete, and a long-distance triathlete could use longer durations than a 5 km runner. Examples follow:

  • Run 6 miles (9.7 km) at zone 2, then 2 miles (3.2 km) alternating every 1/4 mile (0.4 km) between 5% over half marathon goal intensity and at zone 2.

  • Ride 40 miles (64.4 km) at a base intensity level of zone 2. During the final 15 miles (24.1 km) of the ride, alternate 4 miles (6.4 km) at 5% over the race pace of a 70.3 distance triathlon and 1 mile (1.6 km) at zone 1 for recovery.

  • Ride 60 miles (96.6 km) at a base intensity level zone 2. During the final 30 miles (48.3 km) of the ride, maintain a pace ±5% of the race pace of a 70.3 distance triathlon.

▶ *Cooldown:* Reduce to walking intensity during the sport to ease out of the session over the last 5 to 10 minutes, potentially followed by light stretching or relaxing visualization before moving on with the day.

Benchmark Workouts

▶ *Warm-up:* This is sport specific; the aim is to build to workout intensity, potentially including form drills before reaching the target intensity. A warm-up of 10 to 15 minutes is generally adequate. Use a consistent warm-up so it can become a tool to assess readiness for training over time by determining how metrics such as RPE, HR, and pace or power relate.

▸ *Workout:* Perform a duration or distance of 30% to 70% of the race duration at the athlete's goal race pace. During this session, practice race fueling, any specific mental strategies, and specific pacing strategies, and use as much gear as the athlete would use during racing as possible. Use the performance and experience of this workout to help adjust the training approach and race goals to fit actual performance capabilities.

▸ *Cooldown:* Reduce to walking intensity during the sport to ease out of the session over the last 5 to 10 minutes, potentially followed by light stretching or relaxing visualization before moving on with the day.

Table 4.3 provides examples of workouts similar to the concepts just described, which are pulled from athletes' actual training programs, to provide a more detailed example that coaches and athletes can use to help build their workouts for specific situations.

Table 4.3 Examples of Capacity- and Utilization-Themed Workouts

Capacity workout examples	Utilization workout examples
LSD run *Warm-up:* Build strength to help keep healthy and improve readiness to do the running workout) • Joint mobilization (i.e., wiggle, flex, and extend) each major joint. Do 10-15 reps of each action per joint. • Walk backward 20 steps. • Walk sideways 20 steps per side. • Do 10 walking crossover steps per direction. • Build into the first 3 to 5 min of the run (counts to the total) and enjoy the session. *Workout:* Run in zone 2 for 1.75 hr; use HR and RPE. The aim is to learn to run at the lowest intensity possible, calibrating RPE and HR to that point. If possible to do so safely, running on dirt roads or trails is ideal. *Cooldown:* Transition from running to the rest of the day; foster mental and physical rejuvenation after the workout. • Walk 3 to 5 min. • Perform light stretching or yoga.	**Short hill repeat workout** *Warm-up:* Build from zone 1 to zone 2 over about 10 min. *Workout:* Sustain zone 2 for 15 to 30 min to the base of a short steep hill, ideally on a road without too much traffic. Then ride 30 sec up the hill at zone 5 or higher (the highest pace that can be repeated interval to interval through the workout). Safely turn and ride down easily in zone 1, then turn back and repeat. Aim for 8 to 10 intervals of 30 sec in zone 5 or above with a 2- to 3-min zone 1 rest interval between each hill repeat. *Note:* Make this a game. The first interval should be performed solidly but with the knowledge that there are more to go. The athlete should note how far up the hill he or she went on interval number 1, and then try to equal or beat the previous interval as the workout progresses. *Cooldown:* After the last interval, ride home in zone 1 to cool down for 10 to 20 min.

Capacity workout examples	Utilization workout examples
Steady bike to run This session is about building bike to run endurance. *Warm-up:* Build up to zone 2 over 5 minutes, then cruise comfortably in zone 2. *Workout:* Do a 1.5- to 1.75-hr ride in zone 2. Ideally, this ride is done outdoors, which will result in the use of the full range of zone 2 due to variability caused by the hills and wind. If this workout is done on an indoor bike trainer, purposefully alternating between the low end of zone 2 for 5-10 minutes and the high end of zone 2 for 5-10 minutes throughout the ride can help reduce boredom and cause the workout to feel more like an outdoor ride. Then, withing 15 minutes of finishing the ride, do a 25- to 30-minute steady run in zone 2. *Cooldown:* Walk for 5 min. If desired, perform light stretching or yoga.	**Long interval run** This session increases the ability to sustain higher intensities longer without fatigue. *Warm-up:* Build to zone 2 over 10 min, then cruise zone 2 for 5 to 10 min. *Workout:* Do 3 × 12-min intervals such that the first interval is in zone 3, the second interval is roughly half in zone 3 and half in zone 4, and the final interval is in zone 4, with a 2- to 3-min rest interval in zone 1 between each building interval. *Cooldown:* Walk for 5 to 10 min. If desired, perform light stretching or yoga.
Steady aerobic run *Warm-up:* Build strength to help keep healthy and improve readiness to do the running workout) • Joint mobilization (i.e., wiggle, flex, and extend) each major joint. Do 10-15 reps of each action per joint. • Walk backward 20 steps. • Walk sideways 20 steps per side. • Do 10 walking crossover steps per direction. • Build into the first 3 to 5 min of the run (counts to the total) and enjoy the session. *Workout:* Run in zone 2 for 30 min using HR and RPE. The aim is to learn to run at the lowest intensity possible, calibrating RPE and HR at that point. *Cooldown:* Transition from running to the rest of the day; foster mental and physical rejuvenation after the workout). • Walk 3 to 5 min. • Perform light stretching or yoga.	**Micro-interval workout** This session increases the ability to sustain a high work rate despite constant accelerations over the threshold during a race. *Warm-up:* Build to zone 2 over 10 min, then cruise in zone 2 for 10 to 15 min. *Workout:* Do 3 sets of 8 × 40 sec intervals at zone 5 or higher, with 20 sec in zone 1 (soft pedal or even coast) between intervals and a 4-min recovery in zone 1 between sets. Finish the ride with 10 min in zone 2 before fading to zone 1 over 5 min. Pick a route that is easy to ride on steadily. For example, open roads are acceptable as long as they have areas for the intervals that are uphill, flat, or lightly rolling as opposed to an area where the intervals would need to be performed downhill, which would be more dangerous than valuable. *Cooldown:* Ride the last 5 to 10 min in zone 1.

CONCLUSION

Aerobic endurance can be built in endless ways. That said, the approach can be simple, focused on capacity work with lower-intensity steady sessions as the foundation of training over the year, then a shift from less race-like to more race-like utilization-style training as target races approach. The key for coaches and self-coached athletes is to be sure their training approach is centered on the athlete, is adaptable, and fosters well-rounded growth including all levels of work at a load the athlete from which the athlete can consistently recover over the training year. This simple-to-state but complex-to-implement strategy sets the athlete up to adapt and be ready to go on race day.

Exercise Technique

Antonio Squillante
Peter Melanson*

This chapter describes the proper technique for a range of resistance exercises that are commonly performed by aerobic endurance athletes. For all resistance exercises, it is important to follow the general safety suggestions and lifting guidelines presented at the beginning of this chapter. In addition, athletes should always follow the manufacturer's safety and usage instructions for each piece of resistance exercise equipment. Further, before attempting to perform new resistance exercises, an athlete should always receive proper instruction and supervision from a certified strength and conditioning specialist or certified personal trainer. During many free weight resistance exercises, athletes must make sure that they have proper spotting assistance.

LIFTING GUIDELINES

The following guidelines provide basic information that is essential for safe and productive resistance training. Experienced athletes may already know some of this information, but for those who are new to resistance training, understanding these guidelines will be useful whenever they perform resistance training sessions in the weight room.

Technique

Lifters often need to lift a bar or dumbbells off the floor before getting into the starting position for an exercise (e.g., bent-over row, biceps curl, dumbbell flat or incline bench press or fly, upright row, lying triceps extension, stiff-leg deadlift). To avoid excessive strain on the low back, athletes need to place the body in the correct position to lift the weight safely and effectively. Athletes can do this by following these guidelines (5):

  ▶ Use the correct stance in relation to the bar or dumbbells, and properly grasp the bar or dumbbell handles.

*Antonio Squillante was contracted to author this chapter; Peter Melanson's name was added to acknowledge his significant contribution partially retained from the previous edition.

▸ Place the feet between hip- and shoulder-width apart.

▸ Squat down behind the bar or between the dumbbells.

▸ If lifting a bar, position the bar close to the shins and over the balls of the feet, and grasp the bar with a closed grip that is shoulder-width (or slightly wider) apart.

▸ If lifting dumbbells, stand directly between them and grasp the handles with a closed grip and a neutral arm and hand position.

▸ Position the arms outside the knees with the elbows extended.

Before lifting a weight off the floor, athletes must place their body in the correct preparatory position. The following guidelines describe how the body should be positioned immediately before the first repetition of a power exercise (e.g., snatch, power clean) (5).

▸ The back is flat or slightly arched.

▸ The trapezius is relaxed and slightly stretched, the chest is held up and out, and the scapulae are held together.

▸ The head is in line with the spine or slightly hyperextended.

▸ Body weight is balanced between the middle and balls of the feet, but the heels are in contact with the floor.

▸ The shoulders are over or slightly in front of the bar.

▸ The eyes are focused straight ahead or slightly upward.

Weight Belts

The use of a weight belt can help prevent injury during training. The decision on whether to use a belt should be based on the type of exercise and the relative load being lifted. Weight belts are most appropriate in the following situations (1, 2):

▸ During exercises that place stress on the low back (e.g., back squat, front squat, deadlift)

▸ During sets in which near-maximal or maximal loads are being used

The use of a weight belt in these situations may reduce the risk of injuries to the low back—but only when combined with correct exercise technique and proper spotting. Note that some people may have increased blood pressure as a result of wearing a weight belt. Elevated blood pressure is associated with dizziness and fatigue and could result in headaches, fainting, or injury. Additionally, people with hypertension or any preexisting cardiovascular condition should not wear a weight belt because doing so might lead to a heart attack or stroke.

GENERAL SAFETY SUGGESTIONS

Athletes should follow these guidelines to ensure safe exercise technique (5):

- Perform power and explosive exercises in an area that is clean, dry, flat, well-marked, and free of obstacles and people (e.g., on a lifting platform). This guideline also applies to other complex nonpower exercises such as the lunge, deadlift, and step-up. If a repetition in a power or explosive exercise cannot be completed, the athlete should push forward on the bar to move the body backward and then let the bar fall to the floor. Athletes should not attempt to save a missed or failed repetition for this type of exercise.

- Check to see if there is sufficient floor-to-ceiling space before performing exercises that finish with the bar overhead. Athletes should use a bar with revolving sleeves, especially for the power and explosive exercises.

- For the front squat and back squat, use a squat or power rack with the supporting pins or hooks set to position the bar at armpit height. This setting should also be used when the preferred method for an exercise is to begin or end with the bar at shoulder height (rather than begin or end with the bar on the floor).

- When lifting the bar up and out of the supporting pins or hooks of a squat or power rack in preparation for an exercise, always step backward at the beginning of the set and step forward at the end of the set. The athlete should not walk backward to return the bar to the rack. This is a good safety practice that reduces the potential for a misstep when fatigued.

- When using free weights, always use collars and locks to secure the weight plates on the bar.

- For machine exercises, be sure to fully insert the selectorized pin or key (usually L or T shaped) into the weight stack.

- A spotter should assist for safety during free weight exercises.

From NSCA. *Exercise Technique Manual for Resistance Training.* 4th ed. Champaign, IL: Human Kinetics, xii-xiv, 2022.

Grips

Different types of grips are used for different exercises. Two basic positions are used for placing the hands on the bar. In the *pronated* position, the bar is gripped with the palms facing backward. A pronated grip is used for almost all exercises that require the weight to be lifted above the head. In the supinated hand position, the palm is facing forward when grasping the bar. When the thumb is wrapped around the fingers that are grasping the bar, this is referred to as a *closed grip.* On the rare occasion when the bar is gripped with the thumb in line with the fingers, this is referred to as an *open grip.* An open grip is less secure than a closed grip and increases the risk of accidents.

Grip width is also an important variable to consider. It is possible to use a standard grip, a narrow grip, and a wide grip. Although there are recommended grip widths for all exercises, the athlete may have a preference to modify grip width as long as doing so does not affect the performance of the exercise.

TYPES OF EXERCISES

This chapter provides information on three main types of exercises: Olympic lifts, barbell or dumbbell resistance training exercises, and plyometrics (table 5.1).

Olympic lifts use large muscle groups and involve multiple body parts being trained at the same time. These exercises help an athlete develop coordination, strength, and power. They include the snatch, clean and jerk, and their main *derivatives* (variations). Full Olympic lifts are technical and quite challenging. Unless adequate time can be allocated to learning and mastering technique, less technical variations should be used instead. Readers are encouraged to consult the NSCA's *Exercise Technique Manual for Resistance Training* for more information.

Table 5.1 Exercises for Aerobic Endurance Athletes

Exercise	Page number
OLYMPIC LIFTS	
Power Clean	97
Power Snatch	98
BARBELL OR DUMBBELL RESISTANCE TRAINING	
Back Squat	100
Front Squat	100
Bulgarian Squat	101
Forward or Backward Lunge (Barbell or Dumbbell)	102
Step-Up (Barbell or Dumbbell)	103
Romanian Deadlift (RDL)	104
Dumbbell or Barbell Calf Raise	105
Barbell or Dumbbell Bench Press	106
Lat Pulldown (Machine)	107
Bent-Over Row	108
Barbell Shoulder Press	109
Triceps Pushdown (Machine)	110
Dumbbell Biceps Curl	111
PLYOMETRICS	
Depth Jump	112
Countermovement Jump or Broad Jump	113
Squat Jump (With a Pause)	114
Single-Leg Hop	115

Lower and upper body resistance training exercises using a barbell or one or two dumbbells can be used to target large and small muscle groups and involve multiple or isolated muscles or muscle groups. Lower body resistance training exercises include three fundamental movement patterns: squatting, hinging, and lunging. Upper body resistance training exercises include two fundamental movement patterns: pushing (or pressing) and pulling, both on the horizontal and the vertical plane. To prevent muscle imbalances, it is important to incorporate an equal number of exercises for the main muscle groups of the lower and upper extremities. In the essence of time, structural exercises (i.e., multijoint, compound movements with a high amount of axial loading) are often preferred over single-joint exercises. Individuals who are not comfortable or skilled enough to perform barbell exercises or prefer to train at home can use a flat bench and a set of kettlebells or adjustable dumbbells instead.

Plyometric training includes a number of different exercises from jumping to bounding, hopping, and leaping. These are ballistic, explosive exercises used to increase power and promote greater movement economy. Plyometric training can also be used to prevent the risk of common overuse injuries, such as tendinopathy, among aerobic endurance athletes (2).

In a given workout, Olympic lifts and plyometric exercises should be done first because they require the most concentration, skill, and effort (6).

OLYMPIC LIFTS

POWER CLEAN

The athlete stands with the feet between hip- and shoulder-width apart; the toes are pointed forward or slightly outward. The athlete squats and grasps the bar with the hands slightly wider than the shoulders (and outside the knees) using a closed, pronated grip. The elbows are extended and the body is positioned so the back is flat or slightly arched (photo a); the chest is up, the shoulders are over the bar, and the eyes are focused forward or slightly up.

1. The athlete forcefully extends the hips and knees to lift the bar, keeping the torso-to-floor angle constant by maintaining a flat-back position. The elbows should remain fully extended and with the bar kept as close to the shins as possible.

2. As the bar rises to just above the knees, the athlete forcefully extends the hips and knees and also extends the ankles (plantar flexion) and keeps the bar as close to the body as possible. The athlete's back remains flat, and the elbows point out to the sides. The athlete keeps the shoulders over the bar and the elbows extended for as long as possible.

3. When the ankle, knee, and hip reach full extension (triple extension), the athlete shrugs the shoulders upward with the elbows still fully extended. As the shoulders reach their highest elevation, the athlete flexes the elbows to begin pulling the body under the bar; the arms continue pulling as long as possible. The torso is erect, the head is erect or tilted slightly back, and the feet may lose contact with

the floor (photo *b*). After the lower body has fully extended, the athlete pulls the body under the bar and rotates the arms around and under the bar while simultaneously flexing the hips and knees to a quarter-squat position.

4. Once the arms are under the bar, the athlete lifts the elbows so that the upper arms are parallel to the floor to rack the bar across the front of the clavicles and anterior deltoids. When the athlete catches the bar, the torso is nearly erect, the shoulders are slightly ahead of the buttocks, the head is in a neutral position, and the feet are flat.

5. After gaining control and balance, the athlete stands up by extending the hips and knees to a fully erect position (photo *c*).

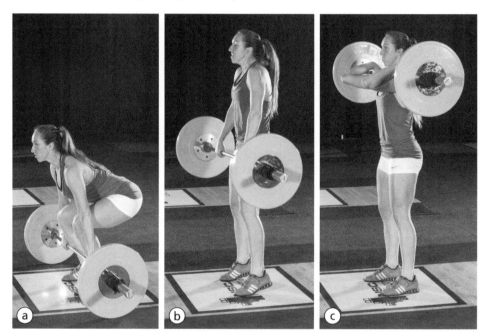

POWER SNATCH

The athlete stands with the feet pointed slightly out and positioned between hip- and shoulder-width apart. With the bar grasped with a closed, pronated, snatch-width grip, the athlete positions the body with the back flat or slightly arched, the trapezius relaxed and slightly stretched, and the chest held up and out. The heels are in contact with the floor, and the shoulders are over or slightly in front of the bar (photo *a*).

1. The athlete lifts the bar by extending the hips and knees while maintaining the flat-back position; the torso-to-floor angle should remain constant. The elbows stay fully extended, and the shoulders remain over or slightly ahead of the bar. The athlete keeps the bar as close to the shins as possible.

2. As the bar rises to just above the knees, the athlete forcefully jumps, performing triple extension, and keeps the bar as close to the body as possible. The back stays flat, the elbows are extended and pointing out, and the shoulders are over the bar.

3. After reaching full triple extension, the athlete rapidly shrugs the shoulders upward with the elbows still fully extended. As the shoulders reach their highest elevation, the athlete flexes the elbows to begin pulling the body under the bar; the arms continue pulling as long as possible (photo b). Because of the explosive nature of this phase, the feet may lose contact with the floor.

4. After the lower body has fully extended, the athlete pulls the body beneath the bar and rotates the hands around and under the bar. Simultaneously, the athlete flexes the hips and knees to a quarter-squat position.

5. Once the body is under the bar, the athlete catches the bar over or slightly behind the head with fully extended elbows, a neutral head position, and flat feet (photo c). After gaining control and balance, the athlete stands up by extending the hips and knees to a fully erect position, and stabilizes the bar overhead.

6. The athlete lowers the bar by gradually allowing a controlled descent of the bar to the thighs while simultaneously flexing the hips and knees to cushion the impact of the bar on the thighs.

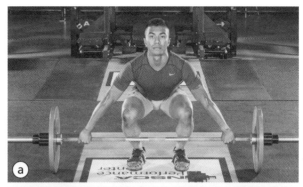

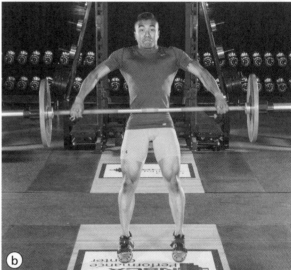

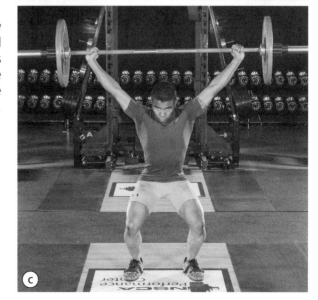

BARBELL OR DUMBBELL RESISTANCE TRAINING

BACK SQUAT

The athlete assumes a shoulder-width stance, holding the barbell on top of the scapulae and trapezius (photo *a*). The hands are slightly wider than the shoulders. The toes may be pointed outward slightly.

1. Keeping the torso erect, the athlete squats by sitting back with the hips until the top of the thighs are parallel to the floor (photo *b*).
2. The athlete then extends the legs at the hips and knees to return to the starting position.

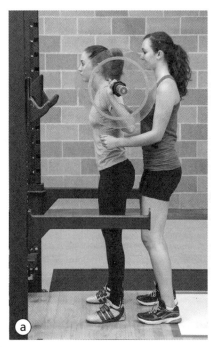
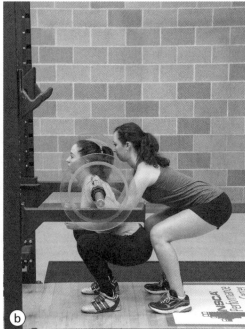

FRONT SQUAT

The athlete assumes a shoulder-width stance, with the toes pointing out slightly. The elbows are positioned high in front of the body as possible so that the barbell rests on the front of the shoulder (photo *a*). The hands are slightly wider than the shoulders.

1. Keeping the torso erect, the athlete squats by lowering the body at the knees and hips until the tops of the thighs are parallel to the floor (photo *b*) with the elbows still kept elevated as high as possible.
2. The athlete then extends the legs at the hips and knees to return to the starting position.

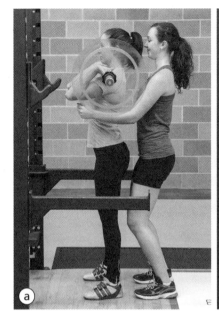
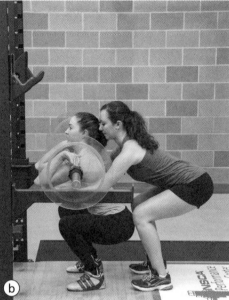

BULGARIAN SQUAT

The athlete starts in a shoulder-width stance and then places the top of one foot on top of a 12- to 18-inch (30-46 cm) box or bench behind the athlete while holding a barbell on top of the scapulae and trapezius (photo *a*).

1. The athlete flexes at the knee and hip of the supporting leg until the top of the front thigh is parallel to the floor (photo *b*). The back knee should be about 1 inch (2.5 cm) above the floor. The athlete should keep the front foot flat on the floor and keep the knee in line with the second and third toe of the lead foot; the lead knee should not excessively extend forward past the toes.

2. The athlete pushes through the supporting leg and returns to the starting position.

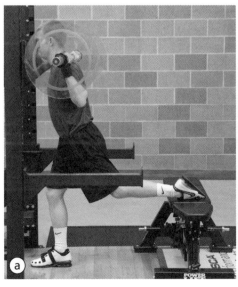
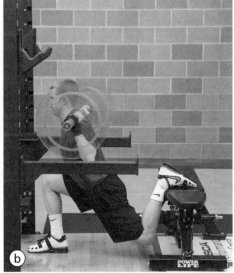

FORWARD OR BACKWARD LUNGE (BARBELL OR DUMBBELL)

The athlete starts in a shoulder-width stance while holding a barbell on top of the scapulae (photo *a*) or holding a pair of dumbbells (one in each hand) at the sides of the body.

1. The athlete begins by stepping forward (the forward lunge exercise) or backward (the backward lunge exercise, sometimes called a *reverse lunge*) with one leg. The step should not be so large that the athlete loses balance.

2. When the entire foot makes contact with the floor, the athlete flexes at the knees and hips until the top of the front thigh is parallel to the floor (photo *b*). The back knee should be about 1 inch (2.5 cm) above the floor. The athlete should keep the front foot flat on the floor and keep the knee in line with the second and third toe of the lead foot; the lead knee should not excessively extend forward past the toes.

3. The athlete forcefully pushes back with the front leg (the forward lunge exercise) or forward with the back leg (the backward lunge exercise) to return to the starting position.

4. The athlete repeats the movement with the other leg.

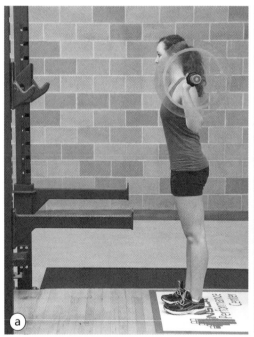

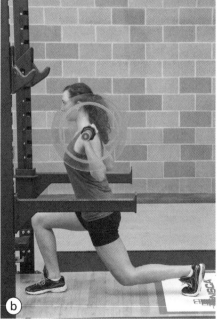

STEP-UP (BARBELL OR DUMBBELL)

The athlete places the lead foot on top of a box that is high enough so that the knee is at a 90-degree angle. The athlete positions a barbell on the upper back (photo a) or holds a pair of dumbbells (one in each hand) at the sides of the body. With one foot on top of the box, the athlete shifts the weight to the lead leg to prevent pushing off the floor with the trail leg.

1. The athlete extends the hip and knee of the lead leg to a standing position on top of the box. The torso is kept erect to avoid flexing forward at the hips.
2. The athlete brings the trail leg up to the box and positions the foot parallel to the lead foot (photo b).
3. The athlete steps down with the trail leg, moving back to the starting position.
4. The athlete repeats this movement for the desired number of repetitions and then switches legs.

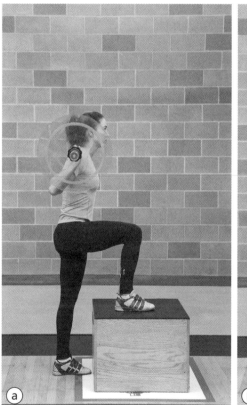
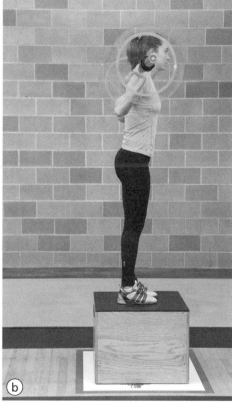

ROMANIAN DEADLIFT (RDL)

The athlete stands with the feet hip-width apart. Using a pronated grip, the athlete holds a barbell against the front of the thighs and unlocks the knees so they are slightly flexed. This position is maintained throughout the duration of the exercise (photo *a*). The athlete should squeeze the scapulae together so that the shoulders do not round during the movement.

1. The athlete begins by pushing the hips back and sliding the bar down the front of the thighs. The torso is kept rigid with the lower back flat or slightly arched (photo *b*). The athlete lowers until the bar is about 1 or 2 inches (2.5-5.0 cm) below the kneecap (or until proper form can no longer be maintained).

2. The athlete returns to the starting position, keeping the shoulders back, the back arched, the head up, and the bar in contact with the legs at all times.

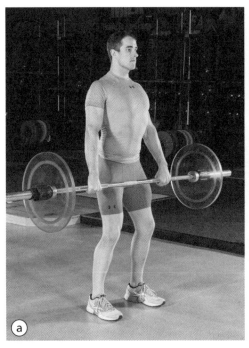
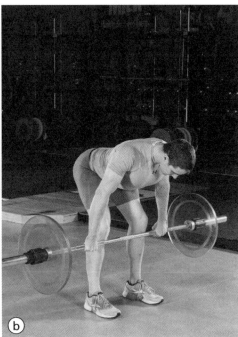

DUMBBELL OR BARBELL CALF RAISE

The athlete stands with both feet side by side near the edge of a raised surface—such as a box, bench, or stair. The athlete holds a dumbbell at each side (photo *a*). (This exercise can also be done alternating legs. In this case, the athlete holds a dumbbell on the side of the working leg. If necessary, the other hand can hold onto something for stability.) *Alternative:* The athlete stands with both feet side by side with the heels hanging off the front edge of a solid raised surface while holding the barbell on top of the scapulae and trapezius (photo *b*). The hands are positioned slightly wider than the shoulders.

1. The athlete rises up on the toes as high as possible while keeping the knees extended or just slightly flexed (photo *c*).
2. The athlete returns to the starting position.

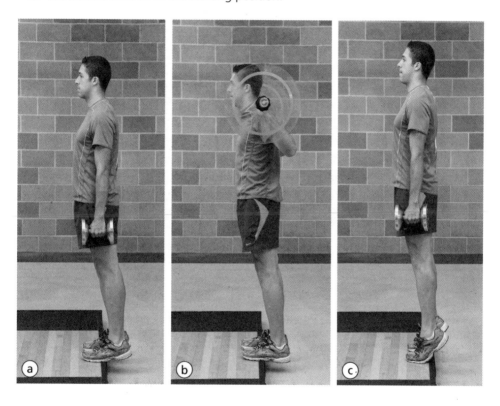

BARBELL OR DUMBBELL BENCH PRESS

Using a flat bench, the athlete assumes a position with the standard five points of contact: The head, shoulders, and glutes are in contact with the bench, and both feet are on the floor. The athlete uses a pronated (overhand) grip on the bar, with the hands positioned slightly wider than shoulder width. The athlete lifts the bar off the rack until it is directly over the chest (photo *a*). *Alternative:* Using a flat bench, the athlete begins with a dumbbell in each hand and lies back on the bench using the standard five points of contact. The athlete places each dumbbell at shoulder width and at just above armpit height (photo *b*).

1. In a controlled manner, the athlete lowers the bar or dumbbells to the chest.

2. The athlete touches the bar against the chest (photo *c*) and then pushes the weight back to the starting position. When using dumbbells, they are lowered to chest level near the armpits, with the elbows slightly abducted (photo *d*).

3. The athlete repeats this movement for the desired number of repetitions, returning the barbell to the rack (or the dumbbells to the floor) on completion of the final repetition.

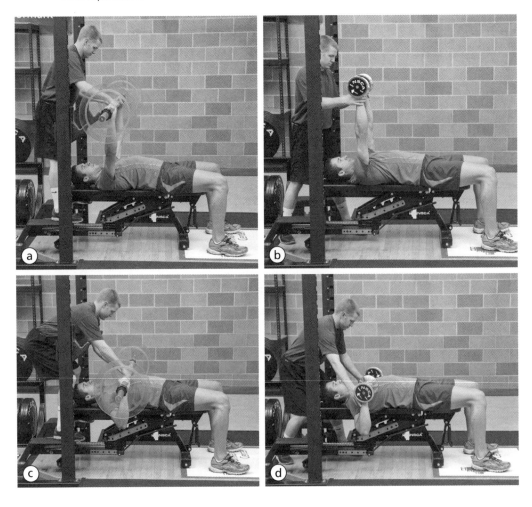

LAT PULLDOWN (MACHINE)

Before starting this exercise, the athlete should adjust the seat and the knee pad of the lat machine to fit his or her body size. The athlete grips the bar with the hands positioned slightly wider than shoulder width (photo *a*), sits down on the seat, and places the knees under the knee pad for support.

1. The athlete leans back slightly at the hips and pulls the bar down to the upper portion of the chest (photo *b*).
2. In a controlled manner, the athlete allows the elbows to extend and return to the starting position.

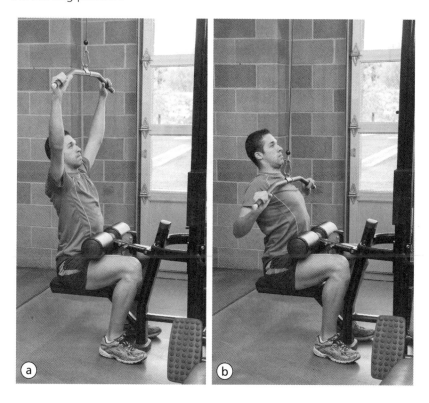

BENT-OVER ROW

The athlete grasps the bar with a closed, pronated grip. The grip should be wider than shoulder width. The athlete positions the feet in a shoulder-width stance with the knees slightly flexed. The torso is flexed forward so that it is slightly above parallel to the floor (photo *a*). Athletes with shorter posterior chain muscles often use a position with cervical extension as shown. Other athletes should use a neutral position for the cervical spine. For the former position, the eyes should be focused ahead, and for the latter, the eyes should be focused a short distance ahead of the feet. The elbows are fully extended so that the bar is hanging down.

1. The athlete pulls the bar toward the torso, keeping the torso rigid, the back flat, and the knees slightly flexed (photo *b*). The athlete should not jerk the torso upward.
2. The athlete touches the bar to the lower chest or upper abdomen.
3. The athlete lowers the bar back to the starting position while maintaining the flat-back position and keeping the torso and knees stationary.
4. At the end of the set, the athlete flexes the hips and knees to place the bar on the floor and then stands up.

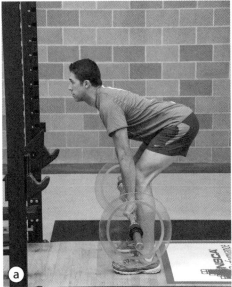
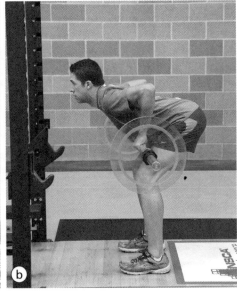

BARBELL SHOULDER PRESS

The athlete sits in a shoulder press bench or a flat bench with the feet shoulder-width apart and flat on the floor and the torso tight and fully erect. Using a grip slightly wider than shoulder-width apart, the athlete holds the barbell on the upper chest and anterior deltoids with the elbows directly below or slightly in front of the bar (photo a).

1. The athlete pushes the barbell directly overhead until the elbows are fully extended while maintaining a rigid torso position (photo b).
2. The athlete allows the elbows to flex slowly, lowering the bar to the upper chest and shoulders.

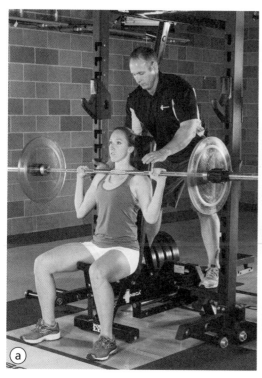
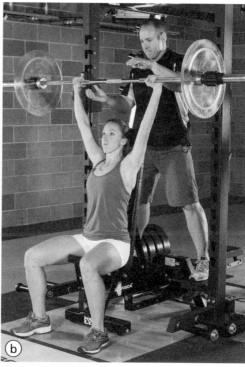

TRICEPS PUSHDOWN (MACHINE)

The athlete grasps the bar using a closed, pronated grip with the hands 6 to 12 inches (15-30 cm) apart and stands erect with the feet shoulder-width apart and the knees slightly flexed. The athlete positions the body close enough to the machine so the cable hangs straight down when the upper arms are held against the sides of the torso and the forearms are parallel to the floor or slightly above (photo *a*). This is the starting position.

1. The athlete pushes the bar down until the elbows are fully extended (photo *b*) but not forcefully locked out. The torso is kept erect and the upper arms are kept stationary.

2. The athlete allows the elbows to flex back slowly to the starting position. The torso, upper arms, and knees remain in the same position. At the end of the set, the athlete returns the bar to its resting position.

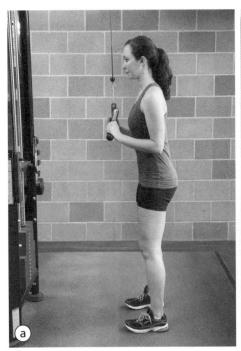 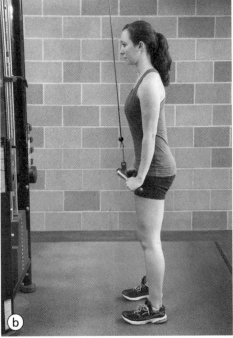

DUMBBELL BICEPS CURL

The athlete grasps two dumbbells using a closed, neutral grip while standing erect with the feet shoulder-width apart and the knees slightly flexed. The dumbbells are positioned alongside the thighs with the elbows fully extended (photo *a*). Repetitions begin from this position.

1. Keeping the dumbbell in a neutral grip, the athlete flexes the elbows until the dumbbells clear the thighs on each side and then supinates the forearms and wrists by turning the hands outward until they are near the anterior deltoids (photo *b*). The athlete keeps the torso erect and the upper arms stationary without jerking the body or swinging the dumbbell upward. (The curls can also be performed by alternating arms. The resting arm stays stationary at the side of the thigh.)

2. The athlete lowers the dumbbells until the elbows are fully extended and pronated, moving them back to the neutral starting position.

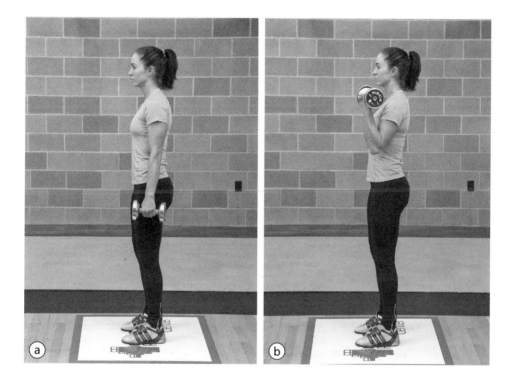

PLYOMETRICS

DEPTH JUMP

The athlete stands tall on a 10- to 20-inch (25-51 cm) box, with the feet between hip- and shoulder-width apart and the toes pointed forward. The athlete takes a step forward (photo a) and, without reaching for the ground, drops from the box. Both feet land at the same time.

1. The athlete lands softly, with knees slightly flexed and feet between hip- and shoulder-width apart. Landing occurs with a moderate degree of hip flexion.

2. As both feet contact the ground, the athlete strives to take off as quickly and as forcefully as possible, with the goal of jumping straight up. Upon taking off, the hips, knees, and ankles should be extended fully (photo b). The lower extremities remain extended while in the air.

3. The athlete lands stably and softly, with a moderate degree of hip and knee flexion. The athlete rests 10 to 15 seconds before repeating a second jump.

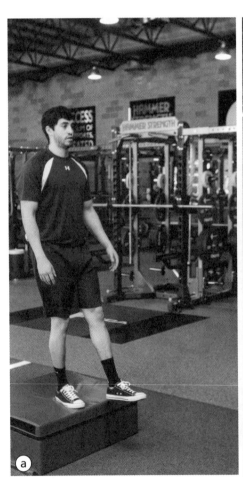
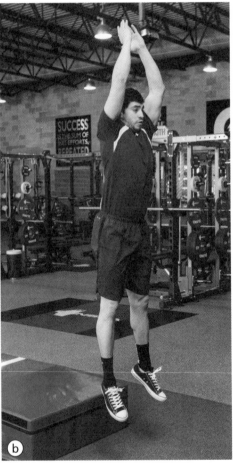

COUNTERMOVEMENT JUMP OR BROAD JUMP

The athlete stands tall with the feet between hip- and shoulder-width apart and the toes pointed forward.

1. The athlete squats to reach about 90 degrees of knee flexion and swings the arms down and back to prepare to take off.

2. Without delay, the athlete takes off with the goal of jumping as high as possible (countermovement jump) or as far as possible (broad jump). Upon taking off, the hips, knees, and ankles should be extended fully. When performing a countermovement jump, the lower extremities remain extended while in the air. When performing a broad jump, the lower extremities swing forward after the initial extension to prepare for landing.

3. The athlete lands stably and softly, with a moderate degree of hip and knee flexion. The athlete may rest for 10 to 15 seconds before repeating a second jump or performing a series of consecutive jumps (rebounds).

Countermovement jumps and broad jumps can be performed using additional load, up to 30% of an athlete's own body weight (4, 7, 8, 9). Dumbbells, kettlebells, or weighted vests are a more suitable option than barbells to increase load dynamic, ballistic-type tasks.

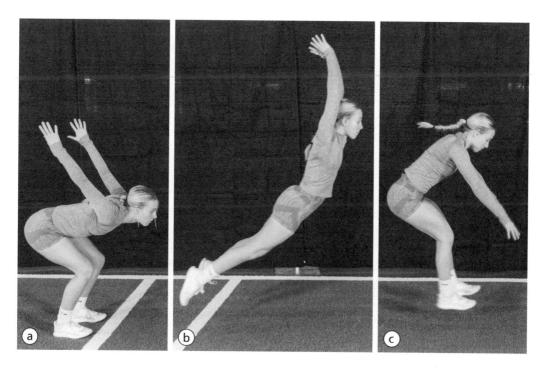

SQUAT JUMP (WITH A PAUSE)

The athlete stands tall with the feet between hip- and shoulder-width apart and the toes pointed forward. Hands are at their sides.

1. The athlete squats to reach about 90 degrees of knee flexion before pausing for 1 second. At the bottom of the squat, the athlete must be motionless (photo *a*).

2. Without further flexing the knees, the athlete takes off with the goal of jumping straight up. Upon taking off, the hips, knees, and ankles should be extended fully. The lower extremities remain extended while in the air (photo *b*).

3. The athlete lands stably and softly, with a moderate degree of hip and knee flexion. The athlete rests for 10 to 15 seconds before repeating a second jump.

   Squat jumps can be performed with additional load ranging between 20% and 100% of an athlete's own body weight (i.e., a loaded squat jump) (3, 7, 8, 9). Using a trap bar, rather than a regular barbell, is a safer and more suitable option in order to avoid the challenge of holding a bar on the shoulder upon landing. A trap bar can also be safely dropped if needed.

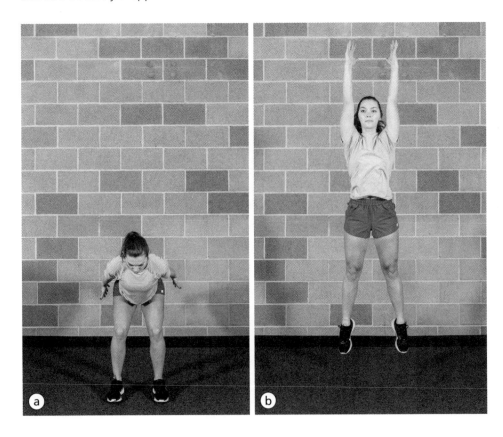

SINGLE-LEG HOP

The athlete stands tall with the feet between hip- and shoulder-width apart and the toes pointed forward. Hands are on the hips.

1. The athlete takes off with one leg only. The goal is to maximize horizontal displacement while minimizing vertical displacement. The athlete can hop forward, laterally, or diagonally.

2. Upon taking off, the hips knees, and ankles should be extended fully. The trail leg swings forward to prepare for or assist with landing.

3. The athlete lands stably on the same foot or the opposite foot and strives to take off immediately, bouncing forward as swiftly as possible.

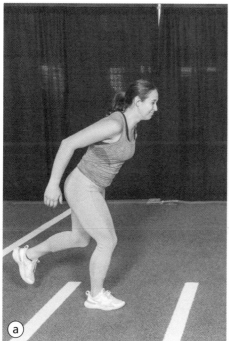 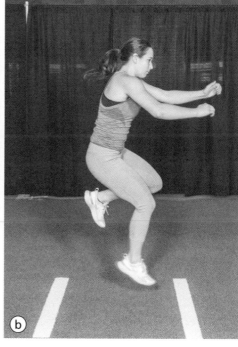

Resistance Training for Endurance Sports

G. Gregory Haff
Kate Baldwin
Stephanie Burgess*

Traditionally, endurance athletes have been reluctant to use resistance training as part of their overall training plan. This reluctance has stemmed from the belief that resistance training will result in substantial hypertrophy and weight gain, which would negatively affect performance. Recent scientific evidence appears to refute this belief and offers a compelling argument that resistance training is essential to the overall development of the endurance athlete (7, 36, 43, 44). Based on this evidence, more endurance athletes are engaging in resistance training, with recent survey data indicating that between 54% and 62% of endurance athletes participate in structured resistance training (1, 45).

Even though endurance athletes have begun to see the benefits of resistance training, the role that it plays in their development causes a lot of confusion. This chapter offers practical information about the implementation of resistance training programs for endurance athletes based on the current research about concurrent resistance and endurance training. A fundamental part of this discussion is the careful, rather than careless, integration of resistance training into the endurance athlete's training plan (36).

The process of integrating training factors involves the concept of *periodization* (31). Although basic periodization concepts are used by endurance athletes and coaches, these concepts are much more developed and scientifically studied in the application of resistance training (12, 41, 60). Additionally, the overall depth of planning is substantially greater and the terminology used is slightly different when discussing resistance training (73). To help endurance coaches develop integrated training programs, this chapter provides a detailed discussion about periodization

*G. Gregory Haff and Kate Baldwin were contracted to author this chapter; Stephanie Burgess' name was added to acknowledge her significant contribution partially retained from the previous edition.

and how resistance training is built into the overall training plan. From this discussion, practical guidelines are established and presented for the development of effective resistance training programs for the endurance athlete. Finally, sample programs are presented for a variety of endurance sports or activities.

RESISTANCE TRAINING'S EFFECT ON ENDURANCE PERFORMANCE

Endurance athletes who are stronger can generally perform at a much higher level than those who lack strength. This suggests that training modalities that stimulate increases in muscular strength without compromising endurance capacity are beneficial for the endurance athlete (57, 58, 61). Support for this contention can be found in the scientific literature; research shows that the appropriate integration of resistance training into the endurance athlete's training plan can result in significantly better performance when compared to classic endurance training plans that focus only on aerobic endurance training (18, 44, 61, 78).

When looking closely at endurance performance, several key factors—including the athlete's maximal aerobic power ($\dot{V}O_2$max), lactate threshold, and movement efficiency—contribute to performance (see figure 6.1) (4, 55). The training modality selected influences these factors by inducing changes to the athlete's

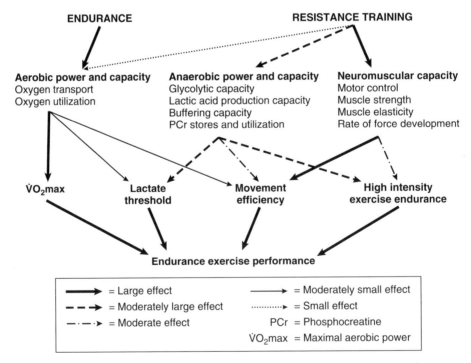

Figure 6.1 The influence of endurance and resistance training on endurance performance.
Adapted by permission from L. Paavolainen., K. Häkkinen, I. Hämäläinen, et al., "Explosive-Strength Training Improves 5-km Running Time by Improving Running Economy and Muscle Power," *Journal of Applied Physiology* 86, no. 5 (1999): 1527-1533.

aerobic power and capacity, anaerobic capabilities, and neuromuscular function. Improvements seen in endurance athletes as a result of resistance training include improved running and cycling economy (43, 44, 45, 81, 85); faster swim, cycle, and run time trials (46, 53, 61, 78, 90); improved run velocity and power at ($\dot{V}O_2$max) (4, 55, 57); reduced heart rate at submaximal intensities (1, 59, 87); and delayed time to exhaustion in cycling and running protocols (1, 38). Additionally, resistance training does not seem to compromise $\dot{V}O_2$max values (57), lactate threshold (57), or body mass (37, 45, 62) in endurance athletes.

Aerobic training exerts a strong influence on both aerobic power and capacity, but it does not exert a great impact on the athlete's anaerobic or neuromuscular abilities (19, 76). Conversely, resistance training exerts a strong influence on the athlete's neuromuscular function and a moderate influence on anaerobic power and capacity, while offering only a minimal influence on aerobic power and capacity (35, 76). By influencing the athlete's anaerobic abilities as well as neuromuscular function, resistance training can elevate the athlete's lactate threshold, movement efficiency, and ability to engage in high-intensity activities (1, 8).

The ability of resistance training to improve endurance performance is likely related to several key factors, including the specific physiological and mechanical adaptations that are stimulated by the resistance training regimen (1, 19). The integration of resistance training into the overall training plan appears to be central to creating these specific performance-enhancing adaptations. Endurance athletes commonly report both time restraints and a lack of knowledge regarding resistance training prescription as prominent barriers preventing them from completing resistance training (1, 45).

These views may be partially explained by design flaws in many of the training programs that include concurrent resistance and endurance training. In many of these instances, resistance training is simply added to the endurance training program, which may result in endurance athletes experiencing excessively high levels of fatigue that can negatively affect overall performance.

If athletes reduce their endurance training load to account for the addition of resistance training and schedule resistance training appropriately, then resistance training can have a positive effect on the athletes' endurance performance. The athlete who performs both resistance and endurance training in an integrated and appropriately planned fashion will perform at a higher level than the athlete who performs only classic endurance training (57).

MODES AND METHODS OF RESISTANCE TRAINING FOR ENDURANCE

Resistance training is an activity in which the body's skeletal muscle system is required to produce force to overcome some external resistance. This resistance can be applied through multiple methods, including free weights, gravity, resistance machines, and weighted objects (80). If the resistance applied to the body is planned correctly, with progressive overload, the musculoskeletal system will adapt and become more efficient at generating forces.

A key to the effectiveness of resistance training is the ability to structure training plans that integrate all training factors and appropriately manage total workloads. If the resistance training portion of the training plan is appropriately structured, specific physiological adaptations can occur that result in quantifiable performance improvements. For example, by increasing muscular strength, the endurance runner generally shows improved running economy that translates into improved performance, as indicated by faster times. The extent to which the adaptations induced by resistance training will translate to specific performance outcomes is largely dependent on the mode (type of equipment) and methods (repetitions, sets, volumes, types of movements) used to construct the training plan.

Modes of Resistance Training

Endurance athletes can use numerous modes of resistance training. These modes can include resistance training (exercise) bands or tubing, medicine balls, core stability or balance training (using a stability ball), weight machines, free weights (barbells, dumbbells, kettlebells, weighted vests), plyometrics, and body-weight exercises such as calisthenics, push-ups, and chin-ups (32, 67, 71, 72). Depending on the training status of the athlete, each of these modes may have a place in the resistance training plan.

Generally, a combination of free weights, weight machines, body-weight exercises, and plyometrics results in the greatest improvements in endurance performance (1, 34). Conversely, training on unstable surfaces or performing core stability exercises has resulted in no improvements in endurance performance (70) and generally mutes the ability to develop force rapidly (49). Total-body resistance training, such as squatting, results in a greater activation of the core muscles (lower back and abdominal muscles) when directly compared to core stability exercise (54). Some modes—such as resistance bands, stability training, and balance training—may be better suited for rehabilitation from injury and should not serve as the primary focus of any resistance training plan for endurance athletes (3). Because most training plans for endurance athletes must balance multiple training factors, the best strategy is to employ activities that are time efficient and have the greatest transfer of training effects; this would include modes such as free weights, weight machines, plyometrics, and medicine balls (1, 3).

Methods of Resistance Training

The methods of resistance training are directly related to the way that the training program is designed. The methods used in the application of resistive loads are largely dictated by the overall goals of the training program or the phase of the periodized training plan. The most effective and time-efficient method for developing strength and power that directly affect athletic performance involves combining several modes of training, such as free weights (e.g., barbells, dumbbell, kettlebells), plyometrics, and medicine ball work (34, 79).

Regardless of the mode used, the training plan must progressively overload the athlete. Progressive overload is accomplished through the manipulation of various training factors, such as varying the frequency of training, the volume load (sets × repetitions × load), the intensity of the exercise or session, the rest interval between sets or repetitions, and the exercises used (34, 79). Too often coaches and sport scientists falsely consider only the variation of volume and intensity of resistance training when attempting to progressively overload the athletes. However, other factors, such as the exercises selected and the order of training, also can significantly influence the effectiveness of the training plan.

Volume

In its most simplistic form, the volume of resistance training is the amount of work accomplished (15, 26). The best method for estimating the amount of work accomplished in a resistance training session is the calculation of the volume load (sets × repetitions × load). The volume load is a far superior method for estimating the amount of work accomplished because it includes the load in the calculation (26). If the load is not included in the calculation (sets × repetitions), the result will often provide a false representation of volume (26, 39).

Table 6.1 presents five scenarios in which an athlete has performed 18 total repetitions in an exercise; at a glance, all five scenarios could falsely be interpreted as having an equal volume of training. Looking at the volume load calculation, the volume of training can differ greatly in response to the load that is lifted. Volume is a representation of work accomplished, so the load should be included in the volume calculation because the load will affect the amount of work undertaken (26, 77).

Table 6.1 Volume Load Calculation Scenarios

Scenario	Sets	Repetitions	% of 1RM*	Load (kg)	Total repetitions	Volume load (kg)
1	1	18	58%	46.0	18	1,037
2	2	9	72%	58.0	18	1,296
3	3	6	81%	65.0	18	1,166
4	6	3	86%	54.0	18	1,231
5	9	2	88%	71.0	18	1,270

*RM = repetition maximum; % of 1RM based off a maximum back squat of 80 kg.

High volume loads generally result in greater caloric expenditure (50) and can stimulate increases in endurance (34). Because of this, many endurance athletes believe that they should always perform high volumes of resistance training (i.e., high number of total repetitions) (45), which may not be the best approach considering the volume of endurance-focused training that they typically undertake. When the volume load is high, it can result in substantial amounts of accumulated fatigue (48), which can create fatigue management prob lems for the endurance athlete (51). When high volume loads are encountered too frequently, an endurance athlete may experience a decrease in performance because of the fatigue that this type of training stimulates. In fact, when lower volumes of resistance training are integrated into the endurance athlete's training program, better improvements in running economy are noted when compared to integrating higher volume resistance training (1, 9, 65). Ultimately, to maximize the effectiveness of training, endurance athletes must consider the relationship between fatigue, performance, and the volume load of training when integrating a resistance training program into their preparation activities.

Intensity

The intensity of an exercise depends on the rate at which energy is used (15, 75). Intensity is typically calculated as a percentage of a specified repetition maximum (RM) (79). For example, in table 6.1, 3 sets of 5 repetitions of the back squat were performed at an intensity of 77% (61 kg) of the heaviest weight that could be lifted one time, or 1RM, which in this case was 80 kilograms. Working from the initial 1RM is the preferred method of establishing training intensity, but this method does have some potential pitfalls (79). As the athlete gets stronger, the 1RM increases, and if testing is not undertaken frequently, the training zones become progressively less effective. To counter this pitfall, an athlete may increase the weight by a small amount, such as 5 pounds (about 2.5 kg) when surpassing the prescribed intensity to ensure progressive overload occurs (79).

Another solution for this issue is to work off of goal 1RM values as shown in table 6.2 (16, 79). However, when using this method, the goal established must be realistic so that the athlete does not overtrain. An additional consideration is that the number of repetitions an athlete can perform at a specific percentage of 1RM varies depending on the exercise and the training experience of the athlete (66, 79).

Another method is to work from the number of repetitions that can be per-formed based on percentages of the 1RM, as shown in table 6.3 (16, 79, 83). For example, if an athlete's 1RM is 80 kilograms, the estimated 3RM is approximately 72 kilograms, and the predicted 6RM is around 68 kilograms. Training zones can then be established based on these numbers, as shown in table 6.4. In other words, athletes find their 1RM and then use table 6.3 and the intensity spectrum presented in tables 6.2 and 6.4 to individualize training intensity zones. This eliminates the need for frequent testing and allows the coach or athlete to use percentages of actual, estimated, or goal RMs.

Table 6.2 Sample Loading Table

Loading	Percentage	% initial 1RM (kg)*	% goal 1RM (kg)*
Very heavy (VH)	95-100	76-80	86-90
Heavy (H)	90-95	72-76	81-86
Moderately heavy (MH)	85-90	68-72	77-81
Moderate (M)	80-85	64-68	72-77
Moderately light (ML)	75-80	60-64	68-72
Light (L)	70-75	56-60	63-68
Very light (VL)	<70	<52	<63

*Goal for an athlete who wants to perform the back squat for 90 kg, who currently can back squat 80 kg for a 1RM.

Adapted from T.O. Bompa and G.G. Haff, *Periodization: Theory and Methodology of Training* (Champaign, IL: Human Kinetics Publishers, 2009) 273; G.G. Haff and E.E. Haff, "Resistance Training Program Design," in *NSCA's Essentials of Personal Training*, edited for the National Strength and Conditioning Association by M.H. Malek and J.W. Coburn (Champaign, IL: Human Kinetics, 2012), 370.

Table 6.3 Load-to-Repetition Relationship

% of 1RM	Number of repetitions for most athletes	Number of repetitions for endurance athletes
100	1	1
95	2	3
90	3	6
85	5	8
80	8	11
75	10	14
70	12	16
65	15	19

Note: The percentage of RM will vary slightly (±0.5%-2.0%).

Adapted from Thibaudeau (2006).

Table 6.4 Sample Loading Ranges Based on Estimated 3RM, 6RM, and 8RM for an Endurance Athlete

Loading	%1RM	3RM zones (kg)*	6RM zones (kg)*	8RM zones (kg)*
Very heavy (VH)	95-100	72-76	68-72	61-64
Heavy (H)	90-95	68-72	65-68	58-61
Moderately heavy (MH)	85-90	65-68	61-65	54-58
Moderate (M)	80-85	61-65	58-61	51-54
Moderately light (ML)	75-80	57-61	54-58	48-51
Light (L)	70-75	53-57	50-54	45-48
Very light (VL)	<70	<53	<50	<45

*Athlete has a 1RM back squat of 80 kg; therefore, based on table 6.3, the athlete's estimated 3RM is 76 kg, 6RM is 72 kg, and 8RM is 64 kg.

Adapted from T.O. Bompa and G.G. Haff, *Periodization: Theory and Methodology of Training*, 5th ed. (Champaign, IL: Human Kinetics Publishers, 2009) 273; G.G. Haff and E.E. Haff, "Resistance Training Program Design," in *NSCA's Essentials of Personal Training*, 2nd ed. edited for the National Strength and Conditioning Association by M.H. Malek and J.W. Coburn (Champaign, IL: Human Kinetics, 2012), 384.

Alternatively, training intensity may be prescribed based on a rating of perceived exertion (RPE) or repetitions in reserve (RIR) (table 6.5) (22, 25, 64). When using the RPE and RIR loading methods, athletes can autoregulate the load to align with their subjective perception of exertion or how many repetitions away from muscular failure they are (91). For example, if an athlete was prescribed 3 sets of 6 repetitions with an RPE of 7, a weight would be selected that corresponds to a very hard effort that leaves 3 repetitions in reserve. While this method of loading does allow the athlete to autoregulate the training and is a useful loading methodology, the farther the athlete will be from muscular failure and the less accurate the prescribed load will be (56, 79), especially if the athlete is less experienced. However, this method may be particularly helpful for endurance athletes who experience large volumes of aerobic training to minimize excessive fatigue.

Table 6.5 Rating of Perceived Exertion (RPE) and Repetitions in Reserve (RIR) Scales

Rating	RPE descriptor	RIR	RIR descriptor
0	Rest	—	Little to no effort
1	Very, very easy		
2	Easy		
3	Moderate	—	Light effort
4	Somewhat hard		
5	Hard	4-6	4-6 repetitions remaining
6	—		
7	Very hard	3	3 repetitions remaining
7.5	—	2-3	2-3 repetitions remaining
8	—	2	2 repetitions remaining
8.5	—	1-2	1-2 repetitions remaining
9	—	1	1 repetition remaining
9.5	—	0	No further repetitions but could increase load
10	Maximal	0	Maximal effort

Adapted from D.A. Hackett, N.A. Johnson, M. Halaki, and C.M. Chow, "A Novel Scale to Assess Resistance-Exercise Effort, *Journal of Sports Sciences* 30 (2012): 1405-1413; M.C. Zourdos, A. Klemp, C. Dolan, et al., "Novel Resistance Training-Specific Rating of Perceived Exertion Scale Measuring Repetitions in Reserve," *Journal of Strength and Conditioning Research* 30 (2016): 267-275.

Repetitions

The number of repetitions that an athlete can perform is determined by the load that is being lifted. The higher the load used, the lower the number of repetitions that can be performed, and vice versa. Many factors may contribute to the number of repetitions that an athlete can perform at a given percentage of 1RM (79). Table 6.3 offers a rough guideline that can be used when creating a training plan.

One concept that must be considered is that the repetition scheme employed can result in specific physiological adaptations (48). As depicted in figure 6.2, repetition schemes of over 20 repetitions can enhance low-intensity endurance, while those of 8 to 15 repetitions can enhance high-intensity endurance. Overall maximal strength is best developed with repetition schemes that range from 1 to 6 repetitions, and power is developed with lower-repetition models of 3 or fewer repetitions (64). While the repetitions schemes and targets presented in figure 6.2 are commonly used, it is important to note that endurance athletes likely do not need to use repetition ranges above 10 because they will receive greater benefits from targeting repetition ranges that allow for them to focus on power, maximal strength, or high-intensity endurance development (1, 4, 82). Based on emerging research, it is likely that the optimal repetition range is between 1 and 8 when programming resistance training for endurance performance (1, 9, 65). Regardless of the repetition ranges implemented as part of the resistance training component of the athlete's training plan, it is important that the coach considers how the resistance training is integrated with the endurance training program as well as how it aligns with the goals and the targeted physiological adaptations established for the periods and phases of the training plan.

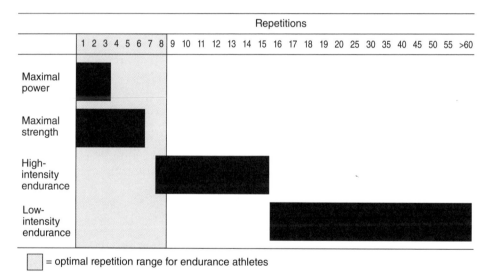

□ = optimal repetition range for endurance athletes

Figure 6.2 Number of repetitions needed to develop four types of strength.
Adapted by permission from T.O. Bompa and G.G. Haff, *Periodization: Theory and Methodology of Training*, 5th ed. (Champaign, IL: Human Kinetics, 2009), 274.

Sets

Sets are a series of repetitions performed continuously followed by a rest interval (86). Multiple-set protocols are significantly more effective than single-set programs because they stimulate greater physiological adaptations and result in greater performance gains (79). The number of sets used in a training program is largely dependent on the training status of the athlete, the phase of training, and the targeted goals of the training plan.

Advanced athletes generally need to perform a greater number of sets (more than 3) per exercise, while novice athletes can achieve performance gains with fewer sets (3 or fewer) (79). Manipulating the number of sets is another method for modifying the volume load of training. Increasing the number of sets increases volume load, while decreasing the number of sets reduces the volume load.

Variation in the number of sets used in the resistance training program is dictated by the phase of training. For example, early in the training year, during the preparatory phase, the number of sets would be greater to increase the overall volume load and to develop muscular endurance. Conversely, during the competitive phase, a lower number of sets is used because of the reduced emphasis on resistance training.

Rest Interval Between Sets

The time allotted between sets, or the rest interval, is a function of the load being lifted, the goal of the training program, and the type of strength being targeted. When targeting the development of muscular strength or power, a long rest interval of 2 to 5 minutes may be warranted (23, 80). Conversely, when attempting to develop high-intensity muscular endurance, shortening the rest interval to 1 to 2 minutes may be advantageous (63). It is important to note that shortening the rest interval (i.e., <1 min) can challenge the athlete's ability to recover between sets and potentially affect the load that can be lifted for a prescribed volume (88). This issue can be minimized if appropriate load prescriptions based on percentages of the target RM zones (table 6.4) are used and training to failure is avoided. Additionally, while short intervals (i.e., <1 min) may be advantageous for developing low-intensity muscular endurance, shortening the rest interval to less than 1 minute will impede the development of power, strength, and high-intensity endurance, all of which have been reported to be important when attempting to maximize endurance performance (14, 63, 80).

Order of Exercises

As a general rule, multijoint exercises that involve a large muscle mass, such as the back squat or power clean, should be performed early in the training session (64). These types of exercises are often technical and require the athlete to be in a state of minimal fatigue to maximize their effectiveness. These exercises should be considered the most important exercises in the resistance training program (64).

Exercises that involve a smaller muscle mass, such as the biceps curl or triceps pushdown, are generally performed after the large-mass exercises have been completed (64). If an athlete chooses to perform the smaller-mass exercises first, this may reduce the effectiveness of the multijoint exercises. For example, if the athlete chooses to perform a triceps exercise (triceps are an accessory muscle for shoulder press exercises) before the bench press, fatigue of the triceps may prevent the ability to overload the anterior deltoid and pectoralis major.

Training Frequency

Training frequency refers to the number of resistance training sessions that will be undertaken during the training plan. As a general rule, the endurance athlete needs no more than three resistance training sessions per week (6). In fact, endurance athletes will likely perform a maximum of two to three resistance training sessions per week during most of the annual training plan (6). Depending on their training schedule, athletes may find it easier to microdose their resistance training across three shorter (20-30 min sessions) compared to two longer (45-60 min) resistance training sessions.

Because resistance training is a supplemental training activity for the endurance athlete, less emphasis is often placed on this type of training; thus, less time is typically scheduled for it (68, 84). The frequency of resistance training for these athletes may be as high as 3 days per week during the preparatory period and as low as 1 day per week during the competitive period of the annual training plan; this has been shown to allow for the maintenance of strength for as long as 20 weeks. Additionally, resistance training may be completely removed from the training plan during the pre-event taper to maximize the removal of accumulated fatigue.

An alternative strategy is to increase the frequency of resistance training while reducing the time allocated to resistance training, which is a microdosing programming strategy (13). For example, if a typical preparatory period has two resistance training sessions per week each lasting 60 minutes in duration (i.e., 120 minutes) per week, a microdosing strategy could be employed where the duration of each session can be reduced to 30 minutes and the frequency increased to four sessions per week. With this strategy the amount of time on a given training day is reduced, potentially allowing for a better integration of resistance training into the endurance athlete's holistic training program (13).

Loading Pattern

Normally, the loading pattern should contain a series of warm-up sets followed by target sets in which a prescribed repetition and intensity scheme is followed (10, 16). For example, if an athlete were to perform target sets in the back squat at 70 kilograms (50% of 1RM) for 3 sets of 6, the athlete would do 2 or 3 warm-up sets before initiating the target sets. The warm-up sets may be structured as follows: 1 set at 20 kilograms, 1 set at 40 kilograms, and 1 set at 60 kilograms. After completing the warm-up sets, the athlete would then perform the target sets. In some instances, a down set may be used as a cooldown, resulting in an increased growth hormone release (21). In the example, the athlete might perform a down set with 52.5 kilograms (or a 25% reduction in load) (10, 16).

Another consideration for the loading pattern involves manipulating the intensity and volume load throughout the training week (see table 6.6). As a general rule, the intensity of training should not be the same every day and should be integrated with the endurance training plan (34). The table depicts a 3:1 loading program. In a 3:1 loading program, intensity (and volume load) increases for 3 consecutive weeks, followed by 1 week of unloading, which is used to induce recovery (16, 24). Within each week, the training load decreases with each training day as fatigue accumulates during the week.

Table 6.6 Sample Loading Pattern for a Training Week of Resistance Training

| Day | Target zone | | Intensities* | | | |
	Sets	Reps	Week 1	Week 2	Week 3	Week 4
LOADING PATTERN FOR A 3-DAY-A-WEEK PROGRAM						
Monday	3	6	ML	M	MH	M
Wednesday	3	6	L	ML	M	ML
Friday	3	6	VL	L	ML	L
LOADING PATTERN FOR A 2-DAY-A-WEEK PROGRAM						
Tuesday	3	6	ML	M	MH	M
Friday	3	6	L	ML	M	ML
LOADING PATTERN FOR A 1-DAY-A-WEEK PROGRAM						
Tuesday	3	6	ML	M	MH	M

*Intensities are based on table 6.4.

Because most endurance athletes perform the greatest volume of endurance work on the weekend, these athletes may want to reverse this loading program so that the light day is at the beginning of the week. This way, the program addresses the fatigue created in response to the higher volumes of endurance training undertaken during the weekend. Ultimately, the major factor that will dictate this manipulation of the resistance training load will be how the endurance training is sequenced and integrated into the overall training plan.

STRUCTURE AND SEQUENCE OF RESISTANCE TRAINING

Once an athlete has decided to use resistance training to improve endurance performance, the athlete and coach must then determine the athlete's overall goals, the specific needs of the athlete, and the target of the training plan. After establishing the athlete's overall goals, the coach and athlete can work together to craft a training program that effectively integrates training factors to facilitate the athlete's progress.

One of the keys to designing an appropriate resistance training program for endurance athletes is the concept of *periodization*. Periodization can be defined as the logical and systematic sequencing and integration of training factors to optimize performance at specific times (24, 29, 31). Periodization should be considered a planning process that serves as the scaffolding from which programmatic decisions are made (31).

Central to this concept is the fact that not every training factor needs to be emphasized at the same time (31). In fact, as the athlete moves through the training year, the focus of the training plan should shift, allowing training factors to be introduced, removed, or reintroduced at predetermined points (29). Thus, for the endurance athlete who has integrated resistance training into a periodized training plan, the plan will include specific time frames for targeting the development of strength, power, or high-intensity muscular endurance. For these factors to be integrated at the appropriate time, the training plan must be broken into specific training periods and phases, which serve as the foundation of the overall training plan.

From a structural standpoint, a periodized training plan can be broken into the six planning structures shown in table 6.7 (29). The largest structure is the multiyear plan, which is usually designed based on a 4-year structure. The multiyear plan provides a general overview of what the athlete is attempting to accomplish in the long term. For example, in a high school setting, the program focus of a freshman cross-country runner will differ greatly from that of a senior who has been engaged in directed training for three consecutive annual training plans or macrocycles (see figure 6.3 on page 143). The foundation of each macrocycle is the competitive schedule, which is used to establish the periods and phases that will be included in the annual training plan (29).

Table 6.7 Defining Specific Levels of the Planning Process

Period	Duration	Description
Multiyear plan	2 to 4 years	Multiple interlinked annual training plans; most common is a quadrennial plan (i.e., 4 years)
Annual	1 year	1 year of training; contains a single or multiple macrocycles
Macrocycle	Several months to a year	Sometimes referred to as an *annual plan*; contains a preparatory, competitive, and transition phase of training
Mesocycle	2 to 6 weeks	Medium-sized training cycle; sometimes referred to as a *macrocycle* or a *block of training*; consists of microcycles that are linked together
Microcycle	Several days to 2 weeks	Small training cycle composed of multiple workouts
Workout	Several hours	Generally consists of several hours of training; more than 30 minutes of rest between bouts would constitute multiple workouts

Sources: Issurin (40); Bompa and Haff (10); Haff (27, 29, 31).

Macrocycles

The multiyear plan serves as the template that is used to establish the individual annual training plans, or macrocycles (28, 29, 31). Generally, the macrocycle can encompass a year in duration, but depending on the sport, an annual plan can be structured to contain several macrocycles, each lasting several months. For example, an endurance athlete at the high school level may have a fall cross-country season and a spring track season. In this scenario, two macrocycles would be designed to address the needs of each season. Regardless of the number of macrocycles, the basic structure of the annual plan contains specific training and performance goals that are sequenced in the context of the multiyear plan (28, 29, 31).

In the example of the cross-country runner in a high school setting, the annual plan for the freshman will be designed with specific goals for establishing a performance foundation; these goals may place a major emphasis on the development of cardiovascular fitness and muscular strength while de-emphasizing the importance of competitive performances. With each successive annual training plan, the athlete will continue to develop these physiological and performance characteristics, but the focus on competitive performances will increase. In the fourth year of the multiyear plan, the annual plan will be designed to result in an optimization of performance, allowing the athletes to achieve the best performance time or competitive success.

Generally, each macrocycle contained within the annual plan is broken into three major periods—preparatory, competitive, and transition (see table 6.8) (28, 29, 31). The preparatory period is the first period of every macrocycle. This period can vary in length depending on the developmental level of the athlete, the requirements of the sport, the length of the macrocycle, and the amount of time before the major competitions. The major focus of this period is the development of the athlete's overall physical capacity with higher-volume training performed with lower intensities (28, 29, 31).

The preparatory period can be subdivided into the *general preparatory* and *specific preparatory* phases (28, 29, 31). The general preparatory phase occurs first and is used to emphasize basic skills, increase working capacity, and elevate overall physical preparation. In the case of resistance training, this phase may target the development of *strength endurance*. In the specific preparatory phase, the training emphasis may shift toward the incorporation of more sport-specific conditioning activities while continuing to increase the athlete's working capacity. In the case of resistance training, a shift from strength endurance to the development of basic strength will occur as the athlete transitions into the specific preparatory phase. As the athlete progresses through this phase, performance levels should rise as the athlete becomes prepared for the competitive phase of the macrocycle (28, 29, 31).

Table 6.8 Periods and Phases of the Annual Training Plan

Phase	Characteristics	
Preparatory	• Contains an overall high volume of training with a lower intensity • Designed to increase overall physical capacity • Cultivates specific psychological traits • Familiarizes the athlete with the basic foundations of the sport	
	Phases	
	General preparatory	• Primary emphasis on basic skills with a lesser emphasis on sport-specific skills • Increases the athlete's working capacity • Elevates overall physical preparation • Improves basic technical elements • High overall volume of training
	Specific preparatory	• Increases the athlete's working capacity • Elevates overall athletic performance
Competitive	• Incorporates competitions of varying levels of importance • Targets the improvement of sport-specific physical attributes • Maximizes performance level • Perfects technical and tactical skills • Maintains sport-specific fitness • Diminishes fatigue and elevates preparedness	
	Phases	
	Precompetitive	• Includes unofficial or minor competitions designed to evaluate the athlete's preparedness • Maintains sport-specific fitness • Increases performance level • Includes decreases in volume along with increases in intensity of training
	Main competitive	• Includes gradual decreases in training volume to reduce fatigue and elevate performance • Designed to maximize performance and peak the athlete at specific times • Contains specific peaking strategies that include modulating the volume and intensity of training
Transition	• Serves as a link between macrocycles • Prepares the athlete for the next macrocycle of training • Is used to induce recovery from training stress and injuries • Includes training at a substantially reduced level to maintain some general fitness • Generally lasts between 2 and 6 weeks	

Adapted from Bompa and Haff (2009); Haff (2019, 2021, 2022).

The second major period of each macrocycle is the *competitive period* (29). The duration of the competitive period is largely dependent on the competition schedule and the relative importance of these competitions. Ultimately, the competitive phase should target a specific major competition in which the athlete's performance will be maximized. As the athlete moves through the competitive period, the training activities become more specific and the emphasis on performance becomes greater (28, 29, 31).

The competitive period is subdivided into the *precompetitive* and *main competitive* phases (28, 29, 31). The precompetitive phase includes activities used to maintain sport-specific fitness while elevating the athlete's level of performance. Additionally, minor competitions or exhibitions are used to evaluate the athlete's progress toward the targeted goals established for the main competitive phase. The main competitive phase includes the major competitions in which the athlete's performance is expected to be maximized. The maximization of performance is accomplished through the manipulation of training variables to help the athlete maintain sport-specific fitness while decreasing the overall level of fatigue. From a resistance training standpoint, the precompetitive and main competitive phases generally contain training activities that are designed to emphasize the development of strength and power.

After the completion of the competitive period, athletes usually move into a transition or active rest period of training (28, 29, 31). This phase serves as a link between macrocycles and is designed to induce recovery from the competitive season. In some cases, this is also a time for the athlete to heal from any injuries that may have occurred during the season. This period is marked by substantially reduced training levels. However, the athlete must be sure to undertake some training activities during this phase to maintain or slow the loss of general fitness. Depending on the needs of the athlete and the time allotted, the transition period will last between 2 and 6 weeks. The transition period is an essential portion of the macrocycle and must be established when constructing the overall annual training plan (28, 29, 31).

Mesocycles, Microcycles, and Workouts

Once the macrocycle is subdivided into periods and phases, smaller training units, known as *mesocycles*, can be designed. Mesocycles consist of 2- to 6-week periods of training that target specific physiological and performance objectives based on the goals established for the specific periods (i.e., general preparatory, specific preparatory, precompetitive, and competitive periods) contained within the macrocycle (28, 29, 31). Depending on the goals established for the macrocycle, various mesocycle structures can be developed (see table 6.9) (5, 28, 29, 31, 74). Each mesocycle contained within the macrocycle should be interlinked or sequenced so that each mesocycle builds on the adaptations established in the previous mesocycle.

For example, in the general preparatory phase, the mesocycle plan for resistance training focuses on the development of muscular strength and performance, which is accomplished by performing lower-repetition, heavier-load resistance. Conversely, during the competitive phase, the goal for the mesocycle is to elevate endurance performance; for endurance athletes, the goal of resistance training may now be to maintain strength and reduce accumulated fatigue. Therefore, the frequency of resistance training may decrease to once per week while maintaining the session intensity. The mesocycle plan addresses the development of fatigue by including a significant decrease in overall training loads 8 to 14 days before the major competition (e.g., the state championships in high school track and field) (30). This decrease allows for a reduction in fatigue and an elevation in performance.

Table 6.9 Sample Mesocycle Structures

Type	Average duration (weeks)	Characteristics
Basic sport specific	6	• Designed to elevate sport-specific fitness where performance is targeted
Buildup	3	• A more general form of training and conditioning that is used to enhance foundational skills or fitness • May be used after a period of specific or high-load training
Competition	2-6	• A mesocycle that specifically targets a competition during that mesocycle • Used in the competitive phase of the annual training plan
Competitive buildup	3	• A period of increasing training loads that occurs during a long competitive phase • Used to reestablish foundational skills or fitness
General	Any duration	• Basic or general education and training that target the development of basic fitness • Often occurs in the preparatory phase of the annual training plan
Immediate preparatory	2	• A training period that occurs before a competition • Targets peaking and recovery • May be considered a taper • May precede a testing period
Precompetitive	6	• A training period used to maximize preparedness and performance for a specific competition or series of competitions • Marked by sport-specific training • Designed to peak fitness, performance, and preparedness
Preparatory	6	• Designed to develop a base necessary for competitive performance • Training moves from extensive to intensive • Fitness is established and used to develop skills
Recovery	1-4	• Has a specific goal of inducing recovery • May occur after a series of competitions • Serves to prepare the athlete for subsequent training
Stabilization	4	• Training used to perfect technique and fitness base • Targets technical errors as well as fitness deficits • Used to develop sport-specific fitness and base of skills

Adapted from Stone, Stone, and Sands (2007); D. Harre, *Trainingslehre* (Berlin, Germany: Sportverlag, 1982).

Each individual week within the mesocycle is referred to as a *microcycle* (28, 29, 31). For the endurance athlete, the structure of a microcycle depends on the location of the microcycle within the larger planning structures (i.e., mesocycle, macrocycle, and annual training plan), the individual athlete's needs, and the time available for structured training. The microcycle is generally 7 days in duration; however, this is not a steadfast rule. The 7-day microcycle structure is most commonly seen during the preparatory period—the period in which no competitions are planned (31). In the competitive period, the microcycle often is less than 7 days. Various types of microcycles can be used to stimulate specific physiological and performance adaptations. In fact, many sport scientists and coaches believe that the microcycle is one of the most important components of the planning process because it is used to structure the individual training days and daily workout schedules (28, 29, 31).

The microcycle is the foundation from which the contents of each individual training day are developed (29). Remember that the number of training days within the microcycle is dependent on many factors, including the athlete's level of development, the time available for training, and the overall period of the meso- and macrocycle (28, 29, 31). For example, during the preparatory period for a novice endurance athlete, the microcycle may contain 3 training days that include resistance training and only 3 or 4 days of specific endurance training. Conversely, during the competitive period, the number of training days that include resistance training could be reduced (fewer than 3 days) or completely removed so that more emphasis can be placed on endurance training. Generally, the more advanced endurance athlete will have more training days within the microcycle, and the novice or recreational athlete will have fewer training days (29).

The training day can be further divided into individual workouts, the smallest training periods (29). The length of the workout can vary, but a workout generally includes several hours of focused training. From a structural standpoint, if 30 minutes or more of rest occurs between two bouts of training in the same day, these bouts are two workouts (29). Thus, multiple training goals may be targeted within the training day by separating sessions by short periods of rest (30 minutes or more) or by spacing multiple workouts throughout the training day. The number of workouts in a training day will depend on the athlete's level of development, ability to tolerate training stress, and time available for training (10).

The sequencing of the workout sessions within the microcycle must be considered because the fatigue generated by one session can affect the athlete's ability to perform during the next workout (8, 29). If the endurance athlete performs two workouts within one training day, the effects of the first workout may result in a reduced training capacity during the second workout (20). This is particularly evident when minimal recovery time is provided between workouts (8).

For example, if the endurance athlete performs a heavy resistance training workout followed by an endurance training session, the overall quality of the endurance training session is significantly reduced as a result of the fatigue generated by the resistance training workout. If the primary target of the training day is the development of strength, this structure would be appropriate; however, the two workouts must be separated to allow the athlete to recover from the resistance training bout before performing the endurance training session. This may be accomplished by scheduling the resistance training workout in the morning and the endurance workout in the afternoon. Ideally, based up emerging research, if possible, a minimum of 6 hours should be placed between resistance and endurance training sessions; this practice enhances the quality of training for both training targets (7, 8, 47). This is particularly important if a run session is completed after a resistance training session, because running is generally more demanding on the body compared to swimming and cycling.

Table 6.10 lists options for how to sequence resistance training and endurance workouts within a training day, along with the likely ramifications of each option.

Table 6.10 Options for the Order of Resistance and Endurance Workouts

Option	Time	Training session focus	Comments
1	a.m.	Resistance training	This order places emphasis on the resistance training and requires a lower intensity and volume of training in the afternoon endurance workout. Ideally, the afternoon endurance training session should be below anaerobic threshold. This order may be best suited for the general preparatory phase.
	p.m.	Endurance training	
2	a.m.	Endurance training	This order places emphasis on the endurance training and requires a lower intensity and volume of training in the afternoon resistance training session. If the endurance athlete is a runner, it may be best to minimize lower-body explosive movements to avoid excessive loading. This order can be used in the specific preparatory or competitive phase.
	p.m.	Resistance training	
3	a.m. or p.m.	Resistance training and endurance training	This order places emphasis on the resistance training. Because the bouts of exercise are performed in close proximity to one another, this order results in a reduced anabolic response being induced by the resistance training. In addition, technical changes resulting from fatigue may occur during the endurance bout.
4	a.m. or p.m.	Endurance training and resistance training	This order places emphasis on the endurance training. Because the bouts of exercise are performed in close proximity to one another, this order results in a magnification of inflammation and greater protein degradation.

It is also important to note that resistance training should not be scheduled on a rest day, because it still induces fatigue and physiological changes, which can hinder recovery. Endurance athletes and coaches should monitor levels of fatigue between resistance and endurance training sessions and make any required modifications to sessions in terms of weights or number of sets as required. It is important to note that these recommendations vary based on an endurance athlete's resistance training, endurance training, and injury history.

SEQUENCING RESISTANCE TRAINING

For any training plan to be effective, the training activities must result in physiological and performance gains that directly translate into improvements in competitive performance. One of the primary factors in achieving this is the sequencing of the various types of training. Four major categories of resistance training exist: *strength endurance*, *basic strength*, *strength power*, and *peaking* or *maintenance* (3, 34). These different goals are achieved by manipulating the training volume, intensity, duration, and number of repetitions or sets (34).

The development of strength endurance is best suited for the early portion of the preparatory period and serves as a tool for developing a training base. In this period, the volume load of training is the highest; thus, a greater reduction in the overall volume and intensity of endurance training is required. Because of this very high-volume load of training, the athlete may only be able to target this category for 1 to 4 weeks. Training for strength endurance is generally undertaken before the development of basic strength.

The second category of training that can be included in the preparatory period is the development of basic strength (33). This category of resistance training is marked by a reduction in volume load along with a significant increase in training intensity, which is designed to increase the athlete's strength levels. Generally, resistance training that targets the development of basic strength is undertaken for 1 to 4 weeks. Although an emphasis on basic strength development is typically seen in the preparatory phase, this type of training may also be used in the precompetitive phase of a long competitive season. The development of basic strength serves as the foundation that allows power-generating capacity to be elevated.

The further development of strength and translation of strength to power generally occurs during the competitive period and is marked by very high intensities and low volumes of training (33). For this category, the training objectives target the continued elevation of muscular strength while maximizing the athlete's power output. Generally, the athlete can target these attributes for 1 to 4 weeks before having to alter the training focus.

The final resistance training category is either a peaking or a maintenance program (29, 30). The decision on whether to use a peaking or maintenance program is largely dictated by the sport. If the sport includes a competitive season that requires a high level of performance over a prolonged period of time, the athlete should use a maintenance program. In most instances, however, the endurance athlete will target a specific competition in which performance will be peaked. When the athlete is attempting to peak for one major competition, the training program includes a 40% to 60% reduction in training load (volume and intensity) 8 to 14 days before the competition, allowing for the dissipation of accumulated fatigue (30). The magnitude of the reduction of training load depends on the length of the taper (period of time before the competition); short tapers (closer to 8 days) include a greater reduction than longer tapers (closer to 14 days) (29, 30). Ultimately, the reduction in training load results in a maximization of performance capacity.

The four categories of resistance training should be viewed as a training continuum on which the appropriate sequencing of training is based. Generally, the basic sequencing pattern is as follows:

Strength endurance → Basic strength → Strength power → Peaking or maintenance

However, some coaches are now forgoing the programming of strength endurance–based resistance training and instead sequencing training as follows:

Basic strength → Strength power → Peaking or maintenance

These general sequences can be used in most situations, but it is not set in stone and can be modified as follows when the preparatory phase is long:

Strength endurance → Basic strength → Strength endurance → Basic strength → Strength power → Peaking or maintenance

or

Basic strength → Strength power → Basic strength → Strength power → Peaking or maintenance

Note that the smallest time frame used for training within one of these specific categories is 1 week and that training should not be done for multiple categories simultaneously. The physiological adaptations achieved in each category facilitate the development that occurs in the next category in the training continuum. For example, in order to tolerate the increased training load encountered during the basic strength category, an athlete must first create an appropriate base of strength endurance. Similarly, basic strength must be developed before the athlete can maximize power-generating ability. Attempting to perform training for all categories in one training session or during one week of training can result in excessive fatigue and an inability to integrate resistance training with the endurance portion of the training plan.

INTEGRATION OF ENDURANCE RESISTANCE TRAINING

As previously noted, an essential part of adding resistance training to an endurance athlete's training plan is to integrate the two types of training successfully. Simply adding resistance training to an existing endurance training plan causes greater levels of fatigue and an overall increased workload. Endurance athletes in this situation often report more fatigue than normal and an inability to sustain the planned training volumes. Special care must be taken to modulate the training loads of both the resistance and endurance portions of the training plan in order to manage the accumulated fatigue appropriately.

The most important integration strategy is to reduce the amount of endurance training to accommodate the addition of resistance training (89). No consensus exists in the scientific literature about the exact amount of reduction required to accommodate the addition of resistance training. Studies reporting improved endurance performance from using a combination of endurance and resistance training reduced the amount of endurance training by 19% to 37% (2, 55, 89).

Determining the proper amount of reduction depends on the phase of training, the amount of resistance training included in the program, and the goals of the annual training plan. For example, during the general preparation phase, the endurance athlete should reduce the amount of endurance training by a greater percent (25%-37%) because of the greater frequency and volume of resistance training. During the competitive phase, however, endurance training could be reduced at a lower percentage (19%-25%) because of the lower workload (frequency and volume) of resistance training within this phase.

Regardless of the training phase, athletes and coaches must pay attention to total workload and the collective effects of both endurance and resistance training. They must consider how the two types of training are integrated. Though reducing the frequency of endurance training when adding resistance training seems to make sense (17), coaches and athletes often view this approach unfavorably. Endurance athletes often believe that they need frequent training sessions usually performed across 5 or 6 days per week to achieve the volumes of training they believe they need to undertake (36).

The scientific literature seems to support the endurance athlete's desire to maintain this volume of training (36, 52). When reducing endurance training loads before a competition (during a taper), the best approach is to decrease the volume and intensity of individual training sessions rather than decrease the frequency of training (11, 30). Using this practice during a taper results in significantly higher performance levels. This approach also allows the athlete to reduce the overall workload of endurance training to accommodate the addition of resistance training (30).

An alternative approach for managing training frequency is to maintain endurance training frequency and use microdosing strategies for the athlete's resistance training interventions (13, 69). With these strategies resistance training sessions are shorter in duration (i.e., 20-30 min) in order to manage fatigue while still providing an effective resistance training dosage (13). In this scenario the athlete may perform 3 resistance training sessions per week that are each 20 minutes long (i.e., 60 total min a week). Through creative programming such as microdosing, resistance training can be integrated more effectively with the athlete's endurance training.

Another important consideration for integration relates to the order of the endurance and resistance training (as discussed previously and highlighted in table 6.10 on page 135). When athletes complete resistance training in the morning and endurance training in the afternoon, a reasonable plan is to complete an easier afternoon workout to accommodate the fatigue from the morning workout (42). This strategy is necessary when targeting strength development and may be best suited for the general preparatory phase. Switching the order of the workouts would negatively affect the resistance training workout. This sequencing may be best suited for the specific preparatory phase or during portions of the competitive phase of the macrocycle.

Regardless of the order of the workouts, athletes and coaches must consider the effects of each training session when constructing a comprehensive training plan that includes both resistance and endurance training. Athletes should avoid performing high-volume, high-intensity resistance and endurance training on the same day if possible. If the volume and intensity of the resistance training are high, the subsequent endurance session should be a low-volume, low-intensity session, ideally below anaerobic threshold. However, if the volume and intensity of the resistance training are low and the athlete is accustomed to resistance training, the endurance session can be of a higher volume and intensity. When integrating resistance training, endurance athletes must ensure that the sessions or workouts are sequenced in the context of the overall workload. Giving careful thought to these factors when designing the training plan will increase the chances of success.

RESISTANCE TRAINING PROGRAM DESIGN FOR ENDURANCE ATHLETES

When developing a resistance training plan, endurance athletes and coaches can employ a sequential planning process as shown in table 6.11. The basic process of integrating resistance training into the endurance athlete's plan should begin with defining the objectives for the training plan. After establishing the objectives, the coach or athlete then define the macrocycle structure, outline the basic structure of the mesocycles, construct the individual microcycle plans, determine the structure of training days, and establish the individual workouts (29).

Table 6.11   Sequential Planning Process for Resistance Training

Step 1	Determine the target objectives for the annual training plan. Planning tasks: 1. Identify the target performance goals. 2. Determine performance tests or standards to target during training. 3. Define the goals and objectives for the resistance training program. 4. Identify the objectives for the endurance training portion of the training plan.

(continued)

Table 6.11 Sequential Planning Process for Resistance Training *(continued)*

Step 2	Define the macrocycle structure. Planning tasks: 1. Define the competition schedule. 2. Determine when the most important competitions will take place. 3. Identify any planned time off (e.g., for student-athletes, identify when classes are not in session). 4. Determine when the athlete may be training without a coach. 5. Specify when the preparatory and competitive phases will occur. 6. Identify when the general and specific preparatory phases will be conducted. 7. Indicate when the precompetitive and competitive phases will occur. 8. Determine when the transition and recovery phases will occur. 9. Establish the specific points when the athlete is planning to peak and indicate this by using the peaking index (see page 143).
Step 3	Outline the basic structure of the mesocycles. Planning tasks: 1. Determine the emphasis of the training phase. 2. Define the length of the mesocycles. 3. Integrate the phases and factors targeted in the training plan with the mesocycle 4. structure. 5. Indicate when performance tests are to be conducted.
Step 4	Construct the individual microcycle plans. Planning tasks: 1. Identify the number of resistance training days, endurance training days, and speed training days in each microcycle. 2. Indicate the volume of resistance, endurance, and speed training in each microcycle. 3. Define the intensity of resistance, endurance, and speed training in each microcycle. 4. Determine the duration and distance of the endurance training in each microcycle. 5. Indicate when recovery microcycles will take place.
Step 5	Determine the structure of training days. Planning tasks: 1. Determine the number of training sessions for each training day. 2. Define the daily training sequence. 3. Identify the intensity and volume of training within each training day.
Step 6	Establish the individual workouts. Planning tasks: 1. Establish the training goals for each workout. 2. Define the warm-up, training, and cooldown activities. 3. Order the training activities according to importance and how fatigue will affect the activities. 4. Sequence the training activities.

Define the Macrocycle Structure

After establishing the athlete's goals and objectives for the annual training plan, the most crucial step in the planning process is to establish the competitive calendar (29). One of the best methods for mapping out the competitive calendar is to use an annual training plan template (28, 29). Using this template, the coach can indicate when each competition is, where the competition is located, and the relative importance of the competition.

For example, when working with a collegiate distance runner who competes in the Big 12 Conference, we would break the annual training plan into two macrocycles; when combined, these macrocycles run from June to June (see figure 6.3 on page 143). The first macrocycle encompasses the cross-country season and culminates with a minor peak for the Big 12 Championships and a major peak on November 26 at the NCAA Championships.

This macrocycle is subdivided into two major periods: the preparatory period and the competitive period. The preparatory period lasts 12 weeks and runs from June until the week ending August 28. This period is subdivided into the two general preparatory phases, which are each 3 weeks, and two specific preparatory phases, which each last 3 weeks. The competitive period lasts 10 weeks and runs from the end of the preparatory period until the competition on the week ending November 4. This period is subdivided into the precompetitive and main competitive phases. The precompetitive phase will include some exhibitions or competitions of minor importance that serve as situational practices where performance is not expected to be peaked. Conversely, performance is expected to elevate across the main competitive phase, resulting in a major peak at the NCAA Championships at the end of the competitive period.

After the major competition, the athlete transitions into the second macrocycle. A 1-week transition period is initiated in which training stress is minimized to allow the athlete to recover from the preceding competitive period. The second macrocycle lasts 14 weeks (November 12 to March 12), including a 4-week preparatory phase and an 8-week competitive period. Because the indoor track season is considered of minor importance for this athlete, a longer preparatory period is used and the athlete is not brought to a major peak.

During the preparatory period the only focus is on specific preparatory activities (29). During the specific preparatory phase, the athlete primarily focuses on developing a foundation for the subsequent competition period. In the competitive period the main competitive phase is designed to last for 8 weeks, with the athlete brought to a minor peak for the Big 12 Championships and the NCAA Championships. As a result of the tight competition schedule, no transition period takes place between the second and third macrocycles.

The third macrocycle is initiated without a transition period, but the first microcycle of the preparatory period contains some recovery sessions, especially early in the week. This preparatory period is relatively short, lasting only 4 weeks; only 2 weeks are dedicated to both the general and specific preparatory phases. The competitive period and the main competitive phase are planned to last 13 weeks in duration and brings the athlete to a major peak at the NCAA Outdoor Championships. After competing in the NCAA Outdoor Championships, this athlete would perform a 3-week transition period before initiating the next annual training plan.

Once the annual training plan is outlined, the coach should identify the important competitions, which are used to establish the individual macrocycles, and define the periods and phases of training (29). This is an essential step because it allows the coach to establish when the athlete will be at peak preparedness. To indicate this, coaches often use a tool called the *peaking index*. The peaking index is a 5-point scale, with 5 indicating the lowest level of preparedness and 1 indicating a peak or maximum level of preparedness (29). As a general rule, the peaking index will be at 4 or 5 during the preparatory period, because this period involves a high volume of training that leads to a lot of cumulative fatigue. Conversely, during the competitive period, the peaking index will be closer to 1; with the lower training volume and appropriate planning, the athlete's level of preparedness will rise as fatigue is dissipated and more emphasis is placed on preparing for competition (29). Figure 6.3 shows the appropriate peaking index to help establish the training objectives for each period.

Some coaches and athletes think that developing an annual training plan is too time-consuming, and they choose to skip this step in the planning process. This is a mistake because a carefully crafted annual training plan allows the coach to better integrate the training factors. Developing the annual plan is of particular importance when resistance training will be included in the endurance athlete's training schedule. The annual training plan can be used to estimate when training stressors will be highest, to determine the targeted peaking times, and to better manage the workloads that the athlete will use in training (28, 29). After the annual training plan is established, the structure and focus of the mesocycles can be added to the planning chart (see figure 6.3).

Outline the Basic Structure of the Mesocycles

Once the competitive calendar, the macrocycles, and the periods and phases have been outlined, the next step is to design the structure of the mesocycles (29). This step is a little more difficult than creating the macrocycle structure because the resistance and endurance training must be considered in relation to the periods and phases that have been established. Continuing with the example of the collegiate distance runner, the first macrocycle (which included a total of 22 weeks) can be broken into six mesocycles. Each mesocycle would have very specific targets (figure 6.3).

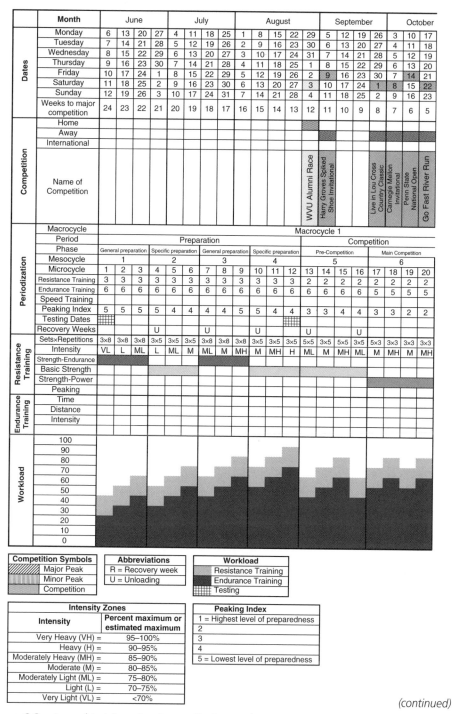

Figure 6.3 Annual training plan for a collegiate endurance runner.

(continued)

	Oct.	November					December				January					February				Mar.
Month	Oct.	November					December				January					February				Mar.
Monday	24	31	7	14	21	28	5	12	19	26	2	9	16	23	30	6	13	20	27	6
Tuesday	25	1	8	15	22	29	6	13	20	27	3	10	17	24	31	7	14	21	28	7
Wednesday	26	2	9	16	23	30	7	14	21	28	4	11	18	25	1	8	15	22	1	8
Thursday	27	3	10	17	24	1	8	15	22	29	5	12	19	26	2	9	16	23	2	9
Friday	28	4	11	18	25	2	9	16	23	30	6	13	20	27	3	10	17	24	3	10
Saturday	29	5	12	19	26	3	10	17	24	31	7	14	21	28	4	11	18	25	4	11
Sunday	30	6	13	20	27	4	11	18	25	1	8	15	22	29	5	12	19	26	5	12
Weeks to major competition	4	3	2	1	0	14	13	12	11	10	9	8	7	6	5	4	3	2	1	0

Competition

- Home
- Away
- International
- Name of Competition:
  - Big 12 Championships
  - NCAA Mid-Atlantic Regional
  - NCAA Championships
  - Canadian National Championships
  - Sharon Colyear-Danville
  - Nittany Lion Challenge
  - Youngstown Invitational
  - Penn State National
  - Sykes & Sabock Challenge
  - BU Valentine
  - Penn State Tune Up
  - Big 12 Championships
  - NCAA Championships

Periodization

Macrocycle	Macrocycle 1						Macrocycle 2													
Period	Competition					Transition	Preparation				Competition									
Phase	Main Competition					Transition	Specific preparation				Main Competition									
Mesocycle	7			8				9			10				11				12	
Microcycle	21	22	23	24	25	26	27	28	29	30	31	32	33	34	35	36	37	38	39	40
Resistance Training	2	2	2	1	1	1	3	3	3	3	3	2	2	2	2	2	2	1	1	1
Endurance Training	5	5	5	5	5	5	5	6	6	6	6	5	5	5	5	5	5	5	5	5
Speed Training																				
Peaking Index	2	3	2	1	2	3	4	4	4	4	3	3	3	2	3	3	2	2	3	2
Testing Dates										▦										
Recovery Weeks	U		U	U							U								U	U

Resistance Training

Sets×Repetitions	3×3	5×3	3×3	3×2	3×2	3×2	5×5	5×5	5×5	3×5	3×5	3×5	3×3	3×3	5×3	3×5	3×3	2×2	3×3	3×3
Intensity	ML	ML	M	L	VL	ML	M	MH	H	M	ML	M	ML	M	MH	M	M	M	L	L
Strength-Endurance																				
Basic Strength																				
Strength-Power																				
Peaking																				

Endurance Training

- Time
- Distance
- Intensity

Workload

(100, 90, 80, 70, 60, 50, 40, 30, 20, 10, 0)

Competition Symbols		Abbreviations	Workload	
▨	Major Peak	R = Recovery week		Resistance Training
▦	Minor Peak	U = Unloading		Endurance Training
▩	Competition			Testing

Intensity Zones			Peaking Index	
Intensity	**Percent maximum or estimated maximum**		1 = Highest level of preparedness	
Very Heavy (VH) =	95–100%		2	
Heavy (H) =	90–95%		3	
Moderately Heavy (MH) =	85–90%		4	
Moderate (M) =	80–85%		5 = Lowest level of preparedness	
Moderately Light (ML) =	75–80%			
Light (L) =	70–75%			
Very Light (VL) =	<70%			

Figure 6.3 *(continued)*

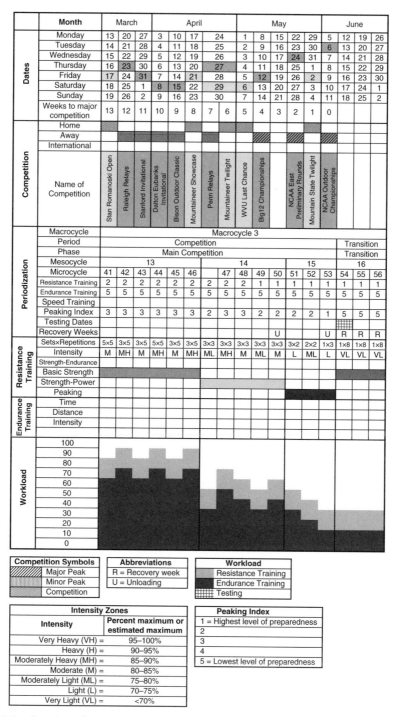

Figure 6.3 *(continued)*

In mesocycle 1, which is part of the preparatory period, resistance training is used to target the development of strength endurance; the endurance portion of the training program involves base work. Because the preparatory period is long, three mesocycles can be established that progress the resistance training from strength endurance in mesocycle 1, to a focus on increasing muscular strength in mesocycle 2, then a return to the development of strength endurance in mesocycle 3, and then return to focusing on increasing muscular strength in mesocycle 4.

The competitive period is also long (a total of 13 weeks), so it can be broken into four mesocycles also (see mesocycles 5 to 8 in figure 6.3). This period begins with the fifth mesocycle, which includes 4 weeks of resistance training that targets strength development. Next, the sixth mesocycle contains 4 weeks of training that targets strength and development with the use of different means. The seventh mesocycle is a four-week mesocycle that focuses on strength and power development. The eighth mesocycle is designed to reduce fatigue and elevate the athlete's preparedness for the NCAA Championships.

The development of the mesocycle structures for the second and third macrocycles progress in a similar fashion. Remember that the various resistance training activities should be sequenced so that the physiological and performance gains are directed toward the specified competitions established in the macrocycle plan.

Construct the Individual Microcycle Plans

After outlining the structure of the mesocycles, the coach can establish the individual microcycles (figure 6.4) (29). The first step in creating the microcycle structure is to define the number of training days or sessions that will be used for resistance, endurance, and other training modalities. The number of sessions contained in each microcycle will largely be a function of the phase of training and the targeted training goals.

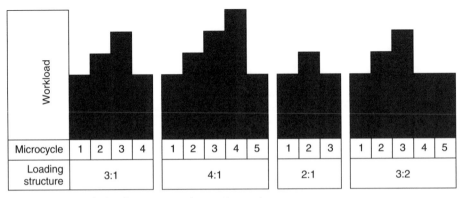

Figure 6.4 Sample loading patterns for a microcycle.

For example, in mesocycle 1, the primary focus of the general preparatory phase is physical development; therefore, a greater focus can be placed on resistance training. During this mesocycle, the resistance training program targets the development of strength endurance and is performed 3 days per week. The athlete performs endurance training activities 6 days a week. A similar breakdown is used for mesocycles 2 through 4. As noted previously, the number of endurance training days stays consistent at 6 days per week during these two mesocycles.

As the athlete begins to shift into the competitive period (mesocycle 5), the amount of resistance training is reduced to only two sessions per week. During this period, the frequency of endurance training remains high, but the types of training vary depending on the targeted goals. During mesocycles 6 and 7 the number of resistance training sessions per week remains at two, with the number of endurance training sessions reduced to five. Finally, during the peaking phase of the first macrocycle, resistance training is reduced to one session per week to allow for the maintenance of muscular strength.

The second step in constructing the microcycle is to determine the general intensity that will be used for the training weeks and to determine when unloading weeks will occur. The loading program for the individual microcycles can be implemented in many ways. In the example annual training plan (figure 6.3) various loading paradigms are implemented including 3:1 loading paradigms. For example, the first mesocycle contains 3 weeks that include a steady increase in training load, and the 4th week is an unloading week. (*Note:* The 4th week is in mesocycle 2.)

When determining the loading pattern, the coach needs to consider all training factors, including total workload because they all contribute to an athlete's fatigue level. Depending on the mesocycle structures, other loading programs can be used, such as a 4:1 or 2:1 pattern (figure 6.4). Ultimately, the coach and athlete have a lot of freedom to manipulate the loading structures based on the competitive schedule and the athlete's needs.

For the resistance training portion of the program, the average intensity during a microcycle is indicated on the plan chart. However, this does not mean that the intensity is constant on each training day. Light and heavy days should both be included, especially when using a combination of training factors such as endurance and resistance training. Remember that the fatigue from one training factor will affect the athlete's ability to perform the other factor. Research indicates that loading structures that include light and heavy days result in significantly better adaptation because they allow for greater variation in the microcycle.

Table 6.12 presents a sample weekly microcycle for a distance runner. By manipulating the intensity of each training day, the coach or athlete can also manipulate the overall volume load, or workload.

Table 6.12 Sample Weekly Microcycle for a Distance Runner

Day	TRAINING FACTOR		
		Resistance training	
	Endurance training	Sets × reps	Intensity (% of 15RM)*
Sunday	Rest day	Rest day	
Monday	45-min fartlek run	Injury risk management exercises	
Tuesday	60-min long slow distance (LSD) run	3 × 6	80%-85% (MH)
Wednesday	45-min interval run	--	
Thursday	60-min easy run	3 × 8	75%-80% (ML)
Friday	45-min repetition run	--	
Saturday	120-min LSD run	--	

*ML is moderately light; MH is moderately heavy. Injury risk management exercises will vary based on each athlete's personal injury history.

Adapted from B.H. Reuter and P.S. Hagerman, "Aerobic Endurance Exercise Training," in *Essentials of Strength Training and Conditioning*, 3rd ed., edited for the National Strength and Conditioning Association by T.R. Baechle and R.W. Earle (Champaign, IL: Human Kinetics, 2008), 490-539.

Note that the workload is multicompartmental and includes contributions from both endurance and resistance training. In figure 6.3 on page 143, this is indicated by two distinct categories being combined to represent the workload. In mesocycle 1, the resistance training targets strength endurance, so the athlete performs a higher volume of resistance training (3 sets of 8 repetitions). This is indicated by larger bars on the workload graph (figure 6.3). As the athlete progresses through the training year, the volume of resistance training varies depending on the targeted outcomes. In the plan shown in figure 6.3, a section for endurance training is also included that allows the coach to indicate distance (mileage), training time, and intensity (e.g., power output and percentage of maximum heart rate) for each microcycle. A complete discussion of how this can be distributed is beyond the scope of this chapter. The important message is that the endurance and resistance training programs need to be treated as a unified and sequenced training load. Refer to chapter 3 for methods of creating endurance training regimens.

Determine the Structure of Training Days

Once the basic structure of the microcycles has been established, the coach can create the daily training structures (29). When establishing the day's training activities, the coach must consider the various training factors and how they affect each other. As noted previously, the fatigue generated from endurance training will compromise the athlete's ability to perform resistance training if the two sessions are in close proximity to one another. This step involves determining the number of training sessions that occur during the day and sequencing them to meet the goals that have been established for the mesocycle.

Additionally, the coach can determine the intensity of the training sessions. For example, if a hard resistance training session is scheduled for the morning, the afternoon endurance session would most likely be less intense (below anaerobic threshold) and may target recovery. Conversely, if a hard endurance workout is planned, the resistance training session that precedes it would need to be of lower intensity. Once the daily training structures are established, the coach can then design the individual resistance training sessions.

Establish the Individual Workouts

The last step in creating a resistance training program is to design the individual workouts (10, 29). In this step, the coach must remember the training targets established for the macrocycle, the mesocycle, and, most important, the microcycle. These targets serve as the guidelines for creating each individual workout. Several items need to be included in an individual workout plan, including the goals for the session, warm-up activities, the body of the session, and the cooldown. Figure 6.5 on page 150 shows a sample plan for an individual workout (10). (This sample training session is based on multijoint exercises that provide a major emphasis on the lower body and only a minor emphasis on the upper body.)

Establishing goals for the workout is essential because the goals will guide the athlete to focus on key points. A sample goal for an endurance athlete may be to focus on using proper form for all exercises or to maintain a consistent rest interval between each set. The goals are generally highly individualized and address specific items that the athlete should focus on during the session.

The first part of every workout is the warm-up. The plan should detail the duration of the warm-up and all activities to be performed. Additionally, any distances for activities should be indicated. The warm-up should involve dynamic activities that increase body temperature and range of motion. Athletes should avoid static stretching during the warm-up because this type of stretching has been shown to compromise strength and power performance.

For an additional warm-up before each exercise, the athlete should perform two or three light sets before starting the target sets. The number of warm-up sets depends on the intensity being used and the type of exercise. For example, in the sample workout (figure 6.5), the squat and press can be used as a warm-up so that fewer warm-up sets are needed for the back squat. In the workout, the target sets should all be completed with the same resistance. This method initiates a greater stimulus for adaptation, which leads to a more substantial improvement in performance. Generally, the more complex exercises that involve a larger muscle mass should be performed first, with less complex exercises that involve a smaller muscle mass being performed later in the training session. For example, the power clean should be performed early in the session, and the leg curl can be performed at the end of the session.

After completing a resistance training session, an athlete should always perform a structured cooldown. The cooldown should include a series of static stretching and last between 10 and 15 minutes. The postworkout period is the ideal time for improving flexibility. Most endurance athletes, especially runners, exhibit poor flexibility. Therefore, flexibility training should be included in the cooldown.

Athlete: ___Kelsey Fowler___   Date: ___2/23/23___

Mesocycle: ___1___   Session time: ___7:00 AM___

Microcycle: ___1___   Sport: ___Cross country___

GOALS

- Focus on the depth of the back squat.
- Maintain technique throughout the session.
- Maintain 2-minute rest intervals between sets.

WARM-UP (20 MINUTES)

- Hip rotations and banded crab walks
- 10 scorpions per side
- 10-20 bodyweight squats
- Lunge and twist for 20 meters
- Spiderman crawl for 20 meters
- 12 bodyweight single-leg seated calf raises

RESISTANCE TRAINING SESSION

Exercise	TARGET SETS			
	Sets	Repetitions	Intensity	Comments
Squat + Press	3	15	VL	Use as a warm-up exercise
Back Squat	3	15	ML	
1-Leg Squat	3	15	ML	Make sure knee is at 90 degrees
Behind the Neck Press	3	15	ML	Maintain control of bar
Dips	3	15		Use body weight
Abdominals	3	25		Your choice of exercises
Notes:	Use 1 minute rest interval between each set Perform 2-3 light warm-up sets until target loads are hit All target sets are performed at the same intensity			

COOLDOWN

Perform 15 minutes of static stretching that include the following areas:

- Shoulders and arms
- Back
- Hips
- Hamstrings
- Groin
- Quadriceps
- Calves

Figure 6.5 Sample workout session.

SAMPLE RESISTANCE TRAINING PROGRAMS FOR ENDURANCE ATHLETES

All resistance training programs should be designed to meet the specific needs of the athlete. While resistance training programs can be constructed in numerous ways, they should always be designed to target the major movement patterns and muscle groups that are essential to the athlete's sport. In the following sections, several sample training programs are presented. These programs are categorized based on the phase of training outlined in the macrocycle plan. Athletes and coaches should use the information about resistance training and planning in this chapter and integrate these concepts with those discussed in chapters 8 through 12 to develop a training program for their particular endurance sport.

Basic Program for Building Strength Endurance

A basic resistance training program for developing strength endurance should be designed to include a larger overall volume: at least 3 sets and greater than 8 repetitions per set; more advanced athletes may choose to use as many as 10 sets for some exercises (including the warm-up sets); however this is not often necessary. As the number of sets increases, the overall intensity (percentage of 1RM) decreases.

For most athletes, three training sessions per microcycle are more than adequate. If the athlete is primarily focused on the development of muscle mass, the overall frequency and volume of training could be increased (the athlete could train more than 3 days per microcycle). However, in most cases, this is not the focus for endurance athletes. Therefore, the sample program presented in table 6.13 on page 152 is designed to include only three resistance training sessions per microcycle.

Each resistance training session in table 6.13 is structured to work the total body in one session. By targeting the total body in one session, this can help the athlete be more time efficient when completing resistance training. This is accomplished through the use of multijoint, large-mass exercises that target movements similar to those seen in most endurance sports. The larger-mass exercises (e.g., squats and hang power clean) are performed early in each session. This ensures that a minimum amount of fatigue is generated before the athlete performs these technical exercises.

This sample program lasts only four microcycles and uses 3 sets of 8 repetitions. Additionally, the intensity varies for each training day and microcycle. Across the four microcycles, the intensity increases for three successive microcycles, and an unloading week takes place during the fourth microcycle. This is the classic 3:1 loading pattern discussed previously. To further increase the focus on the development of strength endurance, the athlete can use 1-minute rest intervals between each set and exercise.

Table 6.13 Sample Basic Program for Building Strength Endurance

Day	Exercises	Target sets*		Intensity			
		Sets	Repetitions	Week 1	Week 2	Week 3	Week 4
Monday	Squat and press	3	8	ML	M	MH	L
	Back squat	3	8	ML	M	MH	L
	Leg curl	3	8	ML	M	MH	L
	Single-leg seated calf raise	3	6	ML	M	MH	L
	Pull-up	3	8	Body weight (add load when possible)			
	Abdominal exercise	5	25				
Wednesday	Hang power clean	3	8	L	ML	M	ML
	Clean pull from floor	3	8	L	ML	M	ML
	Clean-grip Romanian deadlift	3	8	L	ML	M	ML
	Lat pulldown	3	10	L	ML	M	ML
	Three-way shoulder raise	3	10	L	ML	M	ML
	Abdominal exercise	5	25				
Friday	Squat and press	3	8	L	ML	M	ML
	Front squat	3	8	L	ML	M	ML
	Bent-over row	3	8	L	ML	M	ML
	Glute-ham machine	3	10	Body weight (add load when possible)			
	Dip	3	10	Body weight (add load when possible)			
	Abdominal exercise	3	10				

*Two or three warm-up sets should be performed with each exercise. One-minute rest intervals can be used in this block of training.

This basic program can be used to develop strength endurance, to lose body fat, and to increase overall physical fitness. The basic structure can be used to train for any endurance sport, but in order to maximize its effectiveness, it should be integrated into the overall training structure as discussed previously.

Resistance Training Program for a Runner

The resistance training program for a runner should be designed based on the overall macrocycle structure and the targeted training goals for each phase of training. To illustrate the types of resistance training programs that would fit into a macrocycle training plan, three sample programs are presented based on figure 6.3 on page 143. Specifically, the resistance training plans for mesocycle blocks 3 to 5 are presented.

In mesocycle 3, the targeted resistance training goal is the development of strength endurance. Strength endurance is best developed by using an exercise volume of 3 to 10 sets of over 8 repetitions per set. Therefore, for this block of training, the program uses 3 sets of 10 repetitions in order to target the development of strength endurance (see table 6.14). Additionally, the plan for this mesocycle includes only 2 days of resistance training; thus, resistance training will only be performed on Tuesdays and Thursdays. The weekly average training intensity follows the 3:1 loading pattern indicated in the macrocycle plan (figure 6.3). However, this program involves using a heavy day and a light day so that Tuesday is the heaviest resistance training day of each microcycle. This loading structure will allow the runner to have harder endurance workouts at the end of the microcycle (Friday through Sunday).

After 4 weeks, the focus of the resistance training program is altered to target the development of basic strength (as indicated for mesocycle 4 in figure 6.3 on page 143). This sample program is shown in table 6.15. To focus on basic strength, the volume is reduced by decreasing the number of repetitions from

Table 6.14 Sample Strength Endurance Mesocycle Block for a Runner

| Day | Exercises | Target sets* | | Intensity | | | |
		Sets	Repetitions	Week 1	Week 2	Week 3	Week 4
Tuesday	Hang power clean	3	8	ML	M	MH	ML
	Back squat	3	8	ML	M	MH	ML
	Dumbbell incline bench press	3	8	ML	M	MH	ML
	Glute-ham raise	3	10	Body weight (add load when possible)			
	Dip	3	10	Body weight (add load when possible)			
	Abdominal exercise	5	25				
Thursday	Squat and press	3	8	VL	L	ML	VL
	Bulgarian squat	3	8	VL	L	ML	VL
	Single-leg seated calf raise	3	8	VL	L	ML	VL
	Bent-over row	3	8	VL	L	ML	VL
	Snatch-grip Romanian deadlift	3	8	VL	L	ML	VL
	Pull-up	3	10	Body weight (add load when possible)			
	Abdominal exercise	5	25				

*Two or three warm-up sets should be performed with each exercise. One-minute rest intervals can be used in this block.

10 to 5. Because strength is best developed with higher intensities, the intensity is increased in this phase. As with the strength endurance phase, a 3:1 loading pattern is used. Thus, the third microcycle of this block (microcycle 15) contains the most taxing resistance training loads, and it is followed by an unloading microcycle. The exercises selected here are designed to maximize the development of muscular strength while allowing for a transfer of training effects that will result in improved running economy. As noted on the macrocycle planning sheet (figure 6.3), resistance training is performed only 2 days per microcycle. This allows the focus of the overall training plan to shift toward endurance training and more specialized training typical of the precompetition phase.

The next phase of resistance training, shown in table 6.16, is designed to target the optimization of both strength and power-generating capacity as planned in mesocycle 5 (figure 6.3). In this mesocycle, the focus of the overall training plan continues to shift toward more specialized endurance training. Therefore, the emphasis placed on resistance training continues to be reduced. This can be noted by the decrease in the number of resistance training days from 2 in the first microcycle of this block (microcycle 17) to 1 in the subsequent three

Table 6.15 Sample Basic Strength Mesocycle Block for a Runner

Day	Exercises	Target sets*		Intensity			
		Sets	Repetitions	Week 1	Week 2	Week 3	Week 4
Tuesday	Power clean and press	3	3+2	M	MH	H	M
	Back squat	3	5	M	MH	H	M
	Step-up	3	5	M	MH	H	M
	Single-leg seated calf raise	3	5	M	MH	H	M
	Dip (weighted)	3	8	M	MH	H	M
	Abdominal exercise	5	25				
Thursday	Power snatch plus overhead squat	3	2+3	ML	M	MH	ML
	Singe-leg seated calf raise	3	5	ML	M	MH	ML
	Reverse lunge	3	5	ML	M	MH	ML
	Snatch-grip Romanian deadlift	3	5	ML	M	MH	ML
	Chin-up (weighted)	3	8	ML	M	MH	ML
	Abdominal exercise	5	25				

*Two or three warm-up sets should be performed with each exercise. Two-minute rest intervals can be used in this phase.

Table 6.16 Sample Strength Power Mesocycle Block for a Runner

Day	Exercises	Week 1			Week 2			Week 3			Week 4		
		Sets*	Repetitions	Intensity	Sets*	Repetitions	Intensity	Sets*	Repetitions	Intensity	Sets*	Repetitions	Intensity
Tuesday	Push jerk	4	3	M				3	3	MH			
	Power clean	4	3	MH				3	3	H			
	Single-leg seated calf raise	3	3	M				3	3	MH			
	Abdominal exercise	4	25					5	25				
Thursday	Power snatch	5	3	M	3	3	H				3	3	M
	Jump shrug plus split jumps	5	3+3	MH	3	3	H				3	3	M
	Clean-grip Romanian deadlift	5	3	M	3	3	MH				3	3	M
	Abdominal exercise	5	25		5	25							

*Two or three warm-up sets should be performed with each exercise. Three-minute rest intervals can be used in this phase.

microcycles. The overall volume of resistance training also decreases; the athlete performs sets of 3 with more intensive loads. The increased loads and the exercises selected will result in a further elevation of both strength and power-generating capacity. Plyometrics are also included in this block. Box jumps and split jumps have been strategically placed in the program to maximize explosive strength development. The scientific literature suggests that the inclusion of explosive exercises, such as plyometrics and power cleans, help athletes develop the strength characteristics necessary for maximizing running performance.

Resistance training is often excluded from the two microcycles before a major competition. The decision to exclude resistance training at this point largely depends on the overall endurance training plan, the level of fatigue generated, and the individual athlete's tolerance to resistance training. If resistance training is used in this mesocycle (mesocycle 6, figure 6.3 on page 143), the training should involve very minimal loads or volumes and should have a moderate to high intensity until the microcycle immediately before the competition. Generally, endurance athletes respond psychologically better to the removal of resistance training during this phase. Therefore, the sample plan focuses simply on endurance training in the two microcycles leading into the major contest at the end of the macrocycle.

Resistance Training Program for a Cyclist

When developing a resistance training program for a cyclist, coaches need to place the primary emphasis on the development of lower-body and core strength; only a minor emphasis should be placed on the upper body. In programs for these athletes, the upper body needs to be de-emphasized so that the athletes can avoid an increase in frontal area that would result in a decrease in aerodynamic efficiency. However, the upper body must still be trained because it is involved in activities such as sprinting and climbing and is the second most common site of injury for these athletes.

The structure of the resistance training plan is based on the phase of the annual training plan and the goals for the individual mesocycles and microcycles. For example, in the general preparatory phase, the resistance training program contains more training sessions and a larger overall volume of training. Table 6.17 provides an example of a strength endurance block for a cyclist. In this sample program, the athlete performs 3 sets of 8 repetitions for the major exercises, and a 3:1 loading structure is used for four microcycles. Each training session is structured so that the technical, large-mass exercises are done first (when the athlete is the freshest). Additionally, each session is designed to provide a total-body workout that targets the major movement patterns and muscle groups that are used in cycling. To further focus on strength endurance, the athlete can use a short rest interval (1 minute) between sets and exercises in this block.

Table 6.17 Sample Strength Endurance Mesocycle Block for a Cyclist

Day	Exercises	Target sets*		Intensity			
		Sets	Repetitions	Week 1	Week 2	Week 3	Week 4
Monday	Clean pull (from thigh)	3	8	L	ML	M	L
	Back squat	3	8	L	ML	M	L
	Dumbbell incline bench press	3	8	L	ML	M	L
	Dumbbell reverse lunge	3	12	L	ML	M	L
	Clean-grip Romanian deadlift	3	12	L	ML	M	L
	Dip (weighted)	3	12	L	ML	M	L
	Abdominal exercise	5	25				
Wednesday	Squat and press	3	8	VL	L	ML	L
	Quarter back squat (from pins)	3	8	VL	L	ML	L
	Bent-over row	3	8	VL	L	ML	L
	Lat pulldown	3	12	VL	L	ML	L
	Standing good morning	3	12	VL	L	ML	L
	Abdominal exercise	5	25				
Friday	Clean pull (from knee)	3	8	L	ML	M	L
	Squat	3	8	L	ML	M	L
	Dumbbell bench press	3	8	L	ML	M	L
	Bulgarian squat	3	8	L	ML	M	L
	Clean-grip Romanian deadlift	3	8	L	ML	M	L
	Dip (weighted)	3	12	L	ML	M	L
	Abdominal exercise	5	25				

*Two or three warm-up sets should be performed with each exercise. One-minute rest intervals can be used in this block.

When the athlete is transitioning to an emphasis on basic strength (as shown in the sample program in table 6.18), the major modifications to the training program will consist of a substantial decrease in training volume, an increase in the lifting intensity (percentage of 1RM), and an increase in the rest intervals between sets and exercises (2-min intervals). The reduction in volume load should decrease the fatigue typically associated with high volume loads of resistance training. This enables the athlete to focus on developing strength and completing endurance-based training on the bike. In the sample program, the number of training days is reduced to 2 per microcycle, and the number of repetitions is dropped from 8 to 5. During this block, the main focus is still on the development of lower-body strength, which is targeted with exercises such as squats and power cleans. These types of exercises allow the athlete to target the major muscle groups used in cycling while also maximizing the development of core strength without having to perform a wide assortment of exercises.

Table 6.19 presents a sample program designed with an emphasis on strength power. To shift the focus toward power development, the overall training volume is further decreased, the intensity of training is elevated, and the rest interval between sets and exercises is lengthened to 3 minutes. The number of training days in this example is held at 2. The low overall volume load of training and the exercises selected, along with the modifications to the rest interval, should help further develop both strength and power. For example, the use of the power

Table 6.18   Sample Basic Strength Mesocycle Block for a Cyclist

Day	Exercises	Target sets*		Intensity			
		Sets	Repetitions	Week 1	Week 2	Week 3	Week 4
Tuesday	Hang power clean	3	5	M	MH	H	M
	Back squat	3	5	M	MH	H	M
	Single-leg leg press	3	5	M	MH	H	M
	Push press	3	5	M	MH	H	M
	Clean-grip Romanian deadlift	3	5	M	MH	H	M
	Abdominal exercise	5	25				
Thursday	Hang power snatch	3	5	ML	M	MH	ML
	¼ front squat (from pins)	3	5	ML	M	MH	ML
	Reverse lunge	3	5	ML	M	MH	ML
	Snatch pull (from thigh)	3	5	ML	M	MH	ML
	Chin-up	3	5	Body weight			
	Abdominal exercise	5	25				

*Two or three warm-up sets should be performed with each exercise. Two-minute rest intervals can be used in this block.

Table 6.19 Sample Strength Power Mesocycle Block for a Cyclist

Day	Exercises	Target sets*		Intensity			
		Sets	Repetitions	Week 1	Week 2	Week 3	Week 4
Tuesday	Power clean	3	3	MH	H	VH	M
	Back squat plus box jump	3	3+3	MH	H	VH	M
	Push jerk	3	3	MH	H	VH	M
	Dip (weighted)	3	3	MH	H	VH	M
	Abdominal exercise	5	25				
Thursday	Power snatch	3	3	M	MH	H	ML
	Speed squat	3	3	M	MH	H	ML
	Snatch-grip shoulder shrug	3	3	M	MH	H	ML
	Snatch-grip Romanian deadlift	3	3	M	MH	H	ML
	Abdominal exercise	5	25				

*Two or three warm-up sets should be performed with each exercise. Three-minute rest intervals can be used in this block.

clean, power snatch, and speed squat can elevate lower-body power, which should directly translate to power on the bike.

Resistance Training Program for a Swimmer

Like other endurance athletes, swimmers can benefit from the inclusion of resistance training in their training plans. Typically, swimmers undertake large volumes of swim training; thus, effectively incorporating resistance training into their training plans is somewhat challenging. The amount of swim training must be reduced to accommodate the number of resistance training sessions or the amount of training load allotted to resistance training.

In the general preparatory phase, a swimmer will usually perform resistance training on 2 or 3 days per microcycle. As the athlete shifts into the precompetitive and competitive phases, the number of resistance training sessions per microcycle will be reduced to 1 or 2. During the 8 to 14 days before a major competition, resistance training may be completely removed from the program. The reduction in resistance training during these phases will reduce the accumulated fatigue and accommodate the potential increase in swim training.

Table 6.20 presents a sample program for the strength endurance block of resistance training for a swimmer. This sample uses three training sessions per microcycle. The design includes a basic four-microcycle structure that uses a 3:1 loading pattern. Thus, the third microcycle of this block would be the most difficult. In this example, total-body lifting is used in conjunction with several auxiliary exercises that target the muscles used in most swimming strokes. The overall volume load in this block is relatively high because of the high-repetition scheme. The short rest interval of 1 minute is used to create additional physiological stress that targets strength endurance.

As the athlete transitions into the basic strength block, the overall volume load of resistance training is reduced, and the intensity is increased. This is reflected in the sample program provided in table 6.21. These modifications enable the athlete to focus on the development of maximal muscular strength. In this block, the athlete performs more complex lifting exercises, including the

Table 6.20 Sample Strength Endurance Mesocycle Block for a Swimmer

Day	Exercises	Target sets*		Intensity			
		Sets	Repetitions	Week 1	Week 2	Week 3	Week 4
Monday	Back squat	3	8	ML	M	MH	L
	Snatch-grip behind-the-neck press	3	8	ML	M	MH	L
	Straight-arm pull-over	3	10	ML	M	MH	L
	Three-way shoulder raise	3	10	ML	M	MH	L
	Abdominal exercise	5	25				
Wednesday	Clean pull	3	8	L	ML	M	VL
	Clean-grip shrug	3	8	L	ML	M	VL
	Clean-grip Romanian deadlift	3	8	L	ML	M	VL
	Bent-over row	3	10	L	ML	M	VL
	Abdominal exercise	5	25				
Friday	Overhead squat	3	8	VL	L	ML	VL
	Bench press	3	8	VL	L	ML	VL
	Calf raise	3	10	VL	L	ML	VL
	Lat pulldown	3	10	VL	L	ML	VL
	Front raise	3	10	VL	L	ML	VL
	Abdominal exercise	5	25				

*Two or three warm-up sets should be performed with each exercise. One-minute rest intervals can be used in this block.

power clean and power snatch. Additionally, because the athlete will likely have a greater focus on swim training during this block, the number of resistance training sessions is reduced to two. As with the strength endurance block, a 3:1 loading pattern is implemented in which the athlete completes three loading microcycles followed by one unloading microcycle.

After completing the basic strength block, the athlete may undertake a strength power block of training. A sample program for this block is shown in table 6.22. This block is ideal for the addition of plyometric exercises. The overall volume load of training is again reduced, while the intensity of training is increased substantially. Additionally, the overall number of exercises per session is reduced. The rest interval is lengthened to 3 minutes to allow for a more complete recovery before initiating the next set or exercise. This enables the athlete to focus on moving quickly when performing each exercise. The sample program includes two sessions per microcycle, but in some instances, the number of training sessions per microcycle may be reduced to one. The major factor in determining this is the amount of time or effort put into the swim training sessions. If the volume and intensity of swim training are increased during this time frame, the best strategy is to reduce the resistance training to one session per microcycle.

Table 6.21 Sample Basic Strength Mesocycle Block for a Swimmer

Day	Exercises	Target sets*		Intensity			
		Sets	Repetitions	Week 1	Week 2	Week 3	Week 4
Tuesday	Power clean	3	5	M	MH	H	ML
	Back squat	3	5	M	MH	H	ML
	Push press	3	5	M	MH	H	ML
	Good morning	3	5	M	MH	H	ML
	Three-way shoulder raise	3	8	M	MH	H	ML
	Abdominal exercise	5	25				
Thursday	Snatch-grip shoulder shrug	3	5	ML	M	MH	L
	Power snatch	3	5	ML	M	MH	L
	Overhead squat	3	5	ML	M	MH	L
	Chin-up (weighted)	3	8	ML	M	MH	L
	Abdominal exercise	5	25				

*Two or three warm-up sets should be performed with each exercise. Two-minute rest intervals can be used in this block.

Table 6.22 Sample Strength Power Mesocycle Block for a Swimmer

Day	Exercises	Target sets*		Intensity			
		Sets	Repetitions	Week 1	Week 2	Week 3	Week 4
Tuesday	Power clean	3	3	MH	H	VH	M
	¼ back squat plus box jump	3	3+3	MH	H	VH	M
	Straight-arm pull-over	3	3	MH	H	VH	M
	Three-way shoulder raise	3	3	MH	H	VH	M
	Abdominal exercise	5	25				
Thursday	Power snatch	3	3	M	MH	H	ML
	Bench press with medicine ball throw	3	3	M	MH	H	ML
	Snatch-grip Romanian deadlift	3	3	M	MH	H	ML
	Front raise	3	3	M	MH	H	ML
	Abdominal exercise	5	25				

*Two or three warm-up sets should be performed with each exercise. Three-minute rest intervals can be used in this block.

During the peaking portion of the program, resistance training may be reduced to one session per microcycle—or may be removed from the program—for the two microcycles before a major competition. If one session is included per microcycle, the sessions should contain a reduced number of exercises and a decreased training volume (1 to 3 sets of 1 to 3 repetitions). The microcycle before the competition should include a substantial reduction in intensity; this helps induce recovery while allowing the athlete to maintain strength gains. Again, the decision on whether to exclude resistance training during this time frame depends on the choices made in the swim training plan.

Resistance Training Program for a Triathlete

The integration of resistance training into the overall training plan of a triathlete is probably one of the more difficult things to accomplish. The triathlete must effectively periodize the three major activities of swimming, running, and cycling. To further complicate resistance training programming for a triathlete, all three triathlon disciplines use varying muscle groups and movement patterns. Additionally, the swim and cycle disciplines do not involve a ground reaction force like running, meaning it is likely that different muscular contractions take place for each discipline. Generally, the overall volume of training undertaken by these athletes is substantial and difficult to sequence. Because of the large number of training factors being targeted, the resistance training program must be efficient and contain a minimal number of exercises. The goal is to maximize the physiological adaptations targeted by this type of training without creating too much fatigue. To further facilitate these effects, the coach or athlete must consider the integration of the four training factors: swimming, running, cycling, and resistance training.

During the preparatory period for a triathlete, the resistance training program could include 3 days of training per microcycle, but in most instances, 2 days per microcycle would be adequate. Because the triathlete is training for many diverse activities, the best strategy is to divide the daily training into multiple training sessions, as shown in table 6.23. In this example, resistance training is performed on Monday morning and Friday evening.

Table 6.23 Sample Microcycle Structure for a General Preparatory Mesocycle of a Triathlete

Day	Time	Workout
Monday	a.m.	Resistance training
Tuesday	a.m.	Running
Wednesday	a.m.	Swimming
	p.m.	Cycling
Thursday	a.m.	Running
Friday	a.m.	Swimming
	p.m.	Resistance training
Saturday	a.m.	Brick session (cycling and running)
Sunday	a.m.	Running

Table 6.24 provides a sample program for a triathlete in the strength endurance block. This is a general preparatory phase of training, so higher volumes and lower overall intensities of resistance training are incorporated. Short rest intervals (1 min) are used to maximize the development of strength endurance. Because the volume of resistance training is substantial, the volume and intensity of the training sessions that target swimming, running, or cycling can be reduced.

As the athlete shifts into the basic strength block, the program continues to include two resistance training sessions per microcycle. Table 6.25 provides a sample program for a triathlete in the basic strength block. During this block, combination lifts are included, and the overall number of exercises is reduced. Additionally, the overall volume load of training is reduced and the intensity is increased in order to target the development of maximal strength. Because maximal strength is targeted, the rest interval is lengthened to a minimum of

Table 6.24   Sample Strength Endurance Mesocycle Block for a Triathlete

Day	Exercises	Target sets*		Intensity			
		Sets	Repetitions	Week 1	Week 2	Week 3	Week 4
Monday	Back squat	3	8	L	ML	M	VL
	Snatch-grip Romanian deadlift	3	8	L	ML	M	VL
	Seated single-leg calf raise	3	10	L	ML	M	VL
	Bent-over row	3	10	L	ML	M	VL
	Abdominal exercise	5	25				
Friday	Hang power clean	3	8	VL	L	ML	VL
	Split squat	3	8	VL	L	ML	VL
	Dumbbell bench press	3	8	VL	L	ML	VL
	Lat pulldown	3	10	VL	L	ML	VL
	Abdominal exercise	5	25				

*Two or three warm-up sets should be performed with each exercise. One-minute rest intervals can be used in this block.

2 minutes so that the athlete has adequate time to recover between sets and exercises. As the athlete shifts into this block of the resistance training program, the amount of time spent performing swimming, running, or cycling training is likely increased. One factor that must be considered during this time is the sequencing of the training sessions. If the resistance training is particularly difficult, the subsequent endurance session should be a recovery session or a session with a reduced training volume or intensity depending on the athlete's resistance and endurance training history.

After completing the basic strength block, the athlete shifts to a strength power block of resistance training. A sample program for this block is shown in table 6.26; this sample includes one training session per microcycle. In this block, athletes may use one or two resistance training sessions per microcycle; however, most athletes will use only one session per week because of the increased training time spent on the endurance activities. In this example, the rest interval is lengthened to 3 minutes to allow for additional recovery during the training session. Additionally, the number of exercises in each session and the volume load of training are reduced substantially. Volume load is reduced by decreasing the number of sets and repetitions performed during each training session. To ensure that the athlete continues to develop strength and power, the intensity of training is increased. The exercises selected are multijoint, large-mass exercises that provide a very efficient method for enhancing power-generating capacity.

Table 6.25 Sample Basic Strength Mesocycle Block for a Triathlete

Day	Exercises	Sets	Repetitions	Week 1	Week 2	Week 3	Week 4
			Target sets*		Intensity		
Monday	Back squat	3	3+3	ML	M	MH	L
	Split squat	3	5	ML	M	MH	L
	Hip flexion	3	5	ML	M	MH	L
	Lat pulldown	3	8	ML	M	MH	L
	Abdominal exercise	5	25				
Friday	Step-up	3	5	L	ML	M	VL
	Clean-grip Romanian deadlift	3	5	L	ML	M	VL
	Single-leg seated calf raise	3	8	L	ML	M	VL
	Lat pulldown	3	8	L	ML	M	VL
	Abdominal exercise	5	25				

*Two or three warm-up sets should be performed with each exercise. A minimum of two-minute rest intervals can be used in this block.

Table 6.26 Sample Strength Power Mesocycle Block for a Triathlete

Day	Exercises	Sets	Repetitions	Week 1	Week 2	Week 3	Week 4
			Target sets*		Intensity		
Monday	Hang power clean	3	3	M		H	
	¼ squat (from pins) plus vertical jump	3	3+3	M		H	
	Snatch-grip Romanian deadlift	3	3	M		H	
	Abdominal exercise	5	25				
Friday	Single-leg seated calf raise	3	3		MH		ML
	Speed squat	3	3		MH		ML
	Clean-grip Romanian deadlift	3	3		MH		ML
	Abdominal exercise	5	25				

*Two or three warm-up sets should be performed with each exercise. Three-minute rest intervals can be used in this block.

Finally, the triathlete can use a maintenance program. In this type of program, the athlete performs one training session per microcycle. The session would include a minimal number of exercises performed for a low number of sets and repetitions with relatively high intensities. As with the resistance training programs presented for running and cycling, the triathlete may want to remove resistance training from the training plan 8 to 14 days before a major competition. This enhances the pre-event taper by reducing fatigue and facilitating recovery of the legs. Endurance athletes often complain of having "heavy legs" when they are undertaking resistance training programs. Removing resistance training during the taper appears to eliminate this sensation and enables the athlete to feel prepared for competition.

Resistance Training Program for an Obstacle Course Race Athlete

When constructing a resistance training program for an obstacle course race (OCR) athlete, the coach needs to consider that these athletes are required to move their bodies over, around, and under obstacles, as well as hoist or carry heavy objects (40-150 lb [18-68 kg]). To address these demands, a wide array of multijoint training activities including body-weight exercises (e.g., pull-up, burpee, muscle-up), traditional resistance training exercises (e.g., back or front squat, single-leg squat, deadlift, shoulder press, barbell row), and weight-lifting movements (e.g., snatch, clean and jerk) and derivatives (e.g., power clean, power snatch, clean or snatch pull, push press, push jerk) serve as the key components of a comprehensive training program. Additionally, it may be warranted to incorporate exercises with weighted objects (e.g., sandbags, stones, tires) and unevenly loaded dumbbell or kettlebell exercises into the holistic training program.

When constructing the OCR athlete's resistance training program, the 15- to 20-minute warm-up can be designed to incorporate key dynamic body-weight movements such as lunging, step-overs, and single-leg movements (table 6.27). This warm-up uses combinations of stationary and movement-based activities that align with fundamental movements associated with the needs of the OCR athlete. Consider that the warm-up can be a period of the training session when motor literacy can be enhanced while preparing the athlete for the training session.

The coach should consider that a multitude of movement-based exercises can be integrated into the warm-up and that the exercises selected need to align with the athlete's level of development and needs as well as the demands of the training session.

The OCR athlete's resistance training program should be designed to align with the goals and objectives presented in the annual training plan and the peri-

Table 6.27 Sample Dynamic Warm-Up for an OCR Athlete's Resistance Training Session

Exercise	Repetitions
Body-weight squat	15
Speed skater lunge	16 (8 per side)
Lateral lunge	16 (8 per side)
Walking lunge with transverse rotation	16 (8 per side)
Plank with rotation kick-through	16 (8 per side)
Inchworm	16
Mountain climber	16
Lateral roll	16 (8 per side)
Crocodile crawl	16

ods and phases contained within the macrocycle. For example, in the general preparatory phase, the resistance training program contains a greater number of sessions, higher training volumes, and lower training loads to set the foundation for later stages of the annual training plan.

Table 6.28 provides an example of a strength endurance mesocycle for an OCR athlete. In this sample the athlete performs 3 sets of 10 repetitions for all major exercises, and a 3:1 loading structure is used across four microcycles. Each resistance training session in table 6.28 is structured to use a variety of multijoint, large-mass exercises that target movements that underpin key skills required by OCR athletes. More technical large-mass exercises (e.g., front squat plus press, front squat, hang power clean, hex bar deadlift) are placed earlier in each session, while fewer complex exercises are placed later in the session to ensure that the athlete is not fatigued when performing these technical exercises. Typically, a 2-minute rest interval is used during these sessions to allow for heavier loads to be lifted, but if a greater emphasis on endurance is required, the rest interval between each set and exercise can be reduced to 1 minute.

Once the strength endurance mesocycle is completed the training focus can be shifted toward basic strength (table 6.29) to allow the athlete to build the strength required for competition success. In the basic strength mesocycle the number of repetitions per set for the multijoint exercises drops from 10 to 5, and lifting intensity (percentage of 1RM) increases to allow the athlete to focus on maximizing strength development. A variety of multijoint exercises including weightlifting movements and their derivatives, as well as unilateral exercises and sport-specific body-weight exercises, are included. Overall, these types of exercises allow for the development of maximal strength with a variety of movement patterns.

Table 6.28 Sample Strength Endurance Mesocycle Block for an OCR Athlete

Day	Exercises	Target sets*		Intensity			
		Sets	Repetitions	Week 1	Week 2	Week 3	Week 4
Monday	Front squat plus press	3	8	ML	M	MH	L
	Front squat	3	8	ML	M	MH	L
	Weighted box step-over (kettlebell)	3	8	ML	M	MH	L
	Dumbbell bench press	3	8	ML	M	MH	L
	Pull-up (weighted)	3	8	ML	M	MH	L
	Toes to bar	3	12				
Wednesday	Dumbbell power clean plus press	3	8	ML	M	MH	L
	Hex bar deadlift	3	8	ML	M	MH	L.
	Single-leg squat	3	8	ML	M	MH	L
	Clean-grip Romanian deadlift	3	8	ML	M	MH	L
	Muscle-up	3	10	Body weight			
	Dip (weighted)	3	10	ML	M	MH	L
	Russian twist	3	16	Use load when appropriate			
Friday	Back squat and press	3	8	L	ML	M	ML
	Back squat	3	8	L	ML	M	ML
	Farmer's walk (kettlebell)	3	8	L	ML	M	ML
	Dumbbell incline bench press	3	8	L	ML	M	ML
	Pull-up (weighted)	3	10	ML	M	MH	L
	GHD sit-up	3	12	Use load when appropriate			
	Abdominal exercises	3	25				

*Two or three warm-up sets should be performed with each exercise. Two-minute rest intervals can be used in this block. GHD = glute-ham-developer.

Table 6.30 presents a sample program designed with an emphasis on strength power development. This block features a greater emphasis on dynamic exercises that are used to maximize power development as well as exercises that are used to further develop strength. The number of training days is reduced to 2 in order to decrease the overall volume load of training, and rest intervals between sets are increased to 3 minutes, which should help the athlete better manage fatigue and maximize both strength and power development.

Table 6.29 Sample Basic Strength Mesocycle Block for an OCR Athlete

Day	Exercises	Target sets*		Intensity			
		Sets	Repetitions	Week 1	Week 2	Week 3	Week 4
Monday	Hang power clean	3	5	M	MH	H	M
	Back squat	3	5	M	MH	H	M
	Single-leg squat	3	5	M	MH	H	M
	Muscle-up	3	10	Body weight			
	Toes to bar	4	10				
Wednesday	Clean-grip high pull	3	5	M	MH	H	M
	Deadlift	3	5	M	MH	H	M
	Clean-grip Romanian deadlift	3	5	M	MH	H	M
	Pull-up (weighted)	3	10	M	MH	H	M
	Dip (weighted)	3	10	M	MH	H	M
	GHD sit-up	4	10	Use load when appropriate			
Friday	Power clean	3	5	ML	M	MH	L
	Front squat	3	5	ML	M	MH	L
	Single-leg squat	3	5	ML	M	MH	L
	Muscle-up	3	10	Body weight			
	Russian twist	4	16	Use load when appropriate			

*Two or three warm-up sets should be performed with each exercise. Two-minute rest intervals can be used in this block. GHD = glute-ham-developer.

Table 6.30 Sample Strength Power Mesocycle Block for an OCR Athlete

Day	Exercises	Target sets*		Intensity			
		Sets	Repetitions	Week 1	Week 2	Week 3	Week 4
Tuesday	Power clean	3	3	MH	H	VH	M
	Quarter front squat plus box jump	3	3+3	MH	H	VH	M
	Clean high pull	3	3	MH	H	VH	M
	Muscle-up	3	10	Body weight			
	GHD sit-up	3	15	Use load when appropriate			
Thursday	Clean-grip jump shrug	3	3	M	MH	H	M
	Step-up drive-through plus split jump	3	3+3	M	MH	H	M
	Hex bar deadlift	3	3	M	MH	H	M
	Pull-up (weighted)	3	10	M	MH	H	M
	Toes to bar	3	15				

*Two or three warm-up sets should be performed with each exercise. Two-minute rest intervals can be used in this block. GHD = glute-ham-developer.

Warm-Up Methods and Techniques

Rachel Cosgrove

Before beginning a workout or race, athletes need to complete a warm-up to prepare the body for the activity, and, upon finishing, they should perform a cooldown to improve recovery. This chapter covers what to include for the most effective warm-up to ramp up to an effective training session and the most effective cooldown to ramp back down for best recovery. It is a good idea to use the same warm-up in training as what will be used on race or competition day, as supported by the adage of "Do nothing new on race day." The acronym *RAMP* has become a structure of warming up used by many coaches, first coined by Jeffreys (14), and it includes these four stages (see reference 14 for further detail):

R—Raise

A—Activation

M—Movement or Mobilize

P—Potentiate or Preparation

WARM-UP

The purpose of a warm-up is to increase the activation of muscles via the nervous system, increase blood flow to the working muscles, and increase core temperature while gradually ramping up the intensity of activity. This allows the athlete to be physiologically prepared, thereby improving performance and decreasing injury risk during the training session (6, 27, 39).

The total time of the warm-up may be as short as 10 minutes and as long as 30 minutes. Typically, the higher the intensity of the scheduled activity, the longer the warm-up should be. An active warm-up has been shown to improve performance as long as the athlete does not end up too fatigued (5).

Included in the warm-up are four components:

1. Self-myofascial release using a foam roller, massage ball, or other tool to improve tissue quality (4, 7, 10, 15, 16, 32, 37).
2. Flexibility and dynamic stretching including movements to improve and work each joint in a full range of motion (1, 13, 18, 25).
3. Activation exercises to activate the muscles that need to "fire" during the training session (8, 28).
4. Movement preparation exercises including low-intensity aerobic work that is specific to the workout scheduled, progressing into higher-intensity exercises to promote quicker neural recruitment of muscles to be ready to go (40). Performing a sport-specific warm-up after stretching restores any negative effects of static stretching to get the athlete ready to go (6, 33, 38).

For example, before a running workout, an athlete may begin the warm-up with some myofascial release such as foam rolling of the calves, then a hip flexor dynamic stretch followed by a glute-activation exercise to get the posterior chain musculature activated and ready to work. The athlete then could progress into single-leg hops and eventually some running technique drills. Each of the above four categories are explained in more detail here.

Myofascial Release

Myofascial release gives specific attention to muscle tightness or trigger points (knots) in fascial (connective) and muscle tissue. Common tools for myofascial release therapy include the following:

▶ Foam roller
▶ Massage ball, tennis ball, or lacrosse ball
▶ Massage percussion gun
▶ Other tools (e.g., massage stick, vibrating roller, cold roller)

For 5 to 10 minutes, roll out or massage all of the following, or pick two or three areas that feel especially tight. Simply roll the area on the foam roller, use the ball to place pressure on a trigger point or knot, or run the massage device over the area. These are common locations:

▶ Bottom of the feet
▶ Calves
▶ Anterior tibialis (shins)
▶ Quadriceps
▶ Hamstrings
▶ Hip flexors

- Gluteus maximus
- Tensor fascia latae
- Latissimus dorsi
- Thoracic spine (upper back)

Flexibility and Dynamic Stretching

Depending on which activity an athlete is warming up for, he or she should consider what muscles usually become short or tight during the activity. Incorporating stretches and dynamic flexibility to undo some of the shortness and tightness ensures the body is in an optimal state to perform. The following are common questions:

- *Can an athlete be too flexible?* Consider the relationship between muscle length and strength. When working with a very flexible athlete, the most important focus is to ensure that the joint or joints are controlled through the entire movement range. The problem is not too much flexibility; it is too little strength in relation to an athlete's flexibility in the full range of motion.

- *What is the limiting component?* Think outside of the box when troubleshooting flexibility. Lack of range in the hamstrings is often a result of an anterior rotated pelvis (extremely common in triathletes who are constantly shortening their hip flexors), which places too much tension on the hamstrings (20, 22). Therefore, they are already under maximum tension and will not extend further. Tight hamstrings might be corrected with an effective stretch of the hip flexors to realign the pelvic girdle to a neutral position and allow the hamstrings to extend.

- *Is it a neurological or an actual joint limitation?* Structural soft tissue limitations of the joint (e.g., an actual shortness of the muscle) may benefit from static stretching, but neurological limitations need a reeducation of the nervous system (e.g., via some form of proprioceptive neuromuscular facilitation [PNF] stretching).

The following are considerations for the three most common endurance activities: running, cycling, and swimming.

Flexibility for Running

- Chronically tight hip flexors create an anterior pelvic tilt, which can lead to hamstring pulls, low back pain, and knee pain, along with less active gluteal muscles, causing iliotibial band injuries (11). The pelvis can be likened to a bucket full of water. An anterior pelvic tilt will cause the water to spill out the front. In other words, the muscles in the front of the pelvis have shortened. By default, the muscles in the back of the pelvis, mainly the hamstrings, get pulled longer than normal, creating taut hamstrings. A chronically shortened muscle cannot function optimally, and a chronically lengthened muscle is weaker than normal. *Warm-up recommendation:* Include a hip flexor stretch and a drill for posterior chain activation.

▶ Shortened gastrocnemius muscles lead to decreased ankle range of motion from landing step after step with the weight on the front of the foot. Shortened gastrocnemius muscles can potentiate plantar fasciitis and Achilles problems along with other compensatory issues proximally in the kinetic chain (31). *Warm-up recommendation:* Include ankle mobility dynamic stretches along with myofascial release (26).

Flexibility for Cycling

Chronically tight hip flexors are common from the repetitive motion of cycling. If the hip flexors are tight, the knees will start to flare out, resulting in inefficient cycle mechanics and possible injury. In addition to the hip flexor recommendation just discussed, hip internal and external rotation stretches and activating the gluteal muscles are recommended (35). *Warm-up recommendation:* Include a hip flexor stretch, gluteal stretch, and internal and external activation or range-of-motion exercises to create greater hip mobility.

Flexibility for Swimming

Common issues include shortened lats and pecs, contributing to rotator cuff impingement (36). *Warm-up recommendation:* Include foam rolling or massage of the lats and pecs along with upper-body stretches to create greater shoulder mobility and expansion of the chest. Regardless of what method is used to improve flexibility, follow these guidelines when performing flexibility and dynamic stretching:

▶ *Vary the exercises.* In addition to changing the order of the stretches and the types of stretches, the angle of pull for each stretch should be changed. For example, the hamstrings can be statically stretched in several ways: lying supine with the leg straight, with or without the calf being stretched also via ankle dorsiflexion. The leg can be positioned straight up or taken across the midline of the body toward the opposite side, or taken away from the midline of the body on the same side. The foot can be positioned inverted or everted during the stretch. In total, there are two calf positions, times three leg positions, times two foot positions, for a total of 12 variations of a supine hamstrings stretch alone. Each variation elicits subtle differences in the way muscle fibers are stretched. As a general rule, a tight muscle will inhibit the stretch of all other muscles in the surrounding areas. It is a good idea to work on the most limited areas first in the workout.

▶ *Stretch from the hips outward.* The sequence of stretching can dramatically improve results. Stretching the hip flexors and psoas muscles reduces anterior pull on the hips. This in turn improves hamstring range of motion by reducing the tension on the hamstring. This idea saves time and improves results, so always begin with the hip area and work outward.

▶ *Stretch for the proper length of time.* Stretching is perhaps the only training activity where more is better. Static stretches can be held for 2 to 3 minutes. Increase the stretch or change the orientation of the limb slightly every 30 seconds or so. Research has shown a protocol of at least 5 days a week for at least 5 minutes is beneficial in promoting range of motion (34).

Include flexibility as part of a regular routine for endurance athletes. With the repetitive motion done in training, flexibility has to be a priority to keep from getting injured and for muscles to function optimally.

Stretching Techniques

Three types of stretching methods can be used regularly. There are several others, although they have a more limited usage. It is important to keep in mind that stretching can affect the nervous system in addition to the muscle tissue. Stretching can result in neural inhibition, a process where neural activity patterns are suppressed, blocked, or restricted (2). This can help increase the range of motion of a joint.

▶ *Static stretching.* Recently, a growing body of research has reported that static stretching before activity may cause a decrease in power production (12, 24). This decrease in power production could be important in short-distance, high-intensity endurance events or for athletes striving to maximize performance at a very high level. It could also be detrimental for activities of varying intensities, such as a cycling criterium, which requires intermittent periods of high-intensity exercise. Researchers are still exploring the effects of static stretching on performance (3). In the meantime, because these studies are not complete, it is not surprising that muscles express greater force deficits immediately after static stretching, given that the purpose of static stretching is to relax muscles (12, 24). If the athlete needs to develop flexibility, it is usually a higher priority than improving strength with an already limited range. Thus, even if static stretching does make the athlete weaker, for most athletes it is worth the trade-off and may improve performance (19). If a person has a structural limitation (e.g., a physical shortness in the muscle), static stretching is hugely beneficial. After performing static stretching as part of the warm-up, some general and sport-specific movements are indicated to reactivate the muscles from a relaxed state. Following a workout, static stretching may help relieve muscle soreness, promote relaxation, and increase flexibility. In these instances, static stretching primarily should involve major muscle groups, especially those that are least flexible or those that work in a limited range of motion during training or competition. The bottom line is that static stretching is important for endurance athletes and should make up the bulk of their stretching time.

▶ *PNF stretching.* PNF stretching can be done following two methods. An example of the *simple contract-relax* method is stretching the hamstrings by pressing the heel into the floor and isometrically contracting the hamstrings for 5 to 10 seconds. This will override the body's stretch reflex and allow the hamstrings to attain a greater stretch. The second method is *agonist-contract relax, antagonist contract* (ACRAC). Similar to the first method, this involves an active contraction of the antagonists, prior to going into a deeper stretch. Based on *reciprocal inhibition*, when an agonist contracts, the antagonist relaxes and allows for greater range of motion (29).

▶ *Dynamic stretching.* Endurance sports are dynamic activities. Muscles contract concentrically and eccentrically, moving the joints of the body through specific motions. Most of the movements used in endurance activities do not require the full range of motion of the joints. Many athletes, especially as they increase their training volumes, find that some joint motions increase while others decrease because of changes in muscle flexibility. Aging has also been linked to decreases in muscle flexibility.

Traditionally, athletes have performed static stretching to improve muscle flexibility. Recent research has suggested that at least some of the work used to increase muscle flexibility should involve dynamic flexibility. Dynamic flexibility exercises are activities that use sport-specific movements to take the joints through a complete range of motion. This is essentially a form of pendulum-swinging the limbs, torso, and so on (e.g., high leg raises), beginning gradually and increasing range with each repetition. This is not ballistic stretching; the athlete is not using momentum. These sport-specific movements are performed under control and are meant to increase the range of motion of the joints. Before training or competition, a runner who includes dynamic flexibility as part of the warm-up might perform dynamic stretching activities such as walking lunges (for the hip extensors) and walking diagonal lunges (for the abductors). Range of motion and flexibility are more than just muscle length and tension issues. The nervous system is a huge component as well. As mentioned earlier, *neural inhibition* refers to a process where neural activity patterns are suppressed, blocked, or restricted (2).

Activation Exercises

After performing myofascial release and then spending time improving flexibility and range of motion using static stretching, dynamic stretching, PNF stretching, or nervous system stretching, the body is ready to ramp up to train by activating the muscles that will be used. The order of the activities that are part of a warm-up can affect performance; ideally, an athlete should activate the muscles after doing self-myofascial release or static stretching (30). For any endurance athlete the posterior chain, specifically the gluteal muscles and hamstrings, is a key area to activate. Because most people sit a lot, it is common for the gluteal muscles and hamstrings to be neurally inhibited, which leads many endurance athletes to have anterior chain–dominant running or cycling technique (e.g., running that is more like stomping instead of pulling the ground, or cycling by pedaling behind using the posterior chain). By warming up with a movement that activates the posterior chain along with technique drills to focus on form during these activities the gluteal muscles and hamstrings will play a bigger role during movement, making the athlete's movement more efficient.

Movement Preparation Exercises

Finishing the warm-up with activities that continue to increase blood flow, increase neural activation, and start moving specifically for the activity about to happen in training will increase the intensity, heart rate, and body temperature.

Endurance athletes tend to focus on sagittal plane movements, but it is critical to perform movements in all three planes of motion. Movements are noted below in the sagittal plane (e.g., forward and back marching), along with movements in the transverse plane (e.g., lunge walk with a twist or hip rotations) and frontal plane (e.g., wall stretch). Moving the body in a full range of motion in every plane is strongly encouraged during a warm-up to get the body ready.

Movement preparation can include hopping, shuffles, running drills, cycling drills performing single-leg rotations, and can progress into short-sprint, higher-intensity intervals practicing acceleration and deceleration.

SAMPLE WARM-UP ROUTINE

The following is an example of a complete warm-up routine.

1. Self-Myofascial Release

2. Flexibility and Dynamic Stretching

Side quadriceps stretch

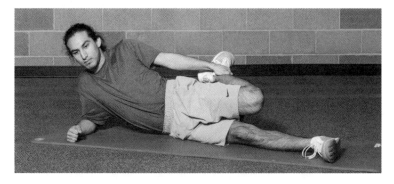

Inverted hamstring stretch

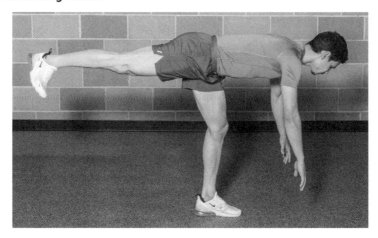

Elbow to instep walk

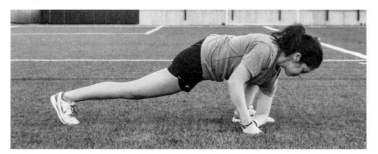

Wall stretch

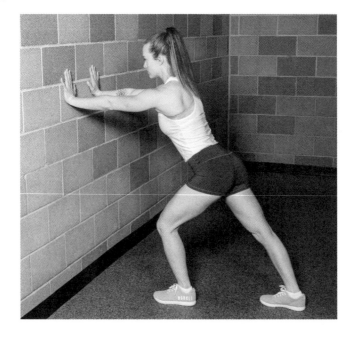

3. Activation Exercises

Stationary and traveling inchworm

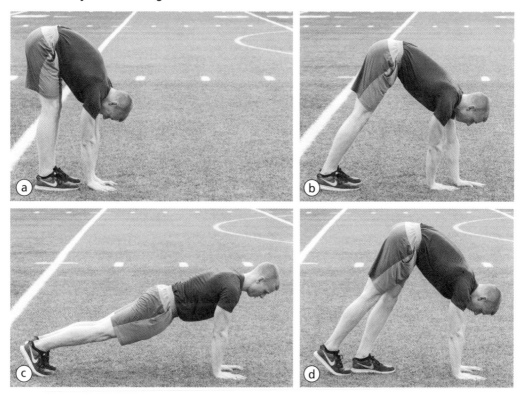

Standing hip external rotation/circumduction

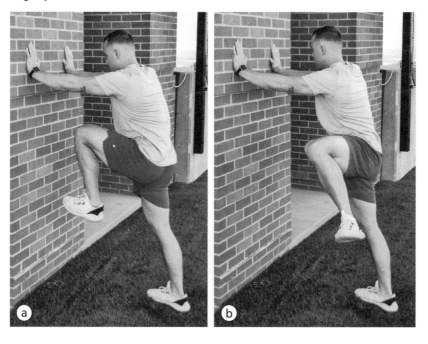

Standing hip internal rotation/circumduction

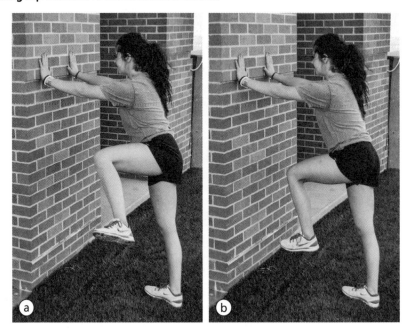

Stationary arm warm-up

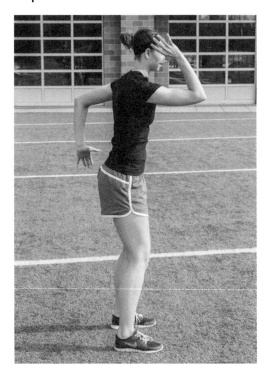

Lateral lunge squat and walk

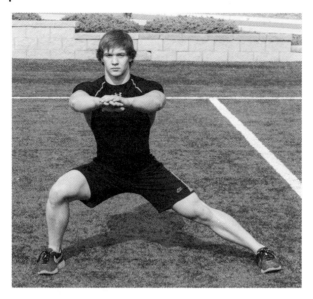

Lunge walk with a twist

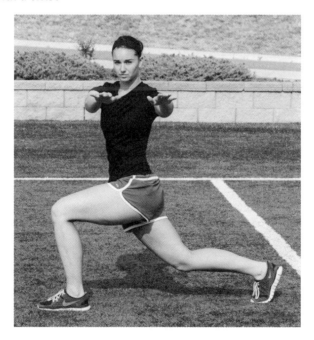

4. Movement Preparation Exercises

Walking high-knee pull

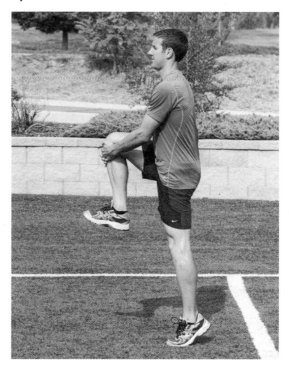

Hop and stick

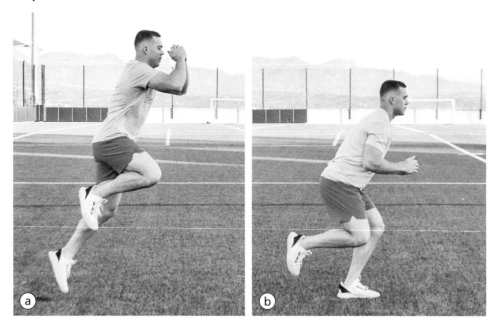

Power skip

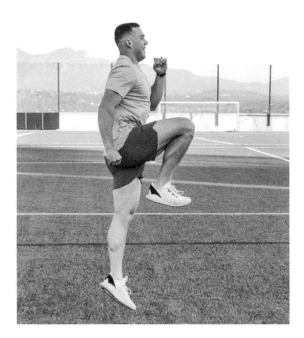

Linear acceleration to deceleration

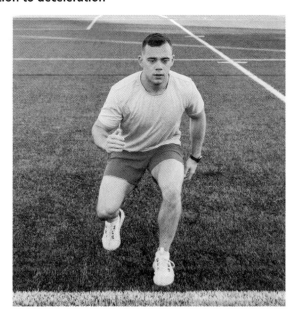

Backward run to deceleration

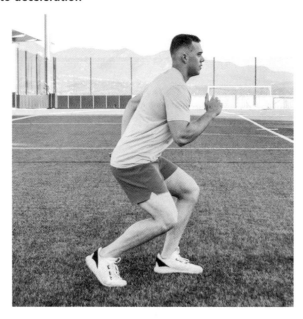

COOLDOWN

Following the training session, performing a cooldown enables the athlete to progress back to a resting state (17, 23). The increased blood flow to the working muscles that occurs during activity is slowly redistributed back to the core of the body. The exercise intensity gradually decreases as the cooldown progresses from sport-specific activity to more general movements. This gradual decrease in intensity allows heart rate and body temperature to begin to return to normal. Perform an activity to bring the heart rate down by essentially reversing the warm-up protocol to finish with static stretching, myofascial release (21), and massage (9).

The total time of a cooldown may be as short as 10 minutes or as long as 30 minutes. Similar to the warm-up, higher-intensity workouts will require a longer cooldown. Activities that last longer will also require a longer cooldown.

Running

Richard C. Blagrove

Endurance running is one of the most popular sports and recreational activities in the world. Over the past decade, participation in endurance running races has increased by more than 50% (3), and finishers in ultraendurance trail running events (>6 hr) have increased exponentially over the last 20 years (85). Success in long-distance (5 km to marathon) and ultraendurance running events is primarily determined by physiological factors, specifically *maximal oxygen uptake* or $\dot{V}O_2max$ (the maximum rate the body can use oxygen during exercise), the fraction of $\dot{V}O_2max$ that can be sustained for the duration of the event, and *running economy* (the energy it takes to run at a submaximal intensity) (52, 69, 72). The middle-distance track events (800 m to 3,000 m) are also heavily reliant on well-developed aerobic factors (12, 47), which is reflected in a bias toward endurance-oriented running sessions for much of the training macrocycle (38, 92). The aim of this chapter is to describe the principles associated with effective training for an endurance runner, covering distances from 800 meters to ultraendurance events. The chapter also provides recommendations for training and event preparation best practice, as well as important behaviors for injury prevention.

TRAINING FOR RUNNING EVENTS

Despite an abundance of scientific research and coaching literature devoted to training for endurance running events, optimal prescription remains as much of an art as it is a science. Training prescription that avoids episodes of injury, illness, and overtraining while maximizing a runner's performance potential within a given time frame depends on a multitude of factors relating to the individual and his or her goals and constraints.

Intuitively, the most specific and relevant type of training to prepare for a given event is training at target event speed for close to the event distance or duration. This approach certainly produces adaptations that are specific to the demands of

The author would like to acknowledge the significant contribution of Suzie Snyder to this chapter.

the event; however, improvements tend to be short lived, performance plateaus quickly, and the risk of staleness and overtraining with this method is high (70). Beyond the phase of training that falls closest to a target event (i.e., 4-8 weeks prior), there should be far less concern with ensuring high specificity with a training approach. Instead, planning training in a manner that provides an appropriate stimulus to develop the various physiological factors that underpin the target event is a more sensible approach. Periodizing training in this manner using a progressive, logical, and sequential strategy will maximize performance long term and reduce the risk of negative health outcomes (54). Examples of training for different event groups (middle-distance, long-distance, marathon, and ultraendurance) using this approach are provided in later sections.

Intensity Domains of Running

A runner's performance over a given distance can be described using the speed–duration relationship (figure 8.1), which is governed by the physiological processes that maintain energy provision and cause fatigue. Although debate exists around the shape of this relationship when brief and very long distances are included (hyperbolic vs. power-law) (27, 36), it appears that the asymptote of the hyperbolic relationship that exists when middle- and long-distance running durations are taken into account defines an important physiological threshold known as *critical speed* (81). Critical speed represents the boundary between the heavy and severe exercise intensity domains above which $\dot{V}O_2$max is eventually reached if exercise continues (severe domain), and below which a metabolic steady state can be achieved whereby exercise can continue for a prolonged time (heavy domain). The mechanisms of fatigue, and consequently the physiological adaptations, associated with training in the heavy versus the severe domain differ considerably (93, 94), which helps inform training prescription for specific events. Critical speed can be estimated mathematically if four recent maximal efforts over any distances completed within 3 and 30 minutes are known. Free online calculators (e.g., https://em-sportscience.com/critical-power-calculator) are available to enable runners to identify their critical speed. In practical terms, critical speed can be maintained for 30 and 40 minutes in well-trained runners (81), which approximates 10-kilometer pace.

Although $\dot{V}O_2$max and volitional exhaustion are always reached during exercise above critical speed, higher intensities of exercise, above speed at $\dot{V}O_2$max, are too brief (i.e., <5 min) to elicit $\dot{V}O_2$max (96). The intensity domain above the maximal speed at which $\dot{V}O_2$max is reached is termed the *extreme domain* (18). Energy in this domain is derived largely from anaerobic sources, and therefore training sessions here are highly suitable for developing middle-distance running performance. To estimate maximal speed at $\dot{V}O_2$max, runners can complete a 5-minute time trial on flat even ground, record the distance they run, and calculate their average speed over the distance (10).

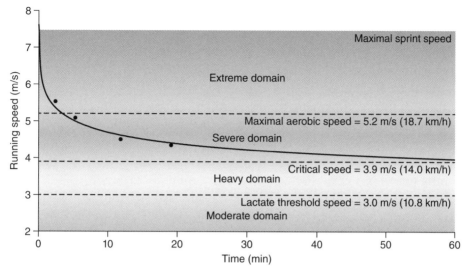

Figure 8.1 An example of a speed-duration relationship based upon four time-trial performances (800 m, 1 mile, 2 miles, 5 km) to identify the critical speed (*second threshold*). Lactate threshold speed (*first threshold*), maximal aerobic speed (fastest speed at maximal oxygen uptake), and maximal sprint speed are also plotted. Using these physiological thresholds, four intensity domains can be identified to be used for training prescription. Causes of fatigue and physiological adaptations differ within each intensity domain and there is overlap between the domains, as illustrated with the blurred bands.

Below critical speed, a steady state of running can be achieved; however, another important threshold exists that separates heavy-intensity exercise from moderate-intensity running (see figure 8.1). In laboratory settings this first threshold is classically denoted first by a rise in blood lactate from resting or baseline levels as speed of running increases, known as the *lactate threshold* *(LT)* (51). In general, this intensity of running approximates marathon pace for a moderately trained runner; however, well-trained runners can operate just above this first threshold for approximately 150 minutes. Again, the physiological limits to performance and mechanisms of fatigue above and below the LT differ considerably; therefore, the adaptations and aerobic factors that training within these domains develops are also quite different (18). The LT corresponds approximately to the first ventilatory threshold, so identifying the separation between the heavy and the moderate domains can be achieved practically with the talk test. If a runner can hold a normal conversation (as they would do at rest) without gasping for air, they can safely say they are operating in the moderate-intensity domain below their lactate or ventilatory threshold.

In training terms, these important physiological thresholds and resultant intensity domains serve as approximate training zones where different types of running sessions can be prescribed to target different aerobic qualities (table 8.1). The three thresholds discussed should not be viewed as switches or borders, whereby a subtle increase in speed moves a runner from one domain instantly into another, but rather represent a phase transition between each intensity domain (80). This is illustrated by the colored shading shown in figure 8.1 with the domain boundaries blurring into one another. Based on this understanding it is prudent for runners to be clear what pace, rating of perceived exertion (RPE; 1-10) (62), and percentage of maximal heart rate (HRmax) they should be running at within each session or repetition based on the desire to develop a specific physiological quality (table 8.1). In a strict physiology sense, only two thresholds have validity and high reproducibility; therefore, a three-zone training model has greatest credibility for training prescription (18, 90). However, the 5-zone and 7-zone models have been used by running coaches and online training guides, so for comparative purposes, these are also shown in table 8.1. Endurance running coaches, running magazines, and online self-help guides tend to use nonscientific terminology to describe the intensity or level of effort that should be elicited for different types of running sessions. The most common training terms along with approximate race paces are also shown for each intensity domain (table 8.1).

Volume of Running

The volume of training that runners perform overall and within each of the training intensity domains should also be individualized. This individualization should consider the event the runner is preparing for; the training phase; the runner's training background, injury history, and lifestyle constraints; and whether the runner tends to respond to a volume- or intensity-driven training approach. Table 8.2 provides an approximate guide for individualizing weekly running volume in preparatory phases based on event category and training or competitive status. Although these volumes are not necessarily targets that runners should aim to reach, they represent typical weekly mileage that runners and coaches report in scientific research studies and practice (24, 25, 38, 39, 50, 54, 68, 92).

There is considerable debate over the optimal means of distributing running training volume across the intensity domains (17, 31). At an elite level, particularly among long-distance and marathon runners, the distribution of training volume across the intensity domains tends to follow a pyramidal design during preparatory periods. That is, approximately 80% of running volume is performed in the moderate domain at easy conversational paces, approximately 15% is run in the heavy domain, and approximately 5% is run in the severe or extreme domain. It is important to recognize that this approach to training may not be suitable for subelite and recreational runners who are unlikely to have reached their genetic ceiling of $\dot{V}O_2$max and run far less overall mileage than highly trained athletes. Therefore, by replicating these proportions of running mileage in recreational and moderately trained runners, the time spent in the

Table 8.1 Physiological and Exercise Characteristics, Training Terminology, and Example Training Prescription for Each Training Intensity Domain

Intensity domain		Moderate		Heavy		Severe			Extreme	
Approximate race pace		Ultraendurance		Marathon	Half marathon	10 km (6.2 mi)	3,000 m (3 km; 1.8 mi)		1,500 m	Maximal
Sustainable duration		>3 hours		~150 min	~60 min	~30 min	~7 min		<5 min	
Equivalent zone models	3-zone	1		2		3				
	5-zone	1	2	3	4	5				
	7-zone	1	2	3	4	5		6	7	
Approx. %HRmax		55%-70%		70%-80%	80%-85%	85%-100%			—	
RPE	(1-10)	1-2	3-4	5	6	7	8	9	10	
	Descriptors	Easy	Moderate	Hard		Very hard	Extremely hard	Nearly maximal	Maximal	
Common training terminology		Warm-up Long slow distance Recovery run		Tempo Steady	Threshold	VO$_2$max Extensive intervals			Intensive intervals Strides, speed, sprints	
Jack Daniels' terminology		Easy		Marathon	Tempo	Intervals			Repetitions	
Main physiological qualities developed		Lactate threshold Running economy		Critical speed Lactate threshold		VO$_2$max Critical speed			Neuromuscular factors Anaerobic capacity	
Interval training	Number of sets	—		1-4		3-8			3-12	
	Repetition duration	—		8-20 min		2-6 min			10-150 sec	
	Work:rest ratio	—		4:1 to 5:1		1:1 to 2:1			1:1 to 1:6	
Example session(s)		30-120+ min at conversational pace		30-60 min hard 4 × 10 min (2 min rec)		6 × 3 min (90 sec rec) 8 × 2 min (60 sec rec)			8 × 30 sec (3 min rec) 4 × 60 sec (6 min rec)	

Note: %HRmax = percentage of maximum heart rate; RPE = rating of perceived exertion (1 = very easy, 10 = maximal); rec = recovery; VO$_2$max = maximal oxygen uptake.

heavy and severe domains, which is known to be a potent stimulus for VO$_2$max improvement (78), is substantially reduced.

It is generally recognized among experienced endurance coaches that the risk of injury and overtraining are increased if more than two hard (severe and extreme intensity domains) interval sessions are scheduled each week. It therefore seems sensible to base weekly training design around these two

Table 8.2 Approximate Weekly Running Volumes During Preparatory Phases for Middle-Distance, Long-Distance, and Marathon and Ultraendurance Runners of Different Training and Competitive Status

Training and competitive status (running history)	Recreational or young runner (0-6 yr)	Moderately trained runner (>2 yr)	Well-trained runner (>3 yr)	Highly trained or elite runner (>6 yr)
Middle distance (800 m to 3 km)	<30 miles (<48 km)	30-45 miles (48-72 km)	45-60 miles (80-96 km)	>60 miles (>96 km)
Long distance (5 km to half marathon)	<40 miles (<64 km)	40-65 miles (64-105 km)	65-90 miles (105-145 km)	>90 miles (>145 km)
Marathon and ultraendurance	<40 miles (<64 km)	40-70 miles (64-113 km)	70-100 miles (113-161 km)	>100 miles (>161 km)

taxing sessions, separated by 2 to 4 days, and build as much moderate-domain easy running around these workouts as possible. For middle-distance runners, additional sessions of strides and short-sprint (80-200 m) repetition sessions should also be included at the expense of long slow distance running (84). For the long-distance runner, in addition to these hard sessions, as training progresses during off-season preparatory phases, nonexhausting tempo runs and long interval sessions in the heavy-intensity domain also can be used sparingly and in a controlled manner.

RESISTANCE TRAINING AND CONDITIONING FOR RUNNERS

Endurance running performance is limited principally by physiological factors related to how effectively oxygen is delivered to working muscles to break down substrates into energy for movement. These largely cardiovascular and metabolic processes, which are developed via consistent prolonged aerobic-based running training, have been the focus of this chapter so far. It therefore seems counterintuitive that an endurance runner would invest valuable training time in high-intensity anaerobic exercise such as resistance training.

The ability of the body to convert metabolic energy from muscles into mechanical movement (i.e., sustained running) is known as *exercise economy*. Endurance runners with exceptional running economy at submaximal speeds have the capability to use less energy to run a given distance compared to their counterparts (2, 22). Whereas $\dot{V}O_2$max is primarily limited by the cardiovascular system, running economy is influenced by a wider range of physiological systems and environmental factors (5), including neuromuscular capabilities (6). This is because the rate at which muscles use energy when running depends on the type of muscle fibers that are being activated, the velocity at which muscles are shortening, and the extent to which they change their length (29). Furthermore, if runners can minimize the amount of work that muscles perform during running, by training tendons to store and release more energy, even greater energy savings can be made.

These neuromuscular contributions to running economy are modifiable with resistance training activities, heavy and explosive resistance training, and plyometrics (11). Specifically, several months of resistance training (2-3 days per week) has been shown to improve running economy by approximately 4% (26), which appears to confer an improvement in endurance running performance and maximal sprint speed (11). Positive changes in running economy and time trial performance have been reported in both sexes and across age groups (11), including young runners (13), suggesting that all endurance runners can benefit from incorporating resistance training into their programs. Importantly for endurance runners, there is little evidence that resistance training causes an increase in muscle or body mass over this time period (11).

Resistance training may also be beneficial for reducing the risk of overuse injury (60). Several prospective investigations have noted that muscular weakness, particularly in muscles around the hips (gluteals), is associated with a higher risk of overuse injury in runners (8, 63, 64). During the stance phase of running, musculoskeletal structures in the lower limb are required to manage high forces (2-9 × body weight depending on muscle or structure). Thus, poor integrity in these tissues as well as an inability to maintain appropriate biomechanical positions under fatigue will place increased strain on musculoskeletal structures, eventually leading to injury. To date, studies that have used a multicomponent approach to strength and conditioning (resistance training, low-intensity plyometrics and running drills, proprioception work, trunk exercises) with endurance runners have tended to show the most positive outcomes for injury incidence (37, 71).

Resistance Training for Runners

Table 8.3 provides an example of a resistance training session that is suitable for a middle- or long-distance runner, including exercise progressions that can be used in subsequent mesocycles. Resistance training sessions should be preceded by a warm-up that includes a range of dynamic fundamental movements (from simple to more complex) that take joints through a full range of motion (e.g., high knee pull, leg swings, lateral and forward lunges, inchworm, squat). Resistance training exercise selection should focus on developing lower-limb maximal strength and structural robustness (using bilateral exercises) and single-leg strength and control (using unilateral exercises). Specific loading for areas vulnerable to injury (e.g., calf–Achilles complex, trunk) should also be

Table 8.3 Example of a Basic Resistance Training Session for an Endurance Runner

Exercise	Progression*	Sets	Repetitions or time	Interset recovery (min)
Goblet squat	Back squat	3	8	2-3
Box jump	Single-leg box jump	3	5	2-3
Barbell step-up	High box step-up	3	6 each leg	2-3
Split squat	Reverse lunge	3	6 each leg	2-3
Push-up	Dumbbell bench press	3	12	2-3
Single-leg calf raise	Calf press hold	3	12	2
Side plank	Single-arm farmer's walk	3	30-45 sec	1

*To be used in future mesocycles of training.

included. Loading on each exercise depends on the runner's level of experience with resistance training. It is recommended that runners do not work to repetition failure on each set but instead choose a load that allows 2 or 3 repetitions in reserve at the end of the prescribed repetitions, or around 7 to 8 out of 10 on an RPE scale (61).

Plyometric Training for Runners

Plyometric exercises, such as hopping, skipping, and bounding, possess high levels of biomechanical similarity to running. Compared to running, plyometrics exercises involve controlling larger amounts of force in shorter amounts of time, making them ideal for developing explosive power capabilities in athletes. Furthermore, higher forces are associated with a greater potential for energy storage in tendons during lengthening of the muscle–tendon unit. Therefore, plyometrics develops a runner's ability to store and return elastic strain energy, which contributes to improvements in running economy and speed (1).

The high magnitude and rates of force application during plyometrics raise the risk of damage to musculoskeletal structures, potentially causing injury if managed inappropriately. Although plyometrics is considered safe and effective, even for novice (35) and young runners (14), it is advised that runners embarking on plyometrics for the first time initially include a small amount (30-50 foot contacts per session) of low-intensity plyometrics (e.g., skips, short range hops, running drills) on two or three occasions per week (11). As runners becomes stronger and more accustomed to plyometrics they should aim to progress to 50 to 80 foot contacts per session and then 80 to 100 foot contacts. Highly trained endurance runners with several years of experience with resistance training may dedicate whole sessions every week to running drills and high-intensity plyometrics with 120-plus foot contacts per session.

Following are examples of low-intensity plyometrics exercises and running drills that progress toward sprinting (see table 8.4). These short plyometrics training units can be incorporated easily into a warm-up before a running or resistance training session. Running drills that place focus on short ground contact times and explosive actions also have the advantage of reinforcing important movement patterns and postures associated with high-speed running. It is best to perform these drills on firm dry grass, rubber matting, or a sprung wooden floor in normal running shoes.

Table 8.4 Plyometric Training Drills for Runners

Drill	Page number
High-Knee Skip	193
B-Skip	194
Straight-Leg Skip	194
Lateral and Backward Skip	195
Power Skip	195
Forward and Backward Line Hop	195
Lateral Line Hop	196
Scissors	196
Lateral Line Hop (Traveling Forward and Backward)	197
High-Knee Run	197
Bounding	198

High-Knee Skip

The runner skips forward normally while emphasizing the use of high knees. The runner should lean forward very slightly and focus on punching the thighs up until the thigh breaks parallel with the ground, and then backward so the foot strikes below or fractionally in front of the hips. The mid- or forefoot strikes the ground, and the runner focuses on a fast ground contact. Toes should be pulled upward, pointing toward the shins, while the foot is off the ground. The drill also helps runners learn to drive their arms explosively and to minimize the vertical motion of the body. Perform 8 to 12 repetitions per leg or over a 10-yard (9.1 m) distance.

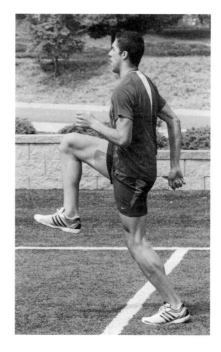

B-Skip

Like the high-knee skip, the runner drives the thigh up aggressively, but instead of the lower leg moving up and down, the drill requires the runner to extend the leg in front of the body immediately after the knee drive phase. In a circular pawing motion, the athlete whips the leg back down to the ground, planting on the ball of the foot under or slightly ahead of the hips. This drill helps runners develop power from hip extension and increases the angular velocity of the foot as it strikes the ground to increase contribution from the gluteal and hamstring muscles. Perform 8 to 12 repetitions per leg or over a 10-yard (9.1 m) distance.

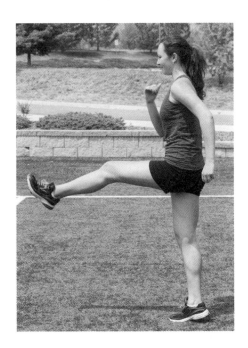

Straight-Leg Skip

The runner skips forward normally but keeps the knees relatively straight, pulling forward and backward only from the hip. The runner should aim to kick the leg up and pull it back down quickly, so the mid- or forefoot strikes beneath or slightly in front of the hips. Toes should be pulled upward pointing toward the shins while the foot is off the ground. The drill develops a runner's hip extension (gluteal and hamstring) contribution to the running stride. Perform 8 to 12 repetitions per leg or over a 10-yard (9.1 m) distance.

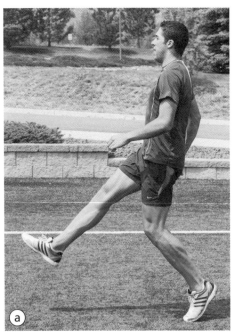

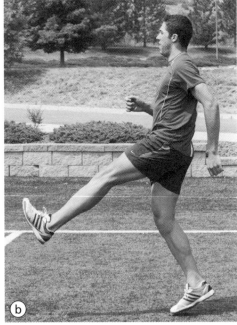

a b

Lateral and Backward Skip

The three types of skips previously outlined can all be performed in a lateral direction (traveling left and traveling right) and also backward. Changing the direction of skips recruits muscles around the hip slightly differently and challenges the athlete's control and stability. As a further progression, these skips can be performed barefoot. This adds greater stress to structures around the foot and ankle but, in small dosages, is an effective way to strengthen this vulnerable area in runners. Perform 8 to 12 repetitions per leg or over a 10-yard (9.1 m) distance of each type and direction of drill.

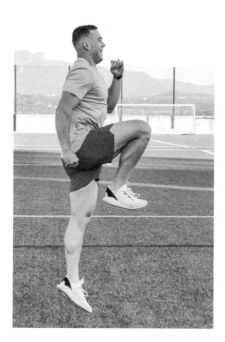

Power Skip

As a progression from the previously described skips, a runner also can use a power skip. To power skip, the runner drives the free knee upward as aggressively as possible and simultaneously uses an aggressive arm action to create an exaggerated skip with more vertical displacement. Toes should be pulled upward toward the shins while the foot is off the ground. The athlete should try to skip as high and as far as possible on each jump or stride, and perform 8 to 12 repetitions per leg or over a 20-yard (18.3 m) distance.

Forward and Backward Line Hop

The runner stands just in front of a line (could be imaginary) and then hops back and forth over the line with the feet together for 8 to 12 repetitions. After the athlete lands for each hop, she should immediately push off again (short ground contact) and hop to the other side of the line without any extra hops or bounces. This exercise can also be progressed to being performed on one leg and then the other.

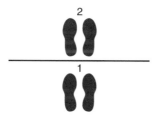

Lateral Line Hop

The runner stands perpendicular to a line and then hops side to side over it for 8 to 12 repetitions. The athlete should aim to spend as little time on the ground as possible while also bouncing with height. This exercise can be performed on one leg as a progression.

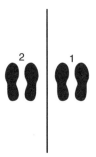

Scissors

The athlete stands in front of a line and then steps across with the right foot, straddling the line with the left foot behind it. The runner jumps up off both feet and shifts the feet rapidly, moving each foot to the opposite side of the line. Each time both feet hit the ground simultaneously the runner should spend as short a time on the ground as possible and continues the drill by changing the position of the feet with a scissor-like motion. Perform 8 to 12 switches per set.

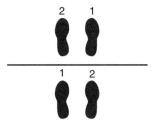

Lateral Line Hop
(Traveling Forward and Backward)

The athlete stands perpendicular to a line and then hops side to side over it with the feet together. The runner moves forward down the line, hopping from side to side, until reaching the end, and then returns to the starting position by hopping backward from side to side. The athlete should keep both feet together for the duration of the drill. Aim to do 6 to 8 hops in each direction. This drill can be progressed to hops on one leg.

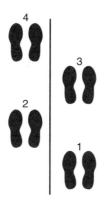

High-Knee Run

Using a sprinting action, the runner remains stationary or progresses forward slowly using an aggressive high-knee and arm action. The athlete should aim to strike the ground on the mid- or forefoot with a slight forward lean with the torso. Toes should be pulled upward, tight toward the shins while the foot is off the ground. Perform 8 to 12 repetitions per leg.

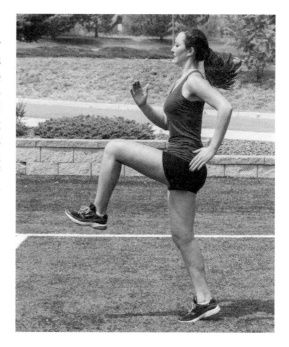

Bounding

Bounding is a high-level plyometric exercise that should only be performed by runners who have at least 6 months experience of plyometric training. The athlete begins by walking or jogging to build momentum. The runner then pushes explosively off the ground with the back leg, driving the opposite knee up and forward to gain height and distance. The athlete keeps the toe cocked up to the shin while the leg is repositioning, and keeps the heel of the driving knee under the hip, ready to land mid- or forefoot. On landing, the athlete immediately drives the other knee up and forward and pushes off the ground with the other leg. The athlete may move the arms in opposition to the legs (as in running) or may use a double-arm swing pattern, pumping with each stride. For this drill, the runner should think about hanging in the air by aiming for height and distance with each step. The more explosive the athlete is, the longer the hang per stride.

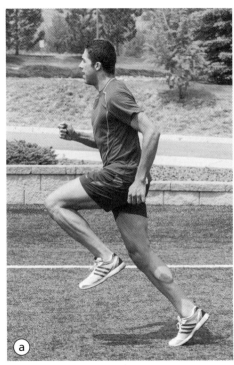 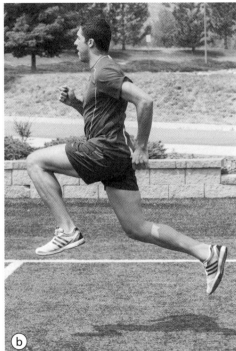

MIDDLE-DISTANCE TRACK RUNNING TRAINING

Middle-distance (800 m to 3 km) runners tend to have a training year comprising of one (outdoor) or two (indoor and outdoor) main track seasons. Beyond approximately 60 seconds of exercise in trained runners, the aerobic contribution to energy metabolism is substantial (33). Thus for middle-distance events a large portion of the training year should be devoted to improving aerobic capabilities, which provide the foundation for developing event-specific anaerobic qualities during the pre- and in-season phases of training (24, 38).

Examples of off-season preparatory, preseason, and in-season phase training weeks for two types of middle-distance runners—recreational or young (<30 miles [48 km] per week) and well-trained or senior runners (>50 miles [80 km] per week)—are provided in tables 8.5 and table 8.6, respectively. During the off-season phase, the priority is on building an aerobic foundation using a mixture of moderate-intensity easy running along with hill strides and extensive interval training (~5 km race speed). Strength and conditioning sessions are also a priority during the off-season for all event categories. In the preseason phase, 1 to 2 months before main competitions, the intensity of key sessions is increased and interval training at race paces is used more frequently. Some volume and tempo-style sessions (heavy-intensity domain) and resistance training are retained during this phase. In-season, preparation for and recovery from races take priority, with intensive interval training focused on racing speeds, tactics; and maintaining form under fatigue. It is also sensible to maintain some resistance training in-season. For the recreational or young runner and for runners who are injury prone, cross-training modalities (e.g., cycling and swimming) can be used to supplement moderate-intensity running. At an elite level, middle-distance runners typically use a similar frequency and prescription of hard interval training sessions (2-3 × per week), but volume of running is even higher (>70 miles [113 km] per week) during the off-season preparatory phase (38). This is achieved by adding runs (twice daily on 1-4 days per week) rather than increasing the duration of individual runs in the example provided (table 8.6).

Table 8.5 One-Week Example Training Program Across Three Phases of the Training Year for a Recreational or Young Middle-Distance Runner

Day	1	2	3	4	5	6	7
Off-season preparatory phase	20 min progression run (M-H), 8 × 30 sec hill strides (jog down) (E), 20 min easy (M)	S&C + optional cross-training (M)	—	20 min easy (M), 6 × 3 min (60 s rec) at 5 km pace (S), 10 min easy (M)	S&C + optional cross-training (M)	45-60 min run (M)	—
Preseason phase	10 min easy (M), 4 × 1 km (3 min jog rec) at 3 km pace (S), 10 min easy (M)	S&C + optional 30 min run (M)	—	10 min easy (M), 6 × 300 m (3 min rec) at 800 m pace (E), 10 min easy (M)	S&C + optional cross-training (M)	15 min easy (M), 3 × 8 min tempo (H) (2 min jog), 15 min easy (M)	—
In-season (track) phase	10 min easy (M), 1000 m-600 m-400 m-200 m (E) (5, 4, 3, 2 min rec), 10 min easy (M)	S&C + optional 30 min run (M)	—	10 min easy (M), 6 × 200 m (E) (3 min jog rec), 10 min easy (M)	Short optional cross-training (M)	10 min easy (M), race or 2 × 600 m or 2 × 1000 m at race pace (10 min rec) (E)	—

Note: M = moderate-intensity domain (RPE 1-4 out of 10); H = heavy-intensity domain (RPE 5-6); S = severe-intensity domain (RPE 7-10); E = extreme-intensity domain (RPE 9-10); rec = recovery; S&C = strength and conditioning.

Table 8.6 One-Week Example Training Program Across Three Phases of the Training Year for a Well-Trained or Senior Middle-Distance Runner

Day	1	2	3	4	5	6	7
Off-season preparatory phase	20 min progression run (M-H), 10 × 45 sec hill strides (jog down), 20 min easy (M)	S&C + 45-60 min run (M)	45-60 min run (M)	20 min easy (M), 6 × 3 min (60 s rec) at 5 km pace (S), 10 min easy (M)	S&C + 45-60 min run or cross-training (M)	75-90 min run (M)	—
Preseason phase	20 min easy (M), 4 × 1 km (3 min jog rec) at 3 km pace (S), 20 min easy (M)	S&C + 45-60 min run (M)	—	10 min easy (M), 6 × 300 m (3 min rec) at 800 m pace (E), 10 min easy (M)	S&C + 45-60 min run or cross-training (M)	15 min easy (M), 3 × 8 min tempo (H) (2 min jog), 15 min easy (M)	60-80 min run (M)
In-season (track) phase	10 min easy (M), 1000 m-600 m-400 m-200 m (E) (5, 4, 3 min rec), 10 min easy (M)	S&C + optional 30 min run (M)	—	10 min easy (M), 6 × 200 m (E) (3 min jog rec) at faster than 800 m pace (E), 10 min easy (M)	Short optional cross-training (M)	10 min easy (M), race or 2 × 600 m or 2 × 1000 m at race pace (10 min rec) (E)	—

Note: M = moderate-intensity domain (RPE 1-4 out of 10); H = heavy-intensity domain (RPE 5-6); S = severe-intensity domain (RPE 7-10); E = extreme-intensity domain (RPE 9-10); rec = recovery; S&C = strength and conditioning.

LONG-DISTANCE TRACK, ROAD, AND CROSS-COUNTRY RUNNING TRAINING

Long-distance (5 km to half marathon) runners may have several major competitions each year (depending on their goals), often over a variety of surfaces such as road, indoor and outdoor track, and cross-country. Compared to the middle-distance runner, longer distance specialists usually complete higher overall volumes of running and include less anaerobic interval sessions (extreme-intensity domain) in their program. At the well-trained and elite level, the vast majority (≥80%) of running volume is easy running performed in the moderate-intensity domain, with a small amount (10%-15%) in the heavy domain and very little in the severe domain (39, 54).

Examples of off-season preparatory, preseason, and in-season phase training weeks for two types of long-distance runners—recreational or young (<40 miles [64 km] per week) and well-trained or senior (>70 miles [113 km] per week)—are provided in tables 8.7 and table 8.8, respectively. For a recreational or young athlete, cross-training sessions (30-40 min) are encouraged on one or two days per week, in addition to four running sessions. For the well-trained runner, twice-daily runs are often used beyond approximately 60 miles (97 km) per week (10 miles [16 km] per day plus rest day) to progress overall training volume (table 8.8). For runners targeting cross-country events it is sensible to perform some of the day 2 (and/or day 6) interval training sessions on undulating soft grassy surfaces to mimic the likely conditions of a race.

Table 8.7 One-Week Example Training Program Across Three Phases of the Training Year for a Recreational or Young Long-Distance Runner

Day	1	2	3	4	5	6	7
Off-season preparatory phase	S&C + optional cross-training (M)	10 min easy (M), 5 × 5 min (90 sec rec) at 10 km pace (H/S), 10 min easy (M)	—	15 min easy (M), 20 min tempo (H), 10 min easy (M)	S&C + optional cross-training (M)	20 min easy (M), 8 × 90 sec hill runs (jog down rec) (S), 10 min easy (M)	50-70 min run (M)
Preseason phase	S&C + optional 30-40 min run or cross-training (M)	10 min easy (M), 6 × 3 min (60 sec jog rec) at 5-10 km pace (S), 10 min easy (M)	—	20 min easy (M), 20 min tempo (H), 10 min easy (M)	S&C + optional cross-training (M)	10 min easy (M), 12 × 400 m (60 sec rec) at 3-5 km pace (S), 10 min easy (M).	50-70 min run (M)
In-season (track) phase	S&C + optional 30-40 min run or cross-training (M)	10 min easy (M), 6 × 800 m (400 m jog rec) at 3 km pace (S), 10 min easy (M)	—	20 min easy (M), 20 min tempo (H), 10 min easy (M)	Optional cross-training (M)	10 min easy (M), race or 5 × 1 km (400 m jog rec) at 5 km pace (S), 10 min easy (M)	50-60 min run (M)

Note: M = moderate-intensity domain (RPE 1-4 out of 10); H = heavy-intensity domain (RPE 5-6); S = severe-intensity domain (RPE 7-10); rec = recovery; S&C = strength and conditioning.

Reprinted by permission from J. Daniels and J. Gilbert, *Oxygen Power: Performance Tables for Distance Runners* (Tempe, AZ: Oxygen Power, 1979).

Table 8.8 One-Week Example Training Program Across Three Phases of the Training Year for a Well-Trained or Senior Long-Distance Runner

Day	1	2	3	4	5	6	7
Off-season preparatory phase	S&C + 60 min run (M) + optional 30 min run (M)	15 min easy (M), 6 × 5 min (90 sec rec) at 10 km pace (H/S), 15 min easy (M)	—	15 min easy (M), 30 min tempo (H), 15 min easy (M) + optional 30 min run (M)	S&C + 60 min run (M)	20 min easy (M), 10 × 90 sec hill runs (jog down rec) (S), 20 min easy (M)	90-120 min run (M)

(continued)

Table 8.8 One-Week Example Training Program Across Three Phases of the Training Year for a Well-Trained or Senior Long-Distance Runner *(continued)*

Day	1	2	3	4	5	6	7
Preseason phase	S&C + 60 min run (M) + optional 30 min run (M)	15 min easy (M), 8 × 3 min (60 sec jog rec) at 5-10 km pace (S), 15 min easy (M)	—	15 min easy (M), 30 min tempo (H), 15 min easy (M) + optional 30 min run (M)	S&C + 60 min run (M)	20 min easy (M), 16 × 400 m (60 s rec) at 3-5 km pace (S), 20 min easy (M)	90-120 min run (M)
In-season (track) phase	S&C + 50-60 min run (M)	15 min easy (M), 8 × 800 m (400 m jog rec) at 3 km pace (S), 15 min easy (M)	—	15 min easy (M), 15 min tempo (H), 20 min easy (M)	Optional cross-training (M)	20 min easy (M), race or 6 × 1 km (400 m jog rec) at 5 km pace (S), 20 min easy (M)	80-100 min run (M)

Note: M = moderate-intensity domain (RPE 1-4 out of 10); H = heavy-intensity domain (RPE 5-6); S = severe-intensity domain (RPE 7-10); rec = recovery; S&C = strength and conditioning.

MARATHON ROAD RUNNING TRAINING

The marathon (26.2 miles [42.2 k]) has become a hugely popular distance for runners ranging from recreational to elite, with participation numbers in big-city marathons growing around the world. A marathon can take 2 to 3 hours for a highly trained runner to complete and upwards of 4 to 5 hours for lesser trained runners. Running volume during off-season preparatory phases appears to be a major determinant of success in long-distance running events, yet in marathon running, the link between mileage and performance is even stronger (30, 83). Furthermore, the distance of the longest run (up to 22 miles [35 km]) is also a major determinant of success in marathon running (30), suggesting runners should prioritize gradually building the distance of their long run during their event preparation.

Examples of training weeks 3 to 4 months before, 1 to 2 months before, and 1 week before a marathon for two types of runners—little experience (<40 miles [64 km] per week and 3:00-4:30 target time) and well-trained (>70 miles [113 km] per week and sub-2:45 target time)—are provided in tables 8.9 and table 8.10, respectively. Because a marathon is run around the first threshold (LT), it may be tempting for runners to prepare for a marathon by only running at easy (moderate domain) intensity. However, clear benefits are seen from higher-intensity sessions for runners of all abilities: to increase $\dot{V}O_2$max and boost their second threshold (critical speed) (78). For the well-trained and elite runner, many long-distance athletes who compete well over the 10-kilometer and the half marathon often find that they perform very well over the marathon distance by gradually increasing their weekly long run. This is likely because they have already developed a large aerobic base from the high volume of easy running over several years.

Table 8.9 One-Week Example Training Program Across Three Phases of Marathon Preparation and Taper for a Runner With Little Experience (3:00-4:30 Target Time)

Day	1	2	3	4	5	6	7
3-4 months before	S&C + optional cross-training (M)	10 min easy (M), 6 × 4 min run (60 sec jog rec) (S), 10 min easy (M)	—	15 min easy (M), 15-20 min tempo (H), 15 min easy (M)	S&C + optional cross-training (M)	45 min run (M)	60-80 min run (M)
1-2 months before	S&C + optional 40-50 min run or cross-training (M)	10 min easy (M), 6 × 1 mile (60 sec jog rec) at 10 km pace (S), 10 min easy (M)	—	20 min easy (M), 4 × 3 km (2 min jog rec) (H), 10 min easy (M)	S&C + optional cross-training (M)	50 min run (M)	20-23 mile run (M/H)
Final week taper	Low volume S&C + optional 30 min run or cross-training (M)	10 min easy (M), 3 × 1 mile (2 min jog rec) (S), 10 min easy (M)	—	10 min easy (M), 15 min tempo (H), 10 min easy (M)	25 min run (M)	Rest or 20 min run (M)	Marathon

Note: M = moderate-intensity domain (RPE 1-4 out of 10); H = heavy-intensity domain (RPE 5-6); S = severe-intensity domain (RPE 7-10); rec = recovery; S&C = strength and conditioning.

Table 8.10 One-Week Example Training Program Across Three Phases of Marathon Preparation and Taper for a Well-Trained Runner (Sub-2:45 Target Time)

Day	1	2	3	4	5	6	7
3-4 months before	S&C + 60 min run (M) + optional 30 min run (M)	15 min easy (M), 6 × 5 min (90 sec jog rec) at 10 km pace (H/S), 15 min easy (M)	—	S&C + 60 min run (M) + optional 30 min run (M)	15 min easy (M), 4 × 3 km at marathon pace (3 min jog rec.) (H), 15 min easy (M)	60 min run (M)	90-120 min run (M)
1-2 months prior	S&C + 60 min run (M) + optional 30 min run (M)	15 min easy (M), 10 × 3 min (60 sec jog rec) at 5-10 km pace (S), 15 min easy (M)	—	S&C + 80 min run (M)	15 min easy (M), 15 km at tempo half marathon pace (H), 15 min easy (M)	60 min run (M)	20-23 mile run (M)
Final week taper	Low volume S&C + 45 min run (M)	15 min easy (M), 3 × 1 mile (2 min jog rec) at 5-10 km pace (S), 15 min easy (M)	—	15 min easy (M), 15 min tempo (H), 15 min easy (M)	30 min run (M)	30 min run (M)	Marathon

Note: M = moderate-intensity domain (RPE 1-4 out of 10); H = heavy-intensity domain (RPE 5-6); S = severe-intensity domain (RPE 7-10); rec = recovery; S&C = strength and conditioning.

ULTRAENDURANCE TRAIL RUNNING TRAINING

Ultraendurance running involves participants covering distances longer than a marathon or a running time exceeding 6 hours, including multiday or multistage events (86). Ultraendurance running events take place over a wide variety of surfaces, terrains, gradients, and altitudes, often in extreme environments, offering a range of physical challenges to participants. *Trail running* is the most popular off-road ultraendurance running sport (85) and has often been used as an umbrella term to describe events that take place in natural environments over a range of distances, terrains, and elevations (86). Strictly speaking, trail running includes several running disciplines that each have unique characteristics with race rules and definitions outlined by various international governing bodies.

A trail running event is defined as a foot race that can include a variety of off-road natural environments (e.g., mountains, desert, forest, coastal paths, grassy plains), without restriction on event distance or elevation change, and with a paved or asphalt surface not exceeding 25% of the course (86). Three other subcategories of trail running exist. First, mountain running events typically take place off-road with distances ranging from 0.6 miles (1 km) to the marathon and with the average incline for classic uphill and classic up and down between 5% and 25%, which is far steeper than typical cross-country running events. In mountain running events in the vertical category, the incline is no less than 25%. Second, fell running (or hill running) shares many similar features to mountain running but can take place over longer distances including multiday events. Ascent categories are also defined differently in fell running, and navigation skills and survival equipment are often a requirement for participation (86). Finally, skyrunning involves events performed 6,562 feet (2,000 m) above sea level, often including extremely technical sections of trail (e.g., glacier, moraine, scrambling over rock).

Risks, Precautions, and Recommendations

Although human beings have evolved to become well suited to covering great distances on foot (15), ultraendurance events place a high physical and cognitive demand on participants, which presents unique risks compared to shorter running distances. Many ultraendurance trail races also take place in demanding environments (mountain, desert, altitude) and challenging conditions (extreme cold or heat), which place additional strain on physiological systems. In multiday events, participants are also required to carry equipment and provisions, creating an additional physiological burden due to the additional mass.

Despite these concerns, adverse and serious events reported during ultraendurance running events are rare (89). Due to the prolonged duration of ultraendurance events, many participants display elevated markers of myocardial, immune function, and acute kidney injury, which usually return to normal levels within a few days (41, 45). It has been speculated that repeated or prolonged participation in ultraendurance sports may cause permanent cardiac damage, myocardial inflammation, and fibrosis (88), but this link has yet to be confirmed. Ultraendurance runners often suffer from upper respiratory-tract infections following an event due to prolonged suppression of immune function. Exercise-associated hyponatremia (plasma sodium level of 135 mmol/L or lower, usually caused by consumption of too much fluid) is common in ultraendurance running participants, particularly those who competed in events in temperate or cool environments (56).

Preparation for ultraendurance events demands a high volume of training, which is associated with illness, overuse injury, and overtraining if workload is not managed appropriately. Indeed, ultraendurance runners have a high incidence of lower limb overuse injuries, particularly to structures around the knee, ankle, and foot (87). Compared to road and track running races, ankle sprains have a high prevalence in trail running events, particularly in those competing for a position or time on a course with uneven surfaces (95). Large elevation changes characterized by prolonged or steep downhill sections place a high demand on muscles to work eccentrically, which can cause structural damage, leading to injury. In training, the prevalence of bone stress injuries are high (66), which is likely the result of inappropriate training workloads and relative energy deficiency in sport syndrome (76).

The following precautions and in-event recommendations are advised for runners preparing for and participating in ultraendurance trail running events (42):

▸ Runners should follow an appropriate training program that gradually and progressively provides exposure to longer distances and the gradients and changes in elevation of the event. This is likely to be the best strategy to avoid exertional rhabdomyolysis and acute kidney injury in the event. Further, for those not participating to achieve a predetermined time or position, reducing running speed on downhill sections is also sensible to avoid excessive muscle damage.

▸ In-event injuries can also be prevented by ensuring an appropriate training program (including resistance training) is followed in the preparatory period for the event.

▸ Runners should research the course including terrain, gradients, topography, obstacles, and other common issues they will face.

▸ Runners should prepare appropriately for extreme and adverse weather and situations (e.g., high winds, snow, hail, insects, wild animals, floods, fires, storms, lightning), follow instructions provided at pre-event safety briefings, and take appropriate protective clothing to wear during the event.

▶ Blisters and chafing are the most common medical problems reported in ultraendurance foot races; therefore, participants should be prepared to prevent and treat these likely issues.

▶ To avoid heat stroke and hypothermia when participating in hot and cold environments, respectively, ultraendurance runners should include a 10- to 14-day heat acclimatization running training period prior to the event.

▶ Altitude illness typically occurs above 8,200 feet (2,500 m), so participants should acclimatize by spending at least one night at an intermediate altitude prior to an event. Gradual ascent and exposure to the event elevation is the best way to prevent altitude illness; however, if this is not possible, the use of prophylactic medication is advised.

▶ In-event, participants should drink to thirst rather than follow a predetermined schedule to avoid exercise-associated hyponatremia.

▶ Energy intakes of approximately 150-400 kcal/hour (e.g., ~40-90 g/hour carbohydrate) depending on what is tolerable, are recommended during ultraendurance events (91). In-event fueling strategy should be practiced prior to the event to train the gut and avoid gastrointestinal issues (49). Race finishers (particularly faster finishers) tend to be able to tolerate the ingestion of higher calories or carbohydrate during an ultraendurance event compared to slower or nonfinishers (67).

▶ Runners can reduce the risk of developing gastrointestinal illness and upper-respiratory infections by maintaining high personal hygiene standards, washing and sanitizing hands at aid stations, and following appropriate caloric intake and hydration.

Training Program

It is advised that endurance runners only embark on training for an ultraendurance event once they have successfully completed a marathon. Table 8.11 shows an example training program for an ultraendurance runner (3:00-4:00 marathon best time) preparing for a 50-mile (80 km) trail race.

Training for an ultraendurance event is not too dissimilar to preparing for a marathon, because the injury and overtraining risk associated with even higher weekly running volumes is increased. The main difference between marathon running preparation and training for an ultraendurance event is the length of the weekly long run. Trained endurance runners preparing for an ultramarathon should aim to run a 2.5- to 4.5-hours-long run most weeks and, once per month, should aim to cover an ultradistance run (31-62 miles [50-100 km]) at a slow speed, if possible (24). Runners new to ultraendurance trail running should aim to complete a weekly long run of 2 to 3 hours on alternate weeks initially and gradually increase duration to 4 or more hours. Long runs on back-to-back

Table 8.11 One-Week Example Training Program Across Three Phases of an Ultraendurance Trail Event (50 Miles [80 km]) Preparation and Taper for a Trained Runner With Marathon Running Experience (3:00-4:00 Personal Best)

Day	1	2	3	4	5	6	7
3-4 months before	—	S&C + 45 min run (M)	15 min easy (M), 10 × 2 min (60 sec jog rec) at 5 km pace (S), 15 min easy (M)	60-75 min run (M)	5 min easy (M), 35 min tempo (H), 5 min easy (M)	S&C + optional cross-training	2.5-3.5 hr run (M)
1-2 months before	—	S&C + 60 min run (M)	80 min run with hard efforts up hills (M/H/S)	80 min run (M)	S&C	15-20 mile run (M)	15-20 mile run (M)
Final week taper	—	Low volume S&C + 30 min run (M)	15 min easy (M), 15 min tempo (H), 15 min easy (M) (M)	—	30 min run (M)	Rest or 30 min run (M)	50-mile (80 km) trail event

Note: M = moderate-intensity domain (RPE 1-4 out of 10); H = heavy-intensity domain (RPE 5-6); S = severe-intensity domain (RPE 7-10); rec = recovery; S&C = strength and conditioning.

days (e.g., 15-20 miles [24-32 km] on both Saturday and Sunday) are also an effective training strategy for runners to use once they have become accustomed to a regular weekly long run. As stated in the previous section, runners should also prepare for the environmental challenges they are likely to face in the event, including regular off-road running on similar surfaces, terrain, and gradients. Like marathon running, ultraendurance running performance is strongly linked to $\dot{V}O_2max$, the fraction of sustainable $\dot{V}O_2max$, and running economy (72), thus interval training, tempo running in the heavy-intensity domain, and resistance training remain important for ultraendurance runners.

RUNNING TECHNIQUE AND GAIT RETRAINING

A wide variety of running styles can be observed when watching any endurance running event. Even at an elite level, the biomechanics and technique of the fastest runners in the world differ considerably (19). Intuitively, coaches and runners often believe there is a correct or perfect way to run, and that one style of running is more economical than others. However, little evidence exists to suggest that many technical factors determine running performance (74) and are associated with injury risk (79). Furthermore, even experienced running coaches are poor at ranking the most and least economical runners based on visual inspection of running form (21). Although coaching runners to adopt a preferential style of running is not recommended, in some scenarios runners should try to change aspects of their running technique.

Gait Retraining for Improving Running Economy

Running economy is defined as how much energy a runner uses to complete a given distance; therefore it seems logical that any unnecessary bodily movements that waste energy should be trained out of a runner. Despite a relatively large number of studies investigating modifiable intrinsic biomechanical factors that might affect running economy, identifying consistent undesirable and suboptimal movements has been problematic (74). Moreover, coaches and biomechanists rarely consider male and female running technique separately despite clear evidence that females have greater stride length (relative to leg length), use higher stride cadence (strides per minute), spend less time on the ground, and have greater anterior pelvic tilt compared to their male counterparts (75). Furthermore, female breast motion during running is known to influence economy and likely interacts with other gait characteristics (73). For female runners, appropriate breast support, which minimizes breast motion, has been shown to eliminate or reduce pain during running and decreases undesirable motion in the trunk and lower limb to improve running economy (75).

Although there is no one-size-fits-all approach to running technique, several modifiable biomechanical factors have been identified as beneficial for running economy in runners (74, 75):

▸ Self-selected stride length (±3%)

▸ Greater leg stiffness (less bend at the ankle, knee, and hip while the foot is on the ground) and less vertical oscillation or bounce between strides

▸ Less leg (knee and hip) extension at toe-off (less terminal stance over-striding)

No evidence currently suggests that resistance training exercises, modification of general movement patterns (e.g., single-leg squats), or isolated running drills alter endurance running gait. These training methods therefore should be used for different purposes, which are outlined in other sections of this chapter. Gait retraining strategies, used during moderate-intensity running training, should be used to modify predetermined gait characteristics. Evidence-based strategies to achieve these outcomes are provided in table 8.12.

Runners and coaches often place a heavy focus on the part of the foot that strikes the ground at initial contact (i.e., rear-foot, mid-foot, or forefoot striker). It has been consistently shown that habitual foot strike does not appear to influence running economy at any speed and that imposing a different foot strike on runners leads to a worsening of economy. Therefore, targeting gait retraining interventions at altering foot strike for performance improvement is misplaced (75).

Rear-foot striking, particularly when the foot hits the ground a long distance in front of a runner's center of mass, is often associated with a large braking (deceleration) force, which subsequently needs to be met by an equally large propulsive force during push-off to maintain running speed. The muscular work required

Table 8.12 Gait Retraining Strategies for Modifying Intrinsic Biomechanical Characteristics Associated With Running Economy, Injury Prevention, and Rehabilitation of Specific Overuse Injuries

Characteristic	Purpose (injury type)	Instruction or cue
Less vertical oscillation	Running economy Injury rehabilitation (plantar fasciitis)	• "Keep your hips up as you run." • "Run tall." • 'Don't bounce as you run."
Less leg extension at toe-off	Running economy	• "Keep your knee and ankle more bent at push-off." • Side-on video feedback
Greater leg stiffness and reduced ground contact time	Running economy	• Run to the beat of a metronome (set 5%-10% higher than normal) • Wearable pod/watch • "Pretend you are running over hot coals or glass."
Increase stride frequency or cadence	Injury rehabilitation (knee pain, chronic exertional compartment syndrome, tibial stress fracture, plantar fasciitis)	• Run to the beat of a metronome (set 5%-10% higher than normal) • Wearable pod/watch • "Hit the ground more often."
Increase step width	Injury prevention (tibial stress fracture)	• "Run along a line (treadmill or track) and keep your feet either side of the line." • "Don't let your knees touch." • "Imagine you are holding a ball between your knees."
Reduce forces on landing	Injury prevention and rehabilitation (knee pain and tibial stress fracture)	• "Run more quietly." • "Run with a soft landing." • "Hit the ground with a flatter foot and forefoot."
Hit the ground with a vertical shin angle and change to mid- or forefoot strike	Injury rehabilitation (knee pain, chronic exertional compartment syndrome)	• "Hit the ground with your foot closer to your body." • "Run on the ball of your foot." • "Imagine you're trying to squash an orange under your foot." • Side-on video feedback
Reduce inward collapse of knees during stance	Injury rehabilitation (iliotibial band syndrome)	• "Point your knees away from you when you run." • Place markers on knees; "keep the markers apart." • Run on a treadmill in front of a mirror
Reduce contralateral hip drop	Injury rehabilitation (knee pain)	• "Run with your knees apart and pointing straight ahead." • "Squeeze your buttocks." • Run on a treadmill in front of a mirror
Upright torso and neutral pelvis	Injury rehabilitation (knee pain, chronic exertional compartment syndrome)	• "Rest your chin on a shelf." • "Run tall."

in the propulsive phase of gait to generate positive impulse incurs a high energy cost; therefore, minimizing the braking (negative) impulse and impact forces theoretically would be more economical. The effect of reducing braking and impact forces on running economy is relatively unexplored, and studies to date have tended to show conflicting results, with differences in findings between males and females. Thus, aiming gait retraining methods at reducing stride length to improve running economy and performance cannot currently be recommended.

Gait Retraining for Injury Prevention and Rehabilitation

The causes of running-related overuse injury are multifactorial yet using a gait retraining approach to injury prevention or rehabilitation assumes that a leading cause of an injury is biomechanical. Gait retraining aims to redistribute the external forces that runners experience during their running stride by shifting stress away from vulnerable or injured areas. However, not all injuries and pains are caused by a biomechanical issue, so employing gait retraining as a universal injury prevention or rehabilitation strategy is inappropriate. If a runner is in pain or sidelined with injury, they are advised to consult with an experienced physical therapist with a specialty in running biomechanics to ascertain whether the running gait is contributing to the issue. In rehabilitation contexts, evidence supports that gait retraining will reduce pain in injured runners (75). A list of common injuries and the gait retraining strategies shown to help rehabilitate runners is shown in table 8.11.

For injury prevention, evidence is weak that gait retraining reduces overall injury incidence; therefore, runners should be cautious taking this approach if they are currently healthy and running pain free. It is important to be aware that successfully altering an aspect of running technique will reduce the loading on some musculoskeletal structures but increase the stress on others that may not be accustomed to repetitive loading. Indeed, in a study that successfully shifted novice runners to a forefoot strike and reduced impact forces, knee and plantar fasciitis injuries were decreased but Achilles tendinopathy and calf strains increased (20). If a runner chooses to use gait retraining in an injury rehabilitation or prevention context, it is important to remain patient and initially reduce the volume and intensity of training for several weeks before progressively increasing workload again.

Extrinsic Biomechanical Factors and Super Shoes

The discussion in this section so far has focused on intrinsic biomechanical factors (i.e., running technique related to running economy and injury). Additionally, several extrinsic biomechanical factors are modifiable and should be considered by runners and coaches to improve performance and reduce injury risk. The shoes that runners choose to wear for running can have a profound impact on their running economy and how forces are distributed through their feet and lower limb. When mass is added to the feet (i.e., heavier shoes), running economy worsens by approximately 1% for every 3.5 ounces (100 g) added (32). Shoes weighing less than 7.8 ounces (220 g) have a negligible effect on running economy compared to running barefoot; therefore, competitive runners should choose lightweight does to race in that weigh ≤7.8 ounces. Shoes heavier than 7.8 ounces (up to ~13 oz. [370 g]) can be worn for moderate-intensity running and tend to provide greater stability, comfort, and cushioning. It should be noted, however, that highly cushioned maximalist shoes actually increase peak impact forces and loading rates rather than attenuate forces because the lower limb is forced to compensate for a more compliant shoe–surface interaction by increasing leg stiffness (59).

Given the repetitive nature of running and the impact forces involved, varying the nature of extrinsic biomechanical stresses may help distribute load via subtle technique alterations and therefore increase musculoskeletal capacity and prevent injury. For example, runners who wear several different pairs of running shoes in parallel for their training have a lower rate of injury compared to those who use just one pair for all running sessions (65). Variability of extrinsic biomechanical factors can also be achieved in other ways, including short bouts of running barefoot and by changing running environment (e.g., terrain and gradient) regularly. Orthotic insoles are often prescribed to runners as a means of modifying a runner's biomechanics to reduce pain and prevent injury. Although the quality of research in this area is weak to moderate, a recent systematic review that looked at more than 5,000 runners concluded that the use of foot orthoses may help reduce the incidence of injuries and pain in runners (77). Despite this finding, it is suggested that runners seek professional advice before investing in a pair of orthoses to address an injury.

Running shoe manufacturers have continuously sought to evolve technology and innovate their shoe designs to give runners a performance advantage. Until 2017 very little differentiated racing shoe brands from one another in terms of running economy or performance. In conjunction with the Breaking2 project, in 2017 Nike unveiled their Vaporfly 4% shoes, which improved running economy by 4% compared to similar racing shoe brands (44). The advanced footwear technology incorporated into the shoes represented a breakthrough in running shoe design, and other shoe brands quickly manufactured their own versions of these super shoes. This new generation of racing shoes, which have consistently been shown to enhance running economy and performance compared to standard racing shoes (82), relies on a very thick and light yet compliant midsole foam and stiff curved carbon fiber plate. The combination of materials acts much like a spring to reduce work at the foot and ankle joint, thereby improving running economy and boosting performance. As a consequence of this new technology, many road running world records have been broken over the last 6 years and performance standards across endurance running events have significantly improved (9). Although the introduction of these new generation racing shoes was initially controversial, any highly trained or elite endurance runner now would be foolish not to invest in a pair of super shoes if they wish to be competitive in races.

REDUCING INJURY RISK IN RUNNERS

Compared to other endurance sports such as road cycling, swimming, rowing, and cross-country skiing, the incidence of overuse injuries in endurance running is high. This is caused by the high magnitudes and rates of loading to lower-limb musculoskeletal structures compared to other endurance activities, many of which are non-weight-bearing. Injury rates in runners new to the sport are approximately 85% for some types of injury, with around half of all runners injured annually (55). The most common injuries tend to be around the knee (~50%), and the lower leg and foot also are injured frequently (34, 55). Specifically, the most common injuries are patellofemoral (knee) pain, Achilles tendinopathy, medial tibial stress syndrome (i.e., shin splints), iliotibial band syndrome, plantar fasciitis, calf strains, and bone stress injuries. In high-performing middle- and long-distance track runners, injuries tend to be more distal (foot, ankle, lower leg), whereas in recreational runners, knee injuries are more common (28, 55).

Injury is the result of an imbalance between the load applied to a runner and the capacity of the runner to withstand that load (53). The load applied to a runner can come in many forms not related to running and other physical training, including psychological and lifestyle demands that can positively or negatively influence biological processes (16). The capacity of a runner to withstand that load is influenced by the resilience of specific musculoskeletal tissues and physical, psychological, and biological factors (23). Scientific investigation has tended to search for individual risk factors that explain why an overuse injury occurs. However, there is a lack of consensus in the literature concerning the modifiable risk factors that should be addressed for specific injuries in runners. Each type of injury has slightly different risk factors, and this should be reflected in preventive measures. Further, the reasons that each individual runner gets injured is likely to be different and rooted in a variety of training, biomechanical, structural, psychological, and biological factors. These factors interact to influence acute and chronic fatigue, tissue damage and repair processes, and perceptions of pain, and therefore the health status of the runner.

Numerous modifiable factors relating to both load application (running training) and a runner's capacity (previous injury, strength, sleep and recovery, lifestyle, nutrition, psychological status) are likely to play a role in injury occurrence. Addressing a single risk factor alone is unlikely to provide a panacea for injury. Indeed, the evidence for any one injury-preventive strategy (e.g., resistance training, nutritional intervention, improved sleep, reducing stress levels, gait retraining) reducing injury risk in endurance runners is weak (4, 7, 57, 97). Therefore, a holistic and multifactorial approach to injury risk reduction is advised (40, 43, 46, 48, 58). Figure 8.2 shows a system of evidence-based risk factors and measures that influence load application or load capacity in a runner. The behaviors and characteristics listed in the light gray box represent measures likely to reduce injury risk. If a runner displays most of these behaviors, an overuse injury is far less likely. The factors listed in the medium gray box represent behaviors and characteristics that elevate risk of injury. Each by themselves are unlikely to cause an injury, but a runner displaying most of these characteristics is at risk of developing an injury in the short to medium term. The behaviors and characteristics listed in the dark gray box are more concerning and leave a runner at a high risk of injury or re-injury. These should be avoided or addressed as priority, wherever possible, with the support of sports medicine professionals and qualified coaches.

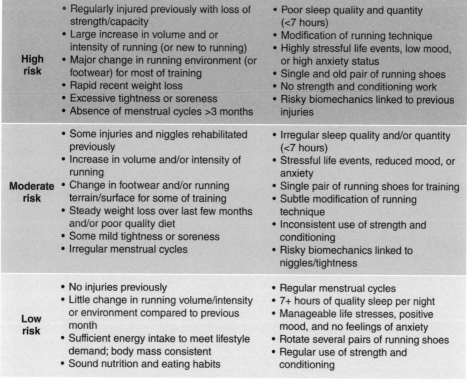

High risk	• Regularly injured previously with loss of strength/capacity • Large increase in volume and or intensity of running (or new to running) • Major change in running environment (or footwear) for most of training • Rapid recent weight loss • Excessive tightness or soreness • Absence of menstrual cycles >3 months	• Poor sleep quality and quantity (<7 hours) • Modification of running technique • Highly stressful life events, low mood, or high anxiety status • Single and old pair of running shoes • No strength and conditioning work • Risky biomechanics linked to previous injuries
Moderate risk	• Some injuries and niggles rehabilitated previously • Increase in volume and/or intensity of running • Change in footwear and/or running terrain/surface for some of training • Steady weight loss over last few months and/or poor quality diet • Some mild tightness or soreness • Irregular menstrual cycles	• Irregular sleep quality and/or quantity (<7 hours) • Stressful life events, reduced mood, or anxiety • Single pair of running shoes for training • Subtle modification of running technique • Inconsistent use of strength and conditioning • Risky biomechanics linked to niggles/tightness
Low risk	• No injuries previously • Little change in running volume/intensity or environment compared to previous month • Sufficient energy intake to meet lifestyle demand; body mass consistent • Sound nutrition and eating habits	• Regular menstrual cycles • 7+ hours of quality sleep per night • Manageable life stresses, positive mood, and no feelings of anxiety • Rotate several pairs of running shoes • Regular use of strength and conditioning

Figure 8.2 A system of training and lifestyle behaviors and characteristics that are associated with a low (light gray), moderate (medium gray), and high (dark gray) risk of developing an overuse running-related injury.

CHAPTER **9**

Cycling

Mike Schultz
Neal Henderson*

The sport of cycling includes a variety of disciplines ranging from extremely short and intense track events, to highly variable cross-country mountain bike events, to multiday transcontinental ultradistance events. There is no single training schedule that will improve all of the skills needed for competing in each of these disparate events, but some concepts of cycling training are universal. In all cases, being able to generate the highest possible power for the duration of the event is critically important. Other factors that cyclists need to develop include handling skills, pacing, strategy, and team tactics. This chapter focuses on improving endurance cycling performance for both the competitive athlete and the recreational cyclist.

TECHNIQUE DEVELOPMENT

Cycling involves various levels of technique. The circular motion of pedaling the bicycle is one aspect of cycling technique that is somewhat constrained. But how a rider achieves that movement can be altered and trained. Proper bike fit (7), biomechanics, and rider position have a great impact on pedaling technique. Additional factors such as crank length, pedal–cleat interfaces, and drive train also affect pedaling technique. Regardless of the type of cycling discipline, riders will need to negotiate a wide variety of pedaling speeds (or cadences), forces, and balance requirements during training and competition.

A cyclist must have a fluid pedaling style at both low and high cadences. Specific drills that include efforts both above and below the preferred cadence should be incorporated into the cyclist's training (see table 9.1). Research shows that most trained cyclists can perform their highest power output during a race, such as in the Tour de France, between 80 and 110 revolutions per minute (rpm) (1). Cycling terrain with long climbs, smooth flatland, or rough roads will ultimately determine the ideal cadence. Athletes attempting to set the hour

---

*Mike Schultz was contracted to author this chapter; Neal Henderson's name was added to acknowledge his significant contribution partially retained from the previous edition.

215

record in cycling (on a track) typically ride at 95 to 105 rpm, while solo cyclists during the Race Across America (RAAM) typically ride at 60 to 80 rpm. Most modern bikes have enough gear options to allow the cyclist to maintain an ideal cadence regardless of speed.

Table 9.1   Cycling Drills

Drill	Page number
Comfort at High Cadences	216
Comfort at Low Cadences	216
Cycling Starts	217
Handling Drill	217
Pack Riding	217

Comfort at High Cadences

This drill helps cyclists improve their comfort level and efficiency at high cadences. The cyclist starts with a preferred cadence and then adds 10 rpm for 30 seconds to 1 minute while maintaining or increasing power and speed. The cyclist then decreases the rpm back to the preferred cadence for 30 seconds to 1 minute to recover and then repeats this cycle with increased rpm until there is a break in form, such as bouncing excessively in the saddle. The following provides an example:

- *Minute 1:* 90 rpm (preferred cadence)
- Minute 2: 100 rpm (adding 10 to the preferred rpm)
- *Minute 3:* 90 rpm (preferred cadence)
- *Minute 4:* 110 rpm (adding 20 to the preferred rpm)
- *Minute 5:* 90 rpm (preferred cadence)
- *Minute 6:* 120 rpm (adding 30 to the preferred rpm)
- *Minute 7:* 90 rpm (preferred cadence)

Comfort at Low Cadences

Low-cadence, high-force drills on the bike are excellent for helping cyclists improve leg and hip strength (4), leading to more comfort when pedaling between 50 and 70 rpm. Low-cadence force efforts are best done on inclines outside or on an indoor trainer with higher resistance. To start, the cyclist pedals the bike into an incline with a preferred cadence, say, 90 rpm (if indoors, increase the resistance). The cyclist then shifts into a harder gear, reducing cadence to 50 to 70 rpm while maintaining the same or increased speed and power. The cyclists should start with 30- to 60-second efforts and work up to a minute or more pedaling with increased force. The cyclist should incorporate both seated and standing efforts to work the full range of motion for cycling. Work up to multiple efforts spaced with 5 to 10 minutes of easier spinning at the preferred cadence to recover from each effort. These efforts are best done early in the workout and in the early season to build cycling-specific strength.

Cycling Starts

Two types of starts are used in cycling events: from a standstill and a controlled rolling start. In many events, cyclists start from a stop, which requires the riders to be able to select an appropriate gear, get into the pedals, and rapidly pedal up to speed. An excellent time to practice starts is during training rides whenever the cyclist stops, whether for traffic signs or a planned stop. Athletes should work to be able to click into the pedals without looking at them. This is also a good time to experiment with gearing, selecting a gear that allows you to get up to training pace at your preferred cadence as quickly as possible.

Handling Drill

Bicycle handling includes being able to ride with the hands on various positions on the handlebars and comfortably corner, or turn, to both sides with equal confidence and speed. An excellent way to practice this is to set up a line of four to six water bottles in a straight line over 50 to 80 yards or meters in a traffic-free area, such as a vacant parking lot on the weekend. The cyclist practices riding down the line and moving in and out of the bottles as if on a slalom course. The cyclist should start off slowly and gradually add speed. To make this drill more difficult, bring the bottles closer together or offset the bottles to require a bigger turning radius at each bottle.

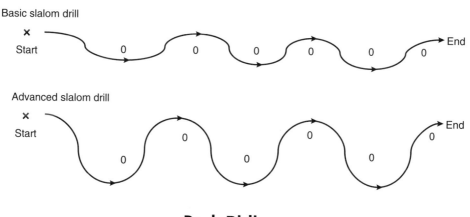

Basic slalom drill

Advanced slalom drill

Pack Riding

In most mass-start cycling events, cyclists need to have the ability to comfortably ride close to other riders. Contact sometimes occurs between riders and their bikes. Being able to react appropriately allows cyclists to stay upright and keeps everyone safe in the pack. To improve their pack-riding skills, cyclists should practice riding in a pack. Cyclists should start in an open field, progress onto gravel roads, and then move onto paved roads. Riding side by side teaches cyclists to be aware of everyone around them at cycling speeds. Cyclists should practice leaning on each other and track standing, or balancing on the bike without moving, ideally in an open field. These skills make cyclists safer and more proficient in any condition. The safest riders are those who have great balance, never overreact, and are always aware of their surroundings.

ENDURANCE CYCLING TRAINING PROGRAMS

This section provides general examples of training programs for cyclists who are preparing for various types of cycling events. The actual amount of training performed is based on age, training history, competitive level, time availability, and cycling discipline. Some elite professional riders spend in excess of 30 hours per week training and competing during the season. National champions in junior and masters racing categories ride between 6 and 12 hours per week.

However, more is not always better. Training is a balancing act of putting appropriate stress on the body and recovering, which leads to improved fitness and performance. Athletes should complete the least amount of training necessary to achieve the greatest response and improvement. Keeping a training log and recording training volume, intensity, perception of effort, and actual performance (including speed, power, and race outcomes) will help determine optimal training levels.

Performing lab or field tests (see chapter 2) is the best way to determine specific ranges of training levels for a cyclist. Coaches and athletes often refer to training zones as a multidimensional evaluation of the training load (see table 9.2) (5). One dimension to use in evaluating training load is rating of perceived effort (RPE). Perception of effort, at a certain intensity, can be related to a scale from 0 to 10, where 0 is no effort and 10 is a maximal effort (6). A submaximal effort could be used as the reference point to see how these three methods of determining training zones relate. The level that is very strongly related to endurance cycling performance is a sustainable power that can be held for 30 to 60 minutes in well-trained cyclists. This point is called the *functional threshold*, and it typically occurs between a 6 and 8 on the RPE scale. This point is also typically between 85% and 94% of actual maximum heart rate (not estimated maximum).

Table 9.2 Recommended Cycling Training Zones using RPE, Heart Rate, and Power

	Zone	RPE (0-10)	Heart rate (% max)	Power (% threshold)	Duration
Active recovery	N/A	0-1	<60%	<55%	20-60 min
Overdistance	1	1-3	65%-80%	55%-75%	1-6+ hr
Endurance	2	3-4	80%-85%	75%-80%	1-3+ hr
Tempo	3	4-6	85%-90%	80%-90%	20-60+ min
Subthreshold	4	6-8	90%-94%	90%-95%	10-30+ min
Threshold	5a	8-9	94%-97%	95%-105%	3-20 min
$\dot{V}O_2$max	5b	9-10	97%-100%	106%-120%	1/2-4 min
Anaerobic capacity (AC)	5c	Variable	Variable	121%-150%	10-60 sec
Peak neuromuscular power (PNP)	5d	Variable	Variable	>150%	3-15 sec

The second measure that is typically used for training zones is heart rate. Generally speaking, the more watts produced, the higher the heart rate. The actual heart rate value at a given effort level varies from one person to the next, and this is not determined by age (8). Defining heart rate ranges from testing makes the use of a heart rate monitor more effective in training.

A third method of determining training zones is to measure power output; a portable power meter is the ideal tool for measuring this (2). Various systems are available, and the most important information that the power meter provides is the athlete's actual instantaneous power output in watts. Speed is a nice measure of the result of power output, but it is affected by wind, temperature, drafting, and road gradient, making speed a relative marker of output and not an absolute. In comparison, a watt is a watt, regardless of the cycling speed.

Another factor to consider when developing a training program is the concept of periodization (3). Generally, a properly designed program begins with more emphasis on general fitness and endurance and then moves toward more specific and intense training. The duration of each phase depends on many factors, but the greatest and most sustainable gains in fitness usually occur when an appropriate early-season foundation or base training phase is incorporated and lasts more than 8 weeks. Approximately 60% to 70% of the potential improvements typically occur during this base phase of training. The more intensive phase of training usually improves fitness by an additional 20% to 30%, and good peaking and tapering yield another 5% to 10% improvement.

Many young and professional athletes do well with a standard 3 weeks of progressive training and then 1 week of a decreased training pattern; however, most masters athletes and athletes with a job, family, and other responsibilities typically achieve greater results with just 2 weeks of progressive training followed by a week of reduced training volume and intensity. There are always exceptions to these rules because at any age, levels of fitness and time available to train ultimately determine periodization structure. The sections that follow provide sample weekly training plans for the preparation (or base) phase of training as well as the intensive build (precompetitive) phase of training. Working with a coach who is certified by USA Cycling is also a good way to devise a personal training schedule that is tailored to strengths, weaknesses, and cycling goals. Joining a local racing club or team is another great way to learn more about the technical and tactical skills necessary to perform better and move up through the racing categories.

Road Cycling Training Programs

Road cycling typically involves a mix of disciplines including time trials, hill climbs, criteriums, and road races (11). Some races include just one of these options, while stage races and omniums involve some combination of these races. Tables 9.3 and 9.4 provide sample weekly plans for the base and intense build phase for riders training to participate in any of these events.

Time trials and hill climbs are the simplest types of races. The distance of a time trial or hill climb may vary, but riders usually use fewer tactics in these race formats than in the others. In these races, the goal is to go as fast as possible from point A to point B. Most time trials are between 10 and 25 miles (16-40 km) in length, though races can be shorter or longer. In a time trial, riders start at specific intervals, typically 20 to 60 seconds apart. Drafting is not allowed during a time trial, and riders often use specialized aerodynamic equipment, clothing, and helmets.

Table 9.3 Weekly Training During the Base or Foundation Phase for Road Cyclists

Monday	Resistance training*; stretching (30-60 min)
Tuesday	Endurance in zone 2; cornering drills (120 min)
Wednesday	Tempo/sub–lactate threshold in zones 3 and 4 (180 min)
Thursday	Endurance/tempo in zones 2 and 3 (90 min)
Friday	Cross-training at active recovery intensity (60 min)
Saturday	Overdistance in zones 1 and 2 (5 hr)
Sunday	Endurance/tempo in zones 2 and 3 (120 min)

*See chapter 6 for guidelines and sample programming.

Table 9.4 Weekly Training During the Intense Build or Precompetitive Phase for Road Cyclists

Monday	Strength maintenance; stretching (30 min)
Tuesday	Endurance in zone 2 with 10 × 30 sec cadence builds from 90 to 120 rpm at $\dot{V}O_2$max intensity (90 min)
Wednesday	Overdistance in zone 1 with 3 × 10 min at tempo to threshold intensity (zone 3-5a); 3 min recovery (120 min)
Thursday	Active recovery (45 min)
Friday	Endurance in zone 2 on time-trial bike (90 min)
Saturday	Team ride at endurance to threshold intensity in zones 2-5d (4 hr)
Sunday	Endurance in zone 2 with 10 × 10 sec anaerobic capacity sprints in zone 5c with 50 sec of recovery between sprints (120 min)

Time-trial riders are typically larger and stronger bike racers who can push a high power output while keeping themselves mentally engaged and motivated for the entire event.

In a hill climb, riders may use some tactics or strategy based on the profile of the race or the presence of teammates, but this event is still primarily a test of muscle endurance. Hill climbs are the ideal race for riders with a slighter build because this race requires the ability to have a high power output along with low body and bike weight. To determine their uphill racing potential, many riders consider their ratio of power output to body weight. Calculating the rate of vertical ascent (in meters or feet per hour) is another way to categorize a rider's hill-climbing fitness and performance. Top-level professional riders often sustain power outputs in excess of 6 watts per kilogram (12.2 W/lb) of body weight during a 20-minute climbing section of a race (10). Top professional cyclists can also ascend at a rate of 1,800 vertical meters per hour during a fast ascent on a steep gradient. That is greater than a vertical mile every hour!

For cyclists who want to improve their performance in time trials or hill climbs, training typically focuses on increasing basic endurance, improving the ability to sustain a hard effort for long periods, and improving lactate threshold and $\dot{V}O_2$max (by performing intervals). Time trialists and hill-climbing specialists have little need for sprint-type training, but if the goal is overall cycling performance, this type of training should also be incorporated into the program.

Athletes who compete in criteriums and road races need to be more comfortable riding in packs. They also need to be able to push more intense efforts and recover rapidly between efforts. These riders should perform aerobic endurance and threshold training (similar to the time trialists and hill climbers), but they also need more emphasis on $\dot{V}O_2$max , anaerobic capacity, and peak neuromuscular training.

Track and Velodrome Cycling Programs

Cycling competitions that take place on cycling-specific banked tracks, called *velodromes*, are typically divided into sprint competitions and endurance competitions.

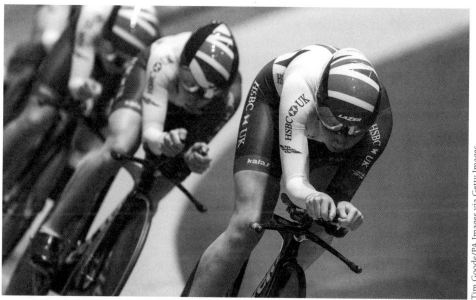

Velodrome cyclists use a combination of high-intensity and endurance training to improve performance.

Tim Goode/PA Images via Getty Images

Many amateur athletes who have access to a track maximize their competitive opportunities by competing in various events ranging from sprint to endurance events. The athletes who are most concerned about performance are likely more specific in their event choices in order to maximize training effect. Track cycling became popular in the late 1800s, and it continues to be an exciting part of the Olympic cycling program. The endurance competitions in track cycling include the individual pursuit, team pursuit, scratch race, points race, and Madison.

For endurance riders, the classic race is the individual pursuit. In international and Olympic competition, men race 4,000 meters (2.5 miles), and women race 3,000 meters (1.9 miles). The pursuit involves a qualifying round and then a final round. The riders with the top four times from the qualifying round are entered in the finals; the riders with the two fastest qualifying times compete for gold and silver, while the third and fourth fastest riders in the qualifying round compete for bronze. The pursuit gets its name from the fact that two riders are on the track at the same time—they start at opposite sides of the track at the same time. In a race final, if a rider overtakes or catches the opposing rider, that rider wins and the competition is over. At the Olympics, the pursuit includes a qualifying, semifinal, and final round of competition; at all other competitions, this event includes just a qualifying and final round. The team pursuit event is similar to the individual pursuit, but a team of four riders covers the race distance.

The scratch race is a mass-start race with more than 30 riders competing to be the first rider across the finish line after a predetermined number of laps. The points race is typically a 40- to 50-kilometer (25-31 mile) race that awards points every 5 or 10 laps to the first 4 riders across the line at each intermediate sprint. Any riders who lap the field also receive a large point bonus. The winner of the points race often does not even contest the final sprint if she has enough points. The Madison is a paired points race in which a team of two riders alternate their position in the race by exchanging places with a hand sling every few laps throughout the race. This is a technically and tactically demanding race format that requires incredible focus and teamwork to achieve success.

Most endurance track riders also compete in road racing events. Tables 9.5 and 9.6 provide sample training programs for sprint and endurance track cyclists during the base and precompetitive training cycles.

Off-Road Training

Proper preparation for mountain and off-road bike competitions includes training to develop cycling power, improve fitness and handling skills, and increase speed on downhill sections (9). Mountain biking is one of the most demanding disciplines in cycling because it requires extremely high levels of fitness as well as highly tuned skills and coordination.

Mountain bike races may be cross-country endurance events that last 2 to 3 hours, marathon-distance events of 5 or more hours, or short and fast short-

Table 9.5 Weekly Training During the Base or Foundation Phase for a Track Cyclist

Day of the week	Sprinter	Endurance rider
Monday	Resistance training[a]; stretching (30-60 min)	Resistance training[a]; stretching (30-60 min)
Tuesday	Overdistance in zone 1 and standing starts (90 min)	Overdistance in zone 1 (120 min)
Wednesday	Anaerobic capacity sprints with overdistance in zone 1 (90 min)	4 × 10 min threshold intervals w/ overdistance in zone 1 (120 min)
Thursday	Endurance in zone 2 (180 min)	Endurance in zone 2 (300 min)
Friday	Active recovery (60 min)	Active recovery (60 min)
Saturday	Flying 200 m practice with overdistance in zone 1 (90 min)	Motorpacing[b] at tempo intensity in zone 3 (180 min)
Sunday	Endurance ride in zone 2 (90 min)	Endurance in zone 2 with PNP sprints in zone 5d (120 min)

[a]See chapter 6 for guidelines and sample programming.
[b]*Motorpacing* refers to drafting behind a vehicle, typically a motorcycle or scooter.

Table 9.6 Weekly Training During the Intense Build or Precompetitive Phase for a Track Cyclist

Day of the week	Sprinter	Endurance rider
Monday	Strength maintenance and stretching (30 min)	Strength maintenance and stretching (30 min)
Tuesday	Endurance in zone 2 with standing starts (90 min)	Endurance in zone 2 with AC sprints (120 min)
Wednesday	Keirin competition simulation (90 min)	10 × 2 min $\dot{V}O_2$max intervals (90 min)
Thursday	Endurance (120 min)	Overdistance in zone 1 with 30 min at tempo in zone 3 (240 min)
Friday	10 × 1 min $\dot{V}O_2$max intervals with overdistance in zone 1 (90 min)	Active recovery (60 min)
Saturday	Team sprint practice (120 min)	Points or Madison race (120 min)
Sunday	Endurance ride in zone 2 (90 min)	Team pursuit practice at threshold intensity with endurance in zone 2 (120 min)

track races (like a criterium on trails) that take 20 to 30 minutes to complete. Mountain biking also includes gravity events such as downhill and four-cross competitions, which typically take 1 to 4 minutes to complete. BMX, a short and fast circuit that includes massive bermed turns and large jumps over a course that takes 30 to 40 seconds to complete, has entered the cycling program as part of the Olympic Games. Cyclocross racing is also a hybrid style of off-road

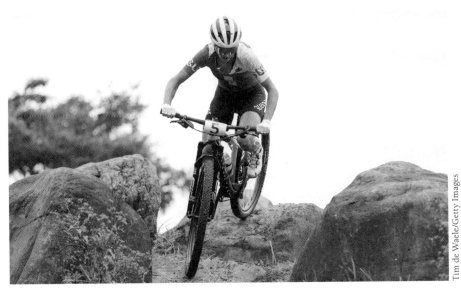

Tim de Waele/Getty Images

Mountain bikers must train endurance, handling skills, and downhill speed.

racing on bicycles that look like a mix between a road bike and mountain bike. These races typically last about an hour.

Most mountain bike riders spend a large portion of their training time on road bikes or on roads because it is easier to control the effort for a ride on roads as opposed to trails. During base and build phases of training, most elite-level mountain bike riders only spend 20% to 30% of their training time riding trails; the remainder is spent on the road developing fitness. During late builds and precompetition phases, training on trails increases to 50% to 60% of the time to improve bike-handling skills, descending ability, balance, and confidence. Most mountain bike events are mass-start events, so being able to start fast and then settle into a rhythm while maneuvering the trail is an important training consideration.

Most cross-country courses are made up of a long loop with steep climbs and descents, or racers may ride multiple laps of a course with uphill and downhill segments. On short-track courses, racers typically only take 3 to 4 minutes to complete a lap. These courses include smaller hills than those found on a cross-country course—but that does not make them any easier.

Cyclocross courses are a mix of dirt, grass, sand, and even paved surfaces. A cyclocross course is interspersed with tight turns and obstacles (called *barriers*) that force riders to dismount and carry their bikes, at times running up short, steep hills. Downhill racers are the daredevils of the mountain biking world. These riders often wear full-body pads and full-face helmets to reduce the chance of serious injury from the inevitable falls that occur in training and racing. BMX is a supercharged sprint that requires incredible acceleration out of the gate, along with confident and skillful bike handling in tight groups. Some of the most powerful riders (measured in sprint power) are BMX riders, and they often score better in peak power output than sprint track cyclists.

Tables 9.7 and 9.8 provide examples of training schedules to be used during the foundation and precompetition weeks for an off-road cyclist preparing for short-track and cross-country mountain bike racing.

Table 9.7 Weekly Training During the Base or Foundation Phase for Off-Road Cyclists

Monday	Resistance training*; stretching (30-60 min)
Tuesday	Overdistance in zone 1 with balance drills and downhill practice (120 min)
Wednesday	Endurance in zone 2 with 30-min sustained climbs at tempo intensity in zone 3 (180 min)
Thursday	Endurance in zone 2 with 4 × 30 starting sprint intensities (AC) with 5 min of rest in between (90 min)
Friday	Cross-training, running, or hiking (60-90 min)
Saturday	Endurance in zone 2 with 30-min sustained climbs at tempo intensity in zone 3 (180 min)
Sunday	Endurance in zone 2 road ride (180 min)

*See chapter 6 for guidelines and sample programming.

Table 9.8 Weekly Training During the Intense Build or Precompetitive Phase for Off-Road Cyclists

Monday	Strength maintenance and stretching (30 min)
Tuesday	Endurance in zone 2 with 6 × 30 sec $\dot{V}O_2$max intensity followed by 10 min at tempo in zone 3 intensity (120 min)
Wednesday	Overdistance in zone 1 with 60-min climb at aerobic endurance in zone 2 intensity (180 min)
Thursday	Active recovery (45 min)
Friday	Overdistance in zone 1 with 8 × 90 sec $\dot{V}O_2$max intensity; 3 min recovery (90 min)
Saturday	Trail ride at endurance to threshold intensity in zones 2-5a (180 min)
Sunday	Endurance in zone 2 (120 min)

Ultradistance Cycling Programs

Ultradistance cycling competitions include single-day set-distance races, 24-hour lap races, and multiday and multistage races. The RAAM is one of the most challenging tests of cycling endurance in the world. It is contested as an individual and team event trying to cover the entire distance (over 3,000 miles [4,830 km]) of the continental United States from West Coast to East Coast. Teams typically take between 6 and 9 days to complete the race, and solo racers finish in 9 to 12 days. Riders sleep very little and average 250 to 350 miles (402-563 km) each day for solo contestants. Other ultradistance events include the Tour Divide, an off-road race from Canada to Mexico, covering 2,700 miles [4,345 km], along with multiday mountain bike races. Many 3- to 7-day mountain bike stage races are held around the world, including in South Africa, the European

Alps, the Canadian Rockies, and the United States. These events attract large crowds of serious competitors.

To properly prepare for an ultradistance cycling competition, athletes must have extreme commitment and training intelligence in order to avoid overtraining. No one prepares for RAAM by riding from one end of the country to the other before the actual race; therefore, the normal strategy of preparing for a race by doing much more than the actual race itself is not used in the preparation for ultradistance events. Instead, proper preparation for ultradistance competitions revolves around building a good endurance base, learning how to pace appropriately, designing a nutrition and hydration plan that can be implemented on race days, and learning to control the mental difficulties of sleep deprivation and extreme fatigue.

The combination of physical and psychological stresses experienced during ultradistance competitions makes for unpredictable race outcomes. Cyclists must be physically and psychologically prepared for the challenges of ultradistance racing. Tables 9.9 and 9.10 provide sample training schedules to be used during the base phase and precompetitive phase for an ultradistance racer preparing for a 24-hour race.

Table 9.9 Weekly Training During the Base or Foundation Phase for Ultradistance Cyclists

Monday	Resistance training*; stretching (30-60 min)
Tuesday	Overdistance in zone 1 with 60-min climb at aerobic endurance at zone 2 (180 min)
Wednesday	Endurance in zone 2 with 30-min sustained climbs at tempo intensity in zone 3 (180 min)
Thursday	Active recovery (30 min)
Friday	Cross-training at overdistance in zone 1 (60 min)
Saturday	Endurance in zone 2 with 30-min sustained climbs at tempo intensity at zone 3 (6-8 hours)
Sunday	Endurance in zone 2 (120 min)

*See chapter 6 for guidelines and sample programming.

Table 9.10 Weekly Training During the Intense Build or Precompetitive Phase for Ultradistance Cyclists

Monday	Strength maintenance and stretching (30 min)
Tuesday	Endurance in zone 2 with 3 × 15 min at tempo intensity in zone 3 (150 min)
Wednesday	Overdistance in zone 1 with 60-min climb at endurance in zone 2 (180 min)
Thursday	Active recovery (45 min)
Friday	Overdistance in zone 1 (120 min)
Saturday	Endurance in zone 2 with 30-min sustained climbs at tempo in zone 3 (6 hr: 3 hr at dusk, 3 hr at night)
Sunday	Endurance in zone 2 (4 hr)

CHAPTER 10

Swimming

Will Kirousis
Dave Joensen
Jason Gootman*

There are close to 750,000 competitive swimmers in the United States today (10, 11). This includes athletes participating in pool and open-water swimming events and multisport racing (triathlon, aqua bike, swimrun [also called an *aquathlon*]). Each of these events takes place in different situations, presents unique challenges to swimmers, and follows different rules. Regardless, each allows swimmers of different ages and abilities to be involved with the sport of swimming. This chapter discusses improving endurance swimming through technique drills, pool-based training, and open-water training. (For guidelines about resistance training for swimming, see chapter 6.)

TECHNIQUE DEVELOPMENT

Swimming is a highly technical sport whose foundational skills must be taught, because swimming movements are not innate. It is unique among endurance sport disciplines because its aquatic environment is roughly 1,000 times denser than air, thus providing much more resistance to athletes' motions (5). This means that a huge fraction of the energy expended during swimming is to overcome the resistance of the water and provide propulsion. Through work to improve swimmers' biomechanics, drag can be reduced, and propulsion increased, enhancing enjoyment and performance. Competitive swimming has four main strokes: freestyle, backstroke, butterfly, and breaststroke. Of these, freestyle and breaststroke are the most common strokes used in long-distance and open-water (in ponds, lakes, rivers, or oceans) swimming events. This includes those who are swim focused and those who are multisport oriented (e.g., triathlon, aqua bike, swimrun). Freestyle is most frequently used because it is the fastest stroke and can be sustained for long distances. Breaststroke, due to

---

*Will Kirousis and Dave Joensen were contracted to author this chapter; Jason Gootman's name was added to acknowledge his significant contribution partially retained from the previous edition.

its head-up and forward-breathing position, is occasionally used during distance swimming as a resting stroke or for sighting (helping the swimmer maintain a straight line in the water by visually verifying the path relative to objects in the distance). Because freestyle is the most used open-water and endurance swimming method, this chapter will focus on drills and practice sessions using freestyle. Technique drills should be a consistent component in a swimmer's workouts. The drills at the end of this section can help athletes improve their freestyle technique through improvements in body position, pulling, kicking, breathing, and stroke coordination (see table 10.1 on page 232). With better technique, athletes will achieve the following benefits:

▶ *Improved hydrodynamics.* Athletes will move through the water with less resistance, allowing them to move more quickly and easily.

▶ *Efficient pull.* Athletes can generate forward propulsion the most effectively and powerfully.

▶ *More proficiency at swimming in open-water races.* Athletes will be able to navigate the most direct path through the water. They will be able to use the draft of other swimmers, reducing energy cost. In addition, athletes will be able to cope with the somewhat chaotic nature of swimming in open-water conditions and swimming with as many as a few thousand other swimmers surrounding them.

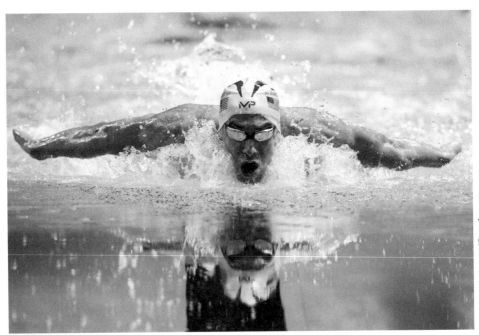

Tom Pennington/Getty Images

Refining swimming technique is vital for improving performance.

The following concepts can help swimmers generally understand and develop good technique in the freestyle:

▶ Maintain a horizontal body position to reduce drag, thereby improving velocity (1, 4).

- The water line should be at the top of the head, much like wearing headphones.
- Eyes should be looking down toward the bottom of the pool.
- The chest presses down while the hips are roughly level with the chest, nearly breaking the surface, and the heels barely break the surface while the swimmer kicks.
- There is a roll along the body's axis, which aids in proportion by allowing the swimmer to apply force to the water better through coordination between the kick's downbeat and the arm pull.

▶ The pull or arm action provides up to 90% of the propulsion during swimming (9). The hand enters the water in front of the shoulder with all four fingers simultaneously, palm facing downward, and elbow bent at entry before extending as the arm reaches forward.

- After the arm is fully extended, the arm pull begins.
- The wrist flexes around 20 to 30 degrees, and the hand reaches deep, so the forearm dives into a vertical position, pointed toward the bottom of the pool (9).
- While the arm moves from in front of the shoulder to the vertical forearm position, the wrist slightly extends, allowing the hand's palm to face back behind the swimmer (7).

▶ This deepest point of the arm pull is referred to as the *catch*. During the catch, the hand is under the elbow.

▶ With the catch achieved, the hand begins to press back, initiating the propulsive phase of the stroke.

- The hand should press straight back along the axillary axis (i.e., essentially along the side of the body) (4, 7, 9).
- During the propulsive phase of the stroke, the palm continues to face back behind the swimmer, requiring a wrist extension. Some swimmers turn the hand inward as it passes the pelvis; it passes under the body but does not cross the midline (4, 7, 9).

▶ At the end of the pull, the arm is not completely extended. Instead, the elbow has a slight bend. When that point has been reached, the stroke recovery phase begins.

▶ The recovery occurs as the arm is lifted from the water through elbow flexion and shoulder rotation.

- During the recovery, the elbow should be outside the body as it swings forward (7).
- Initially, the elbow should lead the hand during the recovery stroke (5).
- As the hand passes the shoulder, the elbow, hand, and shoulder should all be within the transverse plane. Then, with the hand passing the shoulder, the rest of the arm should follow the hand into the next stroke.

▶ The kick during freestyle swimming is referred to as a *flutter kick*.

▶ The importance of the role of the kick during swimming is debated. Some coaches feel the kick supplies up to 30% of the propulsion generated while swimming, while others believe the kick is not significantly propulsive but does help sustain horizontal body position, thus reducing drag (9).

▶ The kick uses the entire leg but covers a relatively short range of motion. Swimmers could imagine kicking inside a tube, only allowing the kick to extend about 6 inches (15 cm) in front of and behind the body. The kick produces an up-and-down beat. Tt the beginning of the downbeat, the knee should be slightly bent, the toe is pointed, and the heel is slightly out of the water. The kick begins by driving toward the bottom of the pool; the shank of the leg and foot will follow. After the downbeat, the ankle dorsiflexes as it is lifted to the surface. The kick is often described as being shallow and fast.

▶ Breathing comfortably is essential for swimming efficiently from a mechanical point of view. Breathing is also vital to sustaining work and fostering recovery should the swimmer need to surge during an event. While breathing, the swimmer's head should stay in line with the body, though it will rotate independently of the body (4). Done well, one goggle eye will remain underwater during the breath as the head turns just enough for the mouth to break the water's surface. In this position, the swimmer's head disturbs the water such that a trough will form along the lower half of the swimmer's face, allowing the swimmer to breathe (4). Exhalation through the mouth should occur as soon as the face enters the water and end when the face exits. Swimmers should work on a comfortable breathing pattern that fits their goal intensity while swimming. Common breathing patterns include taking a breath every second, third, and fourth arm pull. Some athletes and coaches prefer bilateral breathing (alternating breath side); this helps swimmers see other swimmers or terrain features around them while swimming. Breathing should be done in a pattern that feels best to the athlete. However, it is helpful for the athlete to practice breathing to the weak side occasionally to be able to breathe well during a race if waves or a current make breathing harder from one side versus the other.

COORDINATION OF MOVEMENTS IN THE FREESTYLE

Coordination between the arms, legs, and breathing is essential for smooth swimming. This can be tricky, but the benefit is that athletes gain propulsion and a better swim economy.

▶ *Overlap of the arms while swimming.* During most terrestrial sports, the arms swing opposite each other; in swimming, however, the arm positions overlap considerably (3, 7). When one arm enters and extends, it is considered the anchor. The other arm presses back during the propulsive phase of the stroke, then recovers before the anchor arm starts pulling. As one arm recovers, it moves the center of gravity toward the anchor point, further forward. This improves the efficiency of the arm stroke and helps the athlete sustain a horizontally balanced position in the water (7). When the recovery arm passes by the ear, the other arm starts the pull. During the recovery phase, the body rotates toward the anchor am. When the recovery arm enters, the body should be flat, and the face should be in the water.

▶ *Breathing coordination within the stroke cycle.* As mentioned earlier, exhalation occurs when the face is in the water. As the breathing-side hand is passing by the hips, the head should be turned to the side so that the breath can be taken. As the body rolls in the other direction, the face should be turned back, and the face should re-enter the water.

▶ *Kicking coordination within the stroke cycle.* Swimmers can use several kicking patterns. Swimmers should experiment with different styles and find a pattern with which they are comfortable. In addition, swimmers will use different kicking patterns at various points.

- *Two-beat kick.* In a two-beat kick, swimmers use two kicks for every two arm pulls (one-arm cycle) (9). This type of kick conserves energy and postpones fatigue of the leg muscles. The two-beat kick helps maintain a horizontal body position but contributes little to propulsion.

- *Six-beat kick.* This type of kick uses six kicks for every two arm pulls, and it provides the most propulsion but also uses considerable oxygen (9). This kick is prevalent in pool racing, including the 1,500-meter freestyle. More and more world-class distance swimmers are using a six-beat kick. It requires consistent training to maintain this kick for open-water distances.

- *Four-beat kick.* This type of kick uses four kicks for every arm pull (9). This is considered a hybrid of the other kick patterns. This kick provides more propulsion than a two-beat kick but uses less energy than a six-beat kick.

Table 10.1 Swimming Drills

Drill	Page number
Superman	232
Vertical Kicking	233
Kicking With One Arm Leading	233
Belly Button	233
Fingertip Drag	233
Eyes Closed	233
Rotation	234
Fist Swim	234
Downhill	235
Barrel	235
Counting Strokes	235
Sighting	235
Drafting	236
Catch-Up	236
Single-Arm Free	237
Contact	238
Open-Water Starts	238
Open-Water Swim Exits	238

DRILLS TO IMPROVE FREESTYLE SWIMMING SKILL

Drills are an excellent way to focus on one aspect of a technique and master it. Drills may focus on body position, breathing, pulling, the catch, recovery, and coordination. There is no such thing as a perfect swim drill, so it is essential to follow up drills with regular swimming so that bad habits do not appear during other parts of the swim stroke.

Superman

The athlete lies flat on the water's surface with the arms stretched out like Superman flying. The athlete floats in place with the chest slightly pressed into the water. The athlete should experiment to see how leaning with different amounts of pressure changes the balance. The goal is to be as horizontal as possible—the hips are high in the water, nearly level with the chest.

Vertical Kicking

The athlete is in the deep end of the pool. To start the drill, the athlete allows the body to rest vertically as if treading water with the hands crossed in front of the chest. Instruct the athlete to kick while staying in place and trying to hold the head, neck, and part of the shoulders above the water. The kick should be initiated from the hips, with the knees and ankles bending slightly.

Kicking With One Arm Leading

The athlete pushes off the wall and rotates to glide about 45 degrees toward the leading-arm side of the body, with the top arm at the side and the bottom arm reaching out in front of the body. The chin should be against the bottom shoulder, and the head should be rotated so the eyes look straight down at the bottom of the pool. The bottom armpit and ribcage are pressed into the water so that a lift is felt in the body, especially at the hips. The goal is to keep the hips level with the chest. The athlete then kicks the length of the pool smoothly, and when a breath is needed, the athlete should rotate the head only as much as is necessary to clear the mouth from the water. The athlete should then return the head to its original position.

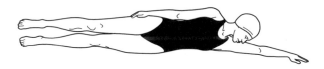

Belly Button

The athlete normally swims, concentrating on rotating from side to side. This cue can be used to help the athlete focus on the rotation: "Point your belly button toward the adjacent lanes or the side walls of the pool."

Fingertip Drag

This drill encourages the swimmer to use a relaxed arm recovery. The athlete swims normally, focusing on dragging the fingertips of the recovery arm across the water during the recovery portion of the stroke. The drill's effectiveness is enhanced if the athlete maintains a high elbow position (recovery arm).

Eyes Closed

This drill helps swimmers move in a straight line, avoid unnecessary wiggling, and get the sense of pulling the body forward over the anchor arm. Additionally, swimmers develop a sense of how the recovery arm aids forward motion. To perform the drill, athletes swim a length of the pool or a specific number of strokes with their eyes closed. Having counted strokes or length previously during sighted swimming helps reduce the odds of accidentally swimming into the pool wall.

Rotation

The athlete pushes off the wall into the home position. Next, the athlete takes a single stroke with the bottom arm, pausing when the pull is finished before the recovery starts. The figure demonstrates the sequence of actions that the athlete should take during the rotation. The athlete is now in the home position on the opposite side from the start of the drill. The athlete repeats the movement, rotating from side to side and pausing momentarily in the home position on each stroke.

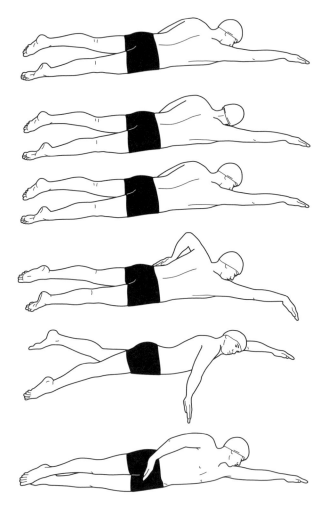

Fist Swim

This drill helps swimmers focus on pulling through the water with a vertical forearm. The athlete swims with a normal stroke but closes the hands into fists. This drill can be used as a game by having the athlete try to minimize the number of strokes per length of the pool. The lower the stroke count per length, the more effective the pull.

Downhill

The athlete swims normally, focusing on slightly pressing the chest into the water as if swimming downhill. Remind the athlete to focus on how the slight pressure keeps the hips high in the water and the body in a horizontal line.

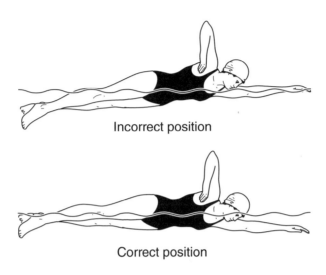

Incorrect position

Correct position

Barrel

The athlete swims with a normal stroke while pretending to reach over a submerged barrel as the hand enters the water, focusing on keeping the elbow high and grabbing and holding onto as much water as possible. The figure shows where the swimmer should imagine the barrel being located. Athletes should not attempt swimming over a barrel.

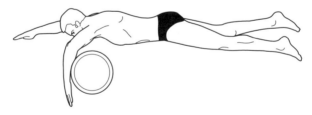

Counting Strokes

This drill aims to improve stroke efficiency by creating a game out of trying to take fewer strokes to cross the pool with the same pace. The athlete swims at the prescribed intensity and counts the strokes used to cover a specific distance with the goal of trying to reduce the number of strokes while maintaining the same speed over that same distance.

Sighting

This drill is best suited for open-water swimming, allowing the swimmer to become familiar with swimming in a straight line. The athlete swims, looking up every 8 to 12 strokes to look for the specified sight objects. Ensure the sight objects chosen are large and easily viewed during a short sight.

Drafting

Learning to draft can allow swimmers to swim faster and with less energy expenditure than they could alone. This drill requires multiple athletes. Begin the drill with the athletes swimming in a line or a small group. The goal is for the swimmers behind the lead swimmer to concentrate on staying as close as possible to the toes of the swimmer in front of them. Swimmers should take turns being the lead swimmer.

Catch-Up

This drill helps the swimmer slow down the pulling phase of the stroke, which helps the swimmer maintain horizontal balance. The athlete begins to swim normally but delays each pull until the opposite recovery hand enters the water. The athlete starts in the first position shown in the figure and then moves sequentially through the remaining positions.

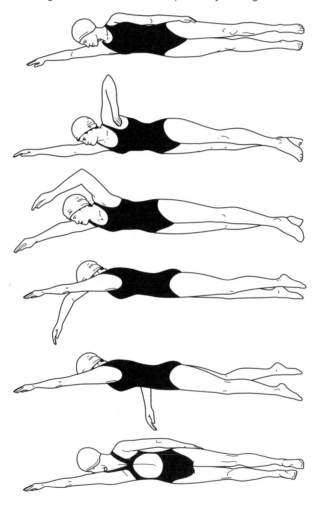

Single-Arm Free

The emphasis of this drill should be on rotating the body before initiating each pull and on pulling as much water as possible with each stroke. The athlete swims the length of the pool with one arm stroking and the other arm stretched out above the head in front of the body. Breathing should be done to the stroke-arm side. The athlete starts in the first position shown in the figure and then moves sequentially through the remaining positions.

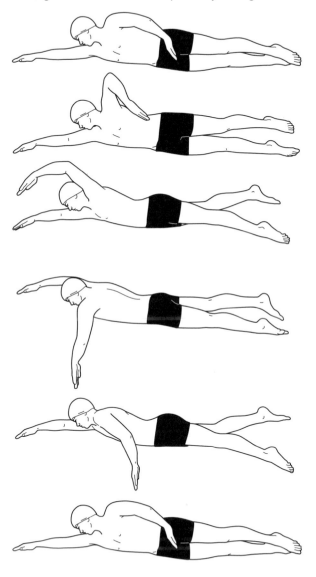

Contact

This drill is excellent preparation for the common contact during open-water swims or the swim segment of a triathlon. This drill requires multiple athletes. The drill begins with the athletes swimming as close as possible to each other. The incidental contact that will occur will mimic the contact between swimmers that may occur during open-water competition. Alternate swimmers in the middle of the group so that each athlete learns to experience contact with other swimmers.

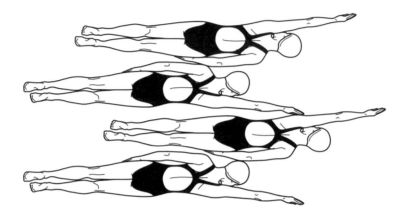

Open-Water Starts

Open-water swims and triathlons may begin on a dock or beach, in shallow water, or in water deep enough to require treading water while waiting for the start of the race. For dock starts, the swimmer should practice diving off a dock and settling into a good swimming pace as soon as possible. When scouting a location for practicing dock starts, check the water depth before diving headfirst. Depending on the season, water levels near docks may vary, and what initially appears to be deep water can turn out to be shallow on closer examination. To practice beach starts, the athlete begins on the beach about 15 feet (4.6 m) from the water and sprints into the water until it is not possible to run any farther. At this point, the athlete begins to swim, settling into a good pace as rapidly as possible. To practice shallow-water starts, the athlete should begin in approximately waist-deep water. The athlete dives or falls forward and begins swimming. Finally, to practice deep-water starts, the athlete begins by treading water for about 30 seconds before beginning to swim and settling into a steady pace.

Open-Water Swim Exits

This exercise begins with the athlete about 20 yards (18 m) from the land. The athlete swims toward the edge of the water. Once the water depth becomes too shallow for swimming, the athlete stands up and runs toward the ground, picking the feet up out of the water to reduce the chance of falling.

POOL-BASED TRAINING

A well-designed pool-based workout includes the following segments: warm-up (which may include drills), pre–main set, main set or sets, and cooldown. As with all workouts, starting with a good warm-up is important. For pool-based swimming workouts, this is accomplished by swimming 200 to 500 yards (183-457 m), building from an easy intensity to an intensity within the moderate domain. In many cases, using a drill set to start a workout is a way to simultaneously work on technique and warm up for the more difficult work.

Table 10.2 provides five examples of freestyle drill sets. Swimmers would perform one of the drill sets at the start of the workout. Because drills are

Table 10.2 Freestyle Drill Sets

Drill set 1	• Superman: 2 × 30 sec with a 10-sec rest interval • Vertical kicking: 2 × 30 sec with a 10-sec rest interval • Single-arm swim: 4 × 25 yards (23 m) alternating sides with no rest interval • 3 × 200 yards (183 m) as follows (with 10-sec rest intervals): - Belly button: 50 yards (46 m) - Fist: 50 yards (46 m) - Downhill: 50 yards (46 m) - Eyes closed: 50 yards (46 m)
Drill set 2	• 4 × 150 yards (137 m) as follows (with 10-sec rest intervals): - Rotation: 50 yards (46 m) - Belly button: 50 yards (46 m) - Regular swimming: 50 yards (46 m) • Vertical kicking: 2 × 30 sec with a 10-sec rest interval
Drill set 3	• Home position: 4 × 25 yards (23 m) alternating sides, no rest interval • 3 × 250 yards (229 m) as follows (with 10-sec rest intervals): - Fist: 50 yards (46 m) - Eyes closed: 50 yards (46 m) - Fingertip drag: 50 yards (46 m) - Regular swimming: 100 yards (91 m) • Single-arm swim: 4 × 25 yards (23 m) alternating sides, no rest interval
Drill set 4	• 3 × 200 yards (183 m) as follows (with 10-sec rest intervals): - Belly button: 50 yards (46 m) - Fist: 50 yards (46 m) - Downhill: 50 yards (46 m) - Eyes closed: 50 yards (46 m) - Sighting: 200 yards (46 m)
Drill set 5	• Open-water starts: 4 × each start type (shallow water, treading water, dock, beach) with 30-sec rest intervals • Open-water swim exits: 4 × exit

done at a moderate intensity, athletes can perform the drills without any prior warm-up. In this instance, the purpose of a drill set is to improve or refine technique and to warm up for the rest of the workout. All athletes can benefit from technique work, regardless of their current ability level. Using technique work as part of the warm-up process is a time-efficient method of organizing and executing workouts.

After the warm-up or drill set, the pre–main set is performed. This set focuses on preparing the athlete for the main set. Next come the main sets (endurance sets), which are the bulk of an athlete's workout and consist of regular, uninterrupted work periods or intervals. Finally, the athlete performs a cooldown. The cooldown should consist of about 200 to 500 yards (183-457 m) of swimming, decreasing from moderate to low intensity.

Descriptive intensity zones can help describe how athletes are to perform workouts. These zones are generally calculated from tests that athletes can perform in the lab or field. In this chapter, the intensity levels described within the example workouts are based on using an analog to critical power or critical speed called *CSS* (critical swim speed). CSS testing helps to calculate target training intensity zones based on the swimmer's current fitness level (2, 6). These swim intensity zones are based on speed, not heart rate.

To perform this CSS test, swim coaches Paul Newsome and Adam Young describe an excellent methodology (6):

- ▶ Swim 500 to 1,200 yards (457-1,097 m) (less well trained, lower end). This should include building from a comfortable pace to an effort that feels close to 80% before finishing with comfortable swimming for 100 to 200 yards (91-183 m).
- ▶ Swim a 400-yard or -meter time trial.
- ▶ Spend 10 to 15 minutes doing some light laps of the pool with 1- to 2-minute rest intervals between each lap.
- ▶ Swim a 200-yard or -meter time trial.
- ▶ Swim an easy cooldown of less than 500 yards or meters at a very comfortable effort.

Done well, CSS testing represents an effort similar to swimming a strong and fast 1,500- to 1,600-yard or -meter time trial (6). To calculate CSS use the following equation (the equation is shown using meters, but yards could be used as well):

$$CSS \text{ (m/sec)} = (400 - 200)/(T400 - T200)$$

T400 and T200 represent the time over those distances in seconds. With that calculated, convert to the time per 100 m segment via the following equation:

$$CSS \text{ (sec/100 m)} = 100/CSS \text{ (m/sec)}$$

Coaches and athletes also can use online calculators for CSS. Table 10.3 provides guidelines for determining intensity zones.

Table 10.3 Determining Swimming Intensity Zones

Intensity zones	Rough % of critical swim speed	Perceived effort
Zone 1	>107% or resting at pool edge	<50%
Zone 2	107%-103%	50%-65%
Zone 3	103%-101%	65%-75%
Zone 4	101%-98%	75%-80%
Zone 5	98%-92%	80%-90%
Zone 6	<92%	>90%

Reprinted by permission from P.F. Skiba, *Scientific Training for Endurance Athletes* (New Jersey, NJ: PhysFarm Training Systems, L.L.C., 2021), 80-81.

Newsome and Young have laid out a solid approach to estimating race times for various distances or events from CSS (6):

▶ 400 m: CSS 2-4 sec / 100 m

▶ 1,500-1,900 m: CSS pace / 100 m

▶ 3.5-5 km: CSS pace + 2-4 sec / 100 m

▶ 10 km: CSS pace + 6-10 sec / 100 m

▶ 20 km: CSS pace + 10-20 sec / 100 m (including fueling stops roughly every 20-30 min through the swim)

Coaches and athletes can design numerous pool workouts using the general workout structure and intensity zones described. Table 10.4 shows several workouts that could work well for shorter sprint or Olympic-distance triathletes, open-water swims up to 1.2 miles (1.9 km), or pool events of 400 to 1,600 meters or yards. The long workouts noted would be excellent for longer triathlons and open-water swimming events over 1.5 miles (2.4 km). The workouts can be tailored to meet the needs of individual athletes by adjusting the distances based on the ability levels and goals of the athlete. Note that this table is broken into sections on capacity and utilization. *Capacity* references improving the athlete's ability to go the distance or extend the distance they can cover and is a foundational quality for all endurance performances. *Utilization* refers to improving the rate an athlete can perform work per unit time (how fast they go) over a given distance. Refer to chapter 4 of this text for a more detailed description of these terms.

Some workouts in the pool can become more complex to cover the swimmer's abilities and create greater variation in the swimmer's program. Table 10.5 shows two examples of such workouts.

Table 10.4 Sample Capacity and Utilization Freestyle Pool Workouts

Capacity workout 1	• 4 × 150 yards (137 m) as follows (with 10-sec rest intervals):
	  - Rotation: 50 yards (46 m)
	  - Belly button: 50 yards (46 m)
	  - Regular swimming: 50 yards (46 m) in zone 2
	• Vertical kicking: 2 × 30 sec with a 10-sec rest interval
	• 6 × 25-yard (23 m) sprints, going as fast as possible with good form (do the first two at 90% and the rest at 100%)
	• Swim 6 × 300 yards (274 m) at zone 2 intensity with 15-sec rest intervals (rest at the wall for the rest intervals)
	• Cooldown: Swim 300 yards (274 m), descending from zone 2 to zone 1 intensity (may use mixed strokes)

Capacity workout 2	• Home position: 4 × 25 yards (23 m), alternating sides, with no rest interval
	• 3 × 250 yards (229 m) as follows (with 10-sec rest intervals):
	  - Fist: 50 yards (46 m)
	  - Fingertip drag: 50 yards (46 m)
	  - Regular swimming: 100 yards (91 m) in zone 2
	• Single-arm swim: 4 × 25 yards (23 m), alternating sides, no rest interval
	• 8 × 50-yard (46 m) sprints, going as fast as possible with good form (do the first two at 90% and the rest at 100%)
	• Swim 600, 500, 400, 300, 200, and 100 yards (549, 457, 366, 274, 183, 91 m) in zone 2 with 15-sec rest intervals
	• Cooldown: Swim 300 yards (274 m), descending from zone 2 to 1 intensity (may use mixed strokes)

Capacity workout 3	• 4 × 150 yards (137 m) as follows (with 10-sec rest intervals):
	  - Rotation: 50 yards (46 m)
	  - Belly button: 50 yards (46 m)
	  - Regular swimming: 50 yards (46 m)in zone 2
	• Vertical kicking: 2 × 30 sec with a 10-sec rest interval
	• 8 × 50-yard (46 m) intervals, starting in zone 4 and building to zone 5 over the set
	• Swim 2 × 500 yards (457 m) in zone 2 with a 15-sec rest interval
	• Swim 5 × 200 yards (183 m) in zone 2 with 15-sec rest intervals
	• Cooldown: Swim 300 yards (274 m), descending from zone 2 to 1 intensity (may use mixed strokes)

Utilization workout 1	• 3 × 200 yards (183 m) as follows (with 10-sec rest intervals):
	  - Belly button: 50 yards (46 m)
	  - Fist: 50 yards (46 m)
	  - Downhill: 50 yards (46 m)
	• Sighting: 200 yards (183 m)
	• 6-8 × 25-yard (23 m) sprints, going as fast as possible with good form (do the first two at 90% and the rest at 100%)
	• Swim 12 × 125 yards (114 m) in zone 4 with 30-sec rest intervals
	• Cooldown: Swim 300 yards (274 m), descending from zone 2 to 1 intensity (may use mixed strokes)

Utilization workout 2	• Superman: 2 × 30 sec with a 10-sec rest interval
	• Vertical kicking: 2 × 30 sec with a 10-sec rest interval
	• Single-arm swim: 4 × 25 yards (23 m), alternating sides, no rest interval
	• 3 × 200 yards (183 m) in zone 2 as follows (with 10-sec rest intervals):
	  - Belly button: 50 yards (46 m)
	  - Fist: 50 yards (46 m)
	  - Downhill: 50 yards (46 m)
	• 5-6 × 25-yard (23 m) sprints, going as fast as possible with good form (do the first two at 90% and the rest at 100%) with 60-sec rest intervals
	• Swim 4 × 300 yards (274 m) starting in zone 3 and building intensity to zone 4 with 30-sec rest intervals
	• Cooldown: Swim 300 yards (274 m), descending from zone 1 to 2 intensity (may use mixed strokes)

Utilization workout 3	• 4 × 150 yards (137 m) as follows (with 10-sec rest intervals):
	  - Rotation: 50 yards (46 m)
	  - Belly button: 50 yards (46 m)
	  - Regular swimming: 50 yards (46 m) in zone 2
	• Vertical kicking: 2 × 30 sec with a 10-sec rest interval
	• 8 × 50 yards (46 m) starting in zone 4 and building to zone 5 as the set progresses
	• Swim 4 × 200 yards (183 m) in zone 4 with 30-sec rest intervals
	• Swim 8 × 75 yards (69 m) in zone 5 with 60-sec rest intervals
	• Cooldown: Swim 300 yards (274 m), descending from zone 2 to 1 intensity (may use mixed strokes)

Long utilization workout 1 (pool)	• Warm-up: Swim 500 yards (457 m), building intensity from zone 1 to 2 • Swim 5 × 500 yards (457 m) with 1-min rest intervals (swim the first two in zone 2 and the last three at race intensity to 5% faster) • Cooldown: Swim 300 yards (274 m), descending from zone 2 to 1 intensity (may use mixed strokes)
Long capacity workout 2 (pool)	• Warm-up: Swim 500 yards (457 m), building intensity from zone 1 to 2 • Swim 4 × 1,000 yards (914 m) with 1-min rest interval (swim in zone 2, practicing sighting every 3-4 breath cycles) • Cooldown: Swim 300 yards (274 m), descending from zone 2 to 1 intensity (may use mixed strokes)

Table 10.5 Sample Complex Pool Swims

WORKOUT #1	
Warm-Up and Drill Set	• 1 × 400 (yards or meters) swim building from zone 1 to zone 2; 30 sec rest interval (RI, resting at the pool wall) • 12 × 50 in zone 2 as 25 kick and 25 drill; 20-30-sec RI • #1-3: 25 Rotation; 25 catchup • #4-6: 25 Kick on side one arm leading (right side); 25 kick on side one arm leading (left side). • #7-9: 25 belly button; 25 fingertip drag • #10-12: 25 barrel; 25 fist
Pre–Main Set	• 5 × 200 swim; 20-sec RI • Start with #1 easy, zone 2, and increase the intensity of each one, so that #4 and #5 are zone 3 increasing to zone 4 effort. Each 200 should be around 3-5 sec faster than the previous one. • 6 × 50 zone 1 increasing to zone 2; 30-sec RI
Main Set	• 4 × 500 swim; 30-sec RI • #1-3: Zone 3; each 500 should be within 3 sec of the others. Focus on equal intensity on each length of the 500. • #4: Start in zone 2 for the first 100, then increase the intensity with each 100, so that the last 100 is in zone 4. First 100: zone 2; second 100: zone 3; third 100: zone 3 increasing to zone 4; fourth 100: zone 3 increasing to zone 4; and the final 100 is zone 4.
Cooldown	• 200 in zone 1
WORKOUT #2	
Warm-Up and Drill Set	• 1 × 500 (yards or meters) swim: Start in zone 1 and build to zone 2; 20 sec RI • 12 × 25 drill • #1-3: Catch up • #4-7: Single arm free, switching arms every length • #8-10: Downhill • #11-12: Push off and swim 10 strokes of eyes closed drill; open eyes and finish the length.
Pre–Main Set	• 12 × 25 with 10-sec RI • #1-4: Zone 2 increasing to zone 3 • #5-8: Zone 3 increasing to zone 4 • #9-12: Zone 4 increasing to zone 5
Main Set	• 20 × 100 swim • Swim in zone 3, maintaining the same time on each as the rest interval decreases. • #1-5: 20-30 sec RI • #6-10: 15-20 sec RI • #11-18: 10 sec RI • #19-20: 30 sec RI, but swim fast at zone 4 or zone 5 • 16 × 25, where each one is half length in zone 5 or zone 6 and half length in zone 1 • RI = same duration as previous interval
Cooldown	• 200 in zone 1

OPEN-WATER TRAINING

Endurance swimmers benefit from open-water training. Specificity is a key component of good training, and because races are in open water, at least some of the swimmer's training should be in open water to allow practice during race like conditions. Open-water swimming is ideal for long workouts and a great opportunity to do specific drills: sighting, drafting, contact, and buoy turning. A good general framework for an open-water workout could include doing a drill set and then performing a continuous swim; the continuous swim could be done via a long steady swim at a low intensity around zone 1 or 2 or could include intervals at higher intensity or pace progressions to build race-specific fitness. Table 10.6 provides several sample open-water workouts that are oriented toward athletes competing in events with swims exceeding 1 mile (1.6 km) in length. For athletes taking part in shorter events, a 10% to 30% reduction in volume is appropriate. Likewise, athletes taking part in swims beyond 3 miles (4.8 km) would need to extend beyond these durations as they approached their peak events.

Table 10.6 Sample Long Open-Water Workouts

Workout 1	• Sighting: 5 min • Drafting: 5 min • Swim 40 min (first 20 min in zone 2, last 20 min at race intensity); throughout the swim, practice the sighting and drafting drills • Swim the final 3-5 min quickly, then, when back on land, walk for 5-10 min to cool down
Workout 2	• Open-water starts: 4 × each start type (shallow water, treading water, dock, beach) with 30-sec rest intervals • Open-water swim exits: 4 reps • Swim 1 hour (at a steady zone 2 intensity) • Back on land, walk for 5-10 min to cool down
Workout 3	• Swim for 1.5 hours at a consistent zone 2 level with a fellow swimmer; practice sighting and drafting throughout the swim • Back on land, walk for 5-10 min to cool down

As mentioned, open-water swimming is ideal for long workouts, but other workouts also can be done in open water. For capacity workouts, athletes swim continuously at a comfortable intensity. Utilization workouts can be less structured than in the pool because there is no pace clock or set distance. *Fartlek* workouts are an excellent option; the athlete swims for a total time or space with random intervals at higher intensity, generally zone 3 or above. A good example of an open-water fartlek workout, is swimming in zone 3 or above to a specific type of tree the swimmer can sight along the shore while swimming, recovering with easy zone 1 swimming or floating between intervals. Another fun fartlek done with a fellow swimmer is to swim 50 fast strokes (zone 4 or above) when the fellow swimmer decides to swim at a faster rate. This involves decision-making skills for both swimmers as they try to anticipate and react to their compatriot's changes in pace. Table 10.7 provides sample fartlek-style utilization workouts. Long workouts should be done in open water whenever possible. Pool workouts can be used when the athlete cannot do an open-water activity.

Table 10.7 Sample Open-Water Utilization-Focused Fartlek Workouts

Workout 1	• Swim for 1 hour • Start in zone 2, but include intervals of 1 to 3 min in zone 4-5 evenly distributed throughout the second half of the swim. Swim easily after each interval until ready to swim in zone 2 before the next higher-intensity interval.
Workout 2	• Swim for 75 min • Start in zone 2. Pick out 4-5 objects along the shore, swim to them in zone 4 or above, recovering quickly before returning to the base zone 2 intensity level.

Note: It is challenging to objectively determine intensity during open-water swimming. Thus, using effort to estimate intensity becomes a focus.

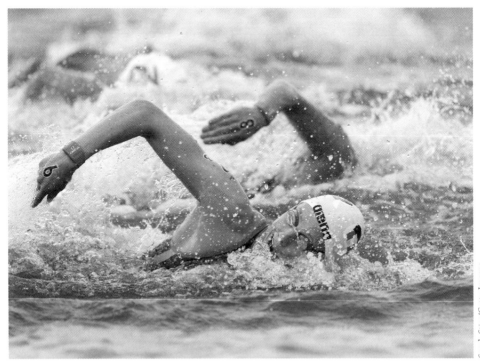

Sarah Stier/Getty Images

Athletes should prepare for the conditions of an open-water race by training in open water.

Cold water is commonly encountered during open-water swimming events. A wetsuit can help improve performance. A neoprene swim cap and booties can also be used in very cold conditions. If athletes expect to wear a wetsuit in a race, they should wear it for at least some of their ongoing training so that they become familiar with swimming in a wetsuit. Swimming in a wetsuit does provide additional flotation and results in faster paces. Additionally, open-water swimming is affected by weather and other natural phenomena such as currents. Within the bounds of safety, athletes should practice swimming in various conditions to ensure well-rounded preparation for their races.

After open-water swims, triathletes can practice swim-to-bike transitions. A mock transition area can be set up, and athletes can swim the final 20 to 100 yards or meters, exit the water, and practice transitioning to the bike. The athlete should also practice wetsuit removal if wetsuits are to be used during competition. Another option could be using a bicycle trainer on the pool deck (if allowed) or at a safe open-water location. This strategy can increase the number of transitions an athlete can perform within a workout.

USE OF VARIOUS WORKOUTS

Long workouts are the most specific workouts that can be used in training for endurance swimmers. These workouts should be considered vital training sessions. Typically, athletes should do one long workout a week (excluding rest weeks and taper phases). The length of these workouts should increase as the athletes approach their key races. Table 10.8 shows a sample progression of long swims for training for a triathlon with a 2.4-mile (3.9 km) swim. The table shows workouts for 11 weeks before the taper phase.

Table 10.8 Long Swims for a Triathlon With a 2.4-Mile (3.9 km) Swim

Week	Total time (min)	Time at race intensity in open water (min)	Pool alternative
1	30	20	4 × 400 yards (366 m), the last one at race intensity
2	40	25	5 × 500 yards (457 m), last two at race intensity
3	50	30	5 × 600 yards (549 m), last three at race intensity
4	Rest week		
5	40	30	5 × 600 yards (549 m), last two at race intensity
6	50	35	4 × 800 yards (732 m), last three at race intensity
7	60	40	4 × 900 yards (823 m), last three at race intensity
8	Rest week		
9	60	30	3 × 1,200 yards (1,097 m), the last one at race intensity
10	70	40	4 × 1,000 yards (914 m), last two at race intensity
11	80	50	4 × 1,200 yards (1,097 m), last three at race intensity

Triathletes typically should do two to four swimming workouts a week, with one utilization session and the remaining sessions various lengths of capacity-style training (see chapter 4 for capacity and utilization areas of focus). Open-water and ultradistance swimmers should do five or more weekly swimming workouts, including two utilization-themed workouts and multiple-length capacity sessions rounding out the weekly swim volume. Capacity workouts are less stressful than utilization workouts, which are higher intensity and require more time to recover. The ideal combination of capacity and utilization training provides an athlete with enough workout stress to stimulate improvement while avoiding underrecovery and potentially overtraining.

Table 10.9 provides a guide to the number and type of workouts that should be performed weekly for certain athletes and events, and table 10.10 includes sample workouts based on these recommendations. The movements presented are for age-group athletes beginning to train for these distances. Athletes who are more advanced or skilled may perform more workouts than shown. As mentioned earlier in the chapter, swim training for shorter-distance triathlons typically are completed a minimum of twice a week (the table indicates three workouts). As the event's distance increases and the athlete's performance level increases, so do the number of activities; this number may increase to as many as 10 to 12 for a high-level ultradistance swimmer.

Table 10.9 Sample Weekly Number and Types of Workouts for Various Athletes

Type of swimmer or event	Number and variety of workouts
Sprint-distance triathlete Race swim distance: Swim 0.2-0.5 miles (0.3-0.8 km)	Three workouts per week • 1 long capacity workout • 1 short capacity workout • 1 utilization workout
Olympic-distance triathlete Race swim distance: Swim 0.93 miles (1.5 km)	3-4 workouts per week • 1 long capacity workout • 1-2 short capacity workouts • 1 utilization workout
Long-distance triathlete Race swim distance: Swim 1.2-2.4 miles (1.9-3.9 km)	3-4 workouts per week • 1 long capacity workout • 1-2 short- to moderate-duration capacity workouts • 1 utilization workout
Ultradistance swimmer Race swim distance: 3-10+ miles (4.8-16+ km)	5 workouts per week* • 1 long capacity workout • 2-3 moderate capacity workouts • 2 utilization workouts

*Any additional workouts would be performed as capacity workouts to ensure recovery.

Table 10.10 Sample Training Weeks for Triathletes (Non-Elite) and Open-Water Swimmers

TYPE OF SWIMMER OR EVENT			
Sprint triathlon	**Olympic triathlon**	**Long-distance triathlon**	**Open-water or ultradistance swimmer***
Long workout			
Pool • Warm-up: Swim 500 yards (457 m), building from easy intensity to zone 2 • Swim 1 × 1,000 yards (914 m) in zone 2 • Cooldown: Swim 200 yards (183 m) easily Total: 1,700 yards (1,554 m)	Pool • Warm-up: Swim 500 yards (457 m), building from easy intensity to zone 2 • Swim 2 × 1,000 yards (914 m) with a 1-min rest interval (RI); first at zone 2, last at race intensity • Cooldown: Swim 300 yards (274 m) easily Total: 2,800 yards (2,560 m)	Open water • Open-water starts: 4 × each start type (shallow water, treading water, dock, beach) with 30-sec RI • Open-water race exits: 4 reps • Swim for 1 hour; first 20 min in zone 2, last 40 min at race intensity • Cooldown: Back on land, walk 10 min	Open water • Sighting: 5 min • Drafting: 5 min • Swim for 40 min; first 20 min in zone 2, last 20 min at race intensity Throughout the swim, practice the sighting and drafting drills • Cooldown: Back on land, walk 10 min
Aerobic intensity workout 1			
Pool • 3 × 150 yards (137 m) as follows (10-sec RI): - Rotation: 50 yards (46 m) - Belly button: 50 yards (46 m) - Regular swimming: 50 yards (46 m) • Vertical kicking: 2 × 30 sec with 10-sec RI • 4 × 25 yards (23 m) in zone 5 with 30-sec RI • Swim 2 × 300 yards (274 m) in zone 2 with 15-sec RI (rest at the wall) • Cooldown: Swim 150 yards (137 m), descending from zone 2 to zone 1 (may use mixed strokes) Total: 1,300 yards (1,189 m)	Pool • 4 × 150 yards (137 m) as follows (10-sec RI): - Rotation: 50 yards (46 m) - Belly button: 50 yards (46 m) - Regular swimming: 50 yards (46 m) • Vertical kicking: 2 × 30 sec with 10-sec RI • 4 × 25 yards (23 m) in zone 5 with 30-sec RI • Swim 3 × 300 yards (274 m) in zone 2 with 15-sec RI (rest at the wall) • Cooldown: Swim 200 yards (183 m), descending from zone 2 to zone 1 (may use mixed strokes) Total: 1,800 yards (1,646 m)	Pool • 4 × 150 yards (137 m) as follows (10-sec RI): - Rotation: 50 yards (46 m) - Belly button: 50 yards (46 m) - Regular swimming: 50 yards (46 m) • Vertical kicking: 2 × 30 sec with 10-sec RI • 6 × 25 yards (23 m) in zone 5 with 30-sec RI • Swim 6 × 300 yards (274 m) in zone 2 with 15-sec RI (rest at the wall) • Cooldown: Swim 300 yards (274 m), descending from zone 2 to zone 1 (may use mixed strokes) Total: 2,850 yards (2,606 m)	Pool • 4 × 150 yards (137 m) as follows (10-sec RI): - Rotation: 50 yards (46 m) - Belly button: 50 yards (46 m) - Regular swimming: 50 yards (46 m) • Vertical kicking: 2 × 30 sec with 10-sec RI • 8 × 50 yards (46 m) in zone 5 with 30-sec RI • Swim 2 × 500 yards (457 m) in zone 2 with 15-sec RI • Swim 5 × 200 yards (183 m) in zone 2 with 15-sec RI • Cooldown: Swim 300 yards (274 m), descending from zone 2 to zone 1 (may use mixed strokes) Total: 3,300 yards (3,018 m)

(continued)

Table 10.10 Sample Training Weeks for Triathletes (Non-Elite) and Open-Water Swimmers *(continued)*

TYPE OF SWIMMER OR EVENT			
Sprint triathlon	Olympic triathlon	Long-distance triathlon	Open-water or ultradistance swimmer*
Aerobic intensity workout 2			
		Pool • 4 × 150 yards (137 m) as follows (10-sec RI): - Rotation: 50 yards (46 m) - Belly button: 50 yards (46 m) - Regular swimming: 50 yards (46 m) • Vertical kicking: 2 × 30 sec with 10-sec RI • 6 × 50-yard (46 m) sprints, going as fast as possible with good form; do the first two at 90% and the rest at 100% • Swim 2 × 400 yards (366 m) in zone 2 with 15-sec RI • Swim 4 × 200 yards (183 m) in zone 2 with 15-sec RI • Cooldown: Swim 200 yards (183 m), descending from zone 2 to zone 1 (may use mixed strokes) Total: 2,700 yards (2,469 m)	Pool • Home position: 4 × 25 yards (23 m), alternating sides, no RI • 3 × 250 yards (229 m) as follows (10-sec RI): - Fist: 50 yards (46 m) - Fingertip drag: 50 yards (46 m) - Regular swimming: 100 yards (91 m) • Single-arm swimming: 4 × 25 yards (23 m), alternating sides, no RI • 8 × 50-yard (46 m) sprints, going as fast as possible with good form; do the first two at 90% and the rest at 100% • Swim 600, 500, 400, 300, 200, and 100 yards (549, 457, 366, 274, 183, 91 m) in zone 2 with 15-sec RI Total: 3,450 yards (3,155 m)

TYPE OF SWIMMER OR EVENT			
Sprint triathlon	Olympic triathlon	Long-distance triathlon	Open-water or ultradistance swimmer*
Anaerobic intensity workout 1			
Pool • 3 × 150 yards (137 m) as follows (10-sec RI): - Rotation: 50 yards (46 m) - Belly button: 50 yards (46 m) - Regular swimming: 50 yards (46 m) • Vertical kicking: 2 × 30 sec with 10-sec RI • 4 × 50 yards (46 m) in zone 5 with 30-sec RI • Swim 3 × 150 yards (137 m) in zone 4 or above with 30-sec RI • Swim 4 × 75 yards (69 m) in zone 4 or above with 30-sec RI • Cooldown: Swim 200 yards (183 m), descending from zone 2 to zone 1 (may use mixed strokes) Total: 1,600 yards (1,463 m)	Pool • 4 × 150 yards (137 m) as follows (10-sec RI): - Rotation: 50 yards (46 m) - Belly button: 50 yards (46 m) - Regular swimming: 50 yards (46 m) • Vertical kicking: 2 × 30 sec with 10-sec RI • 4 × 50 yards (46 m) in zone 5 with 30-sec RI • Swim 4 × 150 yards (137 m) in zone 4 or above with 30-sec RI • Swim 6 × 75 yards (69 m) in zone 4 or above with 30-sec RI • Cooldown: Swim 200 yards (183 m), descending from zone 2 to zone 1 (may use mixed strokes) Total: 2,050 yards (1,875 m)	Pool • Superman: 2 × 30 sec with 10-sec RI • Vertical kicking: 2 × 30 sec with 10-sec RI • Single-arm swim: 4 × 25 yards (23 m), alternating sides, no RI • 3 × 200 yards 183 m) as follows (10-sec RI): - Belly button: 50 yards (46 m) - Fist: 50 yards (46 m) - Downhill: 50 yards (46 m) - Eyes closed: 50 yards (46 m) • 10 × 25 yards (23 m) in zone 5 with 30-sec RI • Swim 4 × 300 yards (274 m) in zone 4 or above with 30-sec RI • Cooldown: Swim 300 yards (274 m), descending from zone 2 to zone 1 (may use mixed strokes) Total: 2,450 yards (2,240 m)	Pool or open water • Swim 1 hour - Start in zone 1 building to zone 2 lightly, but during the swim include 10 intervals of 1 to 3 min in zone 4 or above at the swimmer's discretion, swimming zone 2 after each of them
Anaerobic intensity workout 2			
			Pool or open water • Swim for 1 hour and 15 min - Start aerobically, but during the swim, include 8 intervals of 3 to 5 min in zone 4 or above at the swimmer's discretion, swimming aerobically after each of them

*More than five workouts per week.

In general, all triathlon training should include one long swim. Shorter-distance triathlon training should consist of two additional workouts—one in zone 1-2 and the second in zone 3 or above. At higher performance levels and longer distances, up to three other low-intensity capacity workouts could be included if the athlete can recover well from those sessions within the scope of their broader training program. Chapter 11 of this book provides more information specifically about triathlon training for a variety of events.

ULTRADISTANCE TRAINING

Athletes training for ultradistance swims must consider other training factors in addition to those previously discussed. Because the races can be 3 to 10 or more miles (5-16 km) in length, training must focus on developing high capacity for work, efficiency, and fatigue resistance.

Here are some key training factors for ultradistance swimmers:

1. To complete an ultradistance swim, athletes must use a high training volume at lower intensities (zones 1-2).

2. Achieving a high training volume requires a high training frequency. Athletes may need to complete swims twice a day for most days of the training week.

3. Athletes should use long workouts to prepare them for racing. For example, a swimmer training for a 5-mile (8 km) swim should perform long workouts that build up to very near that distance.

Table 10.11 shows a sample progression of long swims. This table shows the long workouts for the 11 weeks before the taper phase of the race. All of these long workouts should be done at approximately race intensity, which, given duration, will end up between zones 2 and 4 depending on athlete level, course conditions, and competition level. The table focuses on athletes competing in races from 3 miles (5 km) up to ultramarathon or distance races of 6 or more miles (10 km) in duration.

Table 10.11 Sample Progression of Long Swims

Week	Total time
1	1 hour
2	1 hour and 30 min
3	2 hours
4	Rest week
5	1 hour and 30 min
6	2 hours
7	2 hours and 30 min
8	Rest week
9	2 hours
10	2 hours and 30 min
11	3 hours

CHAPTER 11

Triathlon

Krista Schultz

This chapter focuses on training for a triathlon. Triathlon training presents unique differences when compared to training for a single sport, which can make coaching triathletes challenging. However, understanding the differences between single-sport and multisport endurance training helps the coach tie in relevant concepts, drills, and workouts for swimming, biking, and running from previous chapters to simplify triathlon training program design.

HISTORY

First, a brief history of triathlon provides perspective on how particular triathlon distances came about. According to the international governing body for the sport of triathlon and all related multisport, the first official triathlon was held in San Diego, California, in 1974 and featured a 1.5-mile (2.4 km) swim, a 10-mile (16 km) bike ride, and a 3-mile (5 km) run (20). The first-ever Hawaiian Ironman Triathlon was in 1978. The 140.6-mile (226.3 km) event was a combination of three of the toughest endurance races in Hawaii and consisted of 2.4 miles (3.8 km) of swimming, 112 miles (180 km) of cycling, and 26.2 miles (42 km) of running (19). The first triathlon held at an Olympics was in Sydney, Australia, in 2000 and included a 1,500 meter (0.9 mile) swim, 40 kilometer (24.8 mile) bike ride, and 10 kilometer (6.2 mile) run. Since then, the sport has continued to evolve, with the introduction of new distances and formats such as mixed relay, aquabike (swim and bike), off-road triathlon, and separate categories and events for youth and paratriathletes (20).

TRIATHLON DISTANCES

Today triathlons have many distance variations, and athletes compete against others in their age group and sex. Pros often race alongside amateurs too.

Common distances include the short or sprint distance; intermediate distance, which includes the Olympic distance (also referred to as the *international distance*); long distance, which includes the 70.3-mile (113.1 km) distance; and ultradistance, which includes the 140.6-mile (226.3 km) distance, as shown in table 11.1 (18).

Table 11.1 Triathlon Race Distances

Name	Swim distances	Bike distances	Run distances
Short/sprint	0.25-0.62 miles (0.4-1 km)	5-18.6 miles (8-30 km)	1-3.9 miles (1.6-6.3 km)
[a]Intermediate	0.63-1.25 miles (1.1-2 km)	18.7-31 miles (30.1-50 km)	4-8 miles (6.4-12.8 km)
[b]Long	1.26-1.9 miles (2.1-3.1 km)	31.1-62 miles (50.1-99.9 km)	8.1-18.5 miles (12.9-29.9 km)
[c]Ultra	≥2.0 miles (≥3.2 km)	≥62 miles (≥100 km)	≥18.6 miles (≥30 km)

[a]Includes the Olympic or international distance. [b]Includes the 70.3-mile (113.1 km) distance. [c]Includes the 140.6-mile (226.3 km) distance.

From Team USA Triathlon. Available: https://www.teamusa.org/USATriathlon/About/Multisport/Disciplines/Triathlon.

PRINCIPLES OF TRAINING

Before designing a triathlon training program, it is important to understand some key principles that will help guide workout prescription. Table 11.2 summarizes this.

Table 11.2 Key Workout Principles

Principle	Description
Adaptation	Fitness is achieved by adapting to a physical (exercise) stimulus. To progress, an athlete needs to increase the stimulus by progressively overloading through more volume or intensity, or both.
Consistency	Consistency in performing sport-specific exercises is essential for improving.
Individuality	The individual response and individual adaptation to exercise will differ between athletes. As such, the training plan might need adjustment on an individual basis.
Periodization	Periodization means breaking down a training and racing season into distinct blocks of time that each have a specific focus relative to when the target event takes place.
Specificity	Training must stress the body systems critical for optimal performance to achieve the desired adaptations. In other words, as the event gets closer, training becomes more race-like.

Adapted from Herda and Cramer (2016); French (2016); Haff (2007).

DESIGNING A TRAINING PROGRAM

"We are training all the time (whether we realize it or not). The world is our laboratory. We have the opportunity to experiment and learn in every moment."

—David Glover, MS, CSCS

When it comes to triathlon training, designing a training program is critical to achieving success. Overall, creating an effective triathlon training program requires a holistic approach that considers both the big-picture goals and the individual factors that contribute to an athlete's performance. It involves several subcategories that are equally important. Selecting an event is imperative because it determines the specific type of training required and helps assess the practicality of the required training volume based on the athlete's level. Once the event is chosen, developing an annual plan comes next, which entails outlining the training phases leading up to the event, including building aerobic endurance, muscular strength, and speed. Adding other races to the schedule is also essential because it provides opportunities for practice and skill development. Structuring a week to determine which days to do swim, bike, and run sessions, as well as incorporating recovery and rest, is crucial to progress and avoiding injury. Training tools such as heart rate monitors, power meters, and GPS watches are valuable for determining training intensities. Field testing, such as time trials and threshold testing, can help determine fitness levels and set appropriate training zones. In summary, a well-designed training program that incorporates all of these elements is essential for achieving success in triathlon training.

Selecting an Event

Developing a training plan begins with selecting a race and establishing the athlete's goals. Although some of the same considerations apply when goal setting for a single sport, triathlon involves additional considerations. Whether the athlete has a coach, has a training plan, or is self-coached, a goals questionnaire is helpful in determining specific training needs.

When selecting races, it is important for the athlete to consider not only goals but also the practicality of achieving those goals. Athletes should consider things like time availability, family obligations, financial impact, recovery, event locations, and motivation. Some key questions to consider are as follows:

▶ Does the athlete have a busy work schedule and family life, and would training for a triathlon be practical considering life priorities?

▶ Does the athlete need a bike, running shoes, or other equipment that will factor into the cost of training and racing?

> ▶ Does the athlete have the knowledge and motivation to train on their own, or do they need a training plan, coach, group workouts, or training partner?
>
> ▶ Are the events the athlete wants to do local (or within driving distance), or do they require flights and other travel plans?
>
> ▶ Do the race conditions and terrain require specific training? For example, if the bike course in a race is hilly, the athlete will want to be able to train on hilly terrain or train on an indoor bicycle with the ability to add resistance to simulate hills. If they are coming from sea level and racing at a higher altitude, they need to understand how lower levels of oxygen will affect their body (15).

Peak Training Volume for Goal Race Distance

Training week volume (total workout time) will depend on the athlete and a number of factors including their athletic background, triathlon experience, current fitness level, goals, race distance(s), time availability to train, history of injury, and so on. Here are some general guidelines that may need to be adjusted depending on the athlete: Amateur triathletes can expect to train for a sprint distance in 3 to 5 hours per week and for an Olympic distance in 5 to 8 hours a week. While some athletes training for full or half-distance triathlons can handle up 16 to 18 hours a week, this much training is not realistic for most athletes on a sustainable basis. A reasonable target might be 8 to 10 hours per week for a half and 10 to 13 hours per week for a full-on average. An athlete can generally train more distance in a workout than the lengths of the sprint and Olympic distances but should be careful adding extra mileage to the half and full distances. For example, when training for an ultradistance (e.g., 140.6 miles [226.3 km]) triathlon, the athlete does not need to bike more than 100 miles (161 km) or run more than 18 miles (29 km) in training. Athletes may experience psychological benefits from doing the full distance of a 26.2-mile (42.2 km) running marathon in training, for example, but their risk of injury, overtraining, and burnout also increases.

Weekly volume should start with where the athlete is currently at and increase gradually over time. Suddenly increasing training volume from 5 hours per week to 20 hours per week, for example, could be counterproductive and will increase risk of injury (17). For athletes attempting a triathlon or a longer race distance for the first time, it is advisable to prioritize caution and begin with a lower volume and intensity while still ensuring sufficient training to prepare for the event. For example, if the athlete is increasing from an Olympic-distance triathlon to a long-distance triathlon, training at least 8 hours and less than 15 hours per week can significantly decrease the risk for injuries (10).

Coaches should consider the athlete's total training hours year over year when determining the maximum training volume. By gradually increasing training volume over time, athletes can optimize their training and decrease chances of overtraining and injury (17).

A triathlete's training plan is commonly developed at the end of a previous competitive or training year after some time away from the sport and rest from a workout regimen. The typical triathlon race season occurs from late spring to the middle of fall. When structured training resumes, low duration and intensity is recommended during this time (7).

Developing an Annual Plan

To prepare athletes for peak performance, their training will include a cycle of progressive workloads followed by recovery, a concept called *periodization*. The same principles of periodization that were discussed in previous chapters also hold true for triathlon training programs except now three endurance sports need to be balanced appropriately within the program. Periodization is an effective way to improve athletic performance by providing a structured approach to training that helps avoid overtraining, burnout, and injury, and allows for optimal recovery and adaptation (7, 15).

Periodization is a structured approach to training that divides the training program into distinct periods or phases, each with a specific focus and purpose. In triathlon training, these periods include the base period, build period, peak period, taper period, and transition period. The *base period* (also called the *preparatory period* or *off-season*; see chapter 3) is a time for developing a strong foundation of endurance, skill, and technique, typically with lower-intensity and higher-volume training. The *build period* (also called the *precompetition period* or *preseason*; see chapter 3) follows the base period and involves gradually increasing intensity and reducing volume to develop race-specific fitness. The *taper period* involves reducing volume significantly while maintaining intensity to allow for optimal recovery and adaptation leading up to the race. The *peak period* (also called the *competition period*; see chapter 3) is when athletes aim to achieve their highest level of performance, with high-intensity training and race simulations. Finally, the *transition* (also called the *postseason*; see chapter 3) is a period of relative rest after peak form is reached, with a temporary regression of conditioning. Understanding these critical terms and their roles within periodization can help triathletes optimize their training and achieve their race goals (7, 13, 15).

For novice athletes who are preparing for their inaugural event, reaching peak performance may not be their primary goal. Nevertheless, completing the race within a specific time frame or simply finishing the distance necessitates that the body be well-rested and adequately prepared on race day.

The athletes' annual plan, including the training periods or phases leading up to their goal races is called a *macrocycle* and lasts several months or longer. The specific length and frequency of a macrocycle depends on the length of the athlete's race season (7). The macrocycle is broken down into smaller training periods called *mesocycles*, which focus on different aspects of training performance and normally lasts about 3 to 6 weeks. For example, a mesocycle can focus on aerobic endurance, strength endurance, or power endurance and for triathletes can be discipline specific such as developing run endurance or cycling power (13). Mesocycles are broken down into *microcycles*, which are smaller training phases that represent a training week. The details of the microcycle or week plan depend on the focus of the mesocycle (13).

Think of training like a funnel based on the principle of *specificity* as depicted in figure 11.1. The further away from an event the athlete is, the more nonspecific the training can be. As the athlete gets closer, the training becomes more focused on that event.

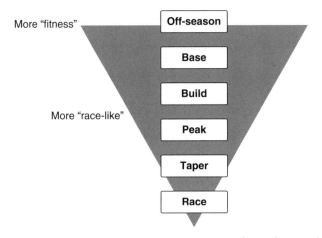

Figure 11.1 The "funnel" concept describing the principles of specificity and periodization.

High-level athletes such as Olympic competitors have a goal of continuous improvement over several years based on their goal event and would follow a bigger-picture, multiyear plan. The annual or year plan in this case would be designed to align with the multiyear plan (13).

Adding Other Races to the Schedule

Ideally, athletes should plan to do shorter distance training races before a goal race. A training race allows athletes to practice race-day execution and to prepare the body for the demands of racing while giving them an idea of their current fitness. Athletes can also use races such as 10-kilometer runs and sprint triathlons as speed workouts leading up to longer races and can substitute a race for one of their weekend workouts. Athletes should do a mini taper (1-3 days of reduced training volume) leading up to a race and take a recovery day after if needed. Table 11.3 gives examples of when to add training races based on the goal race distance.

Table 11.3 When to Add Training Races

Goal race distance	Training race distance	Weeks before goal race
[a]Ultra	[b]Long	5-8
[a]Ultra	Olympic	2-4
[b]Long	Olympic or sprint	2-6
Olympic	Sprint	2-6

[a]Includes the 140.6-mile (226.3 km) distance. [b]Includes the 70.3-mile (113.1 km) distance.

Another helpful chart for event planning is figure 11.2, which depicts race-to-race spacing guidelines based on race distance.

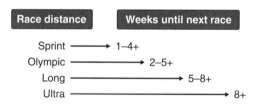

Figure 11.2 Race-to-race spacing guidelines.

An example of race spacing for an ultradistance triathlete is shown in figure 11.3.

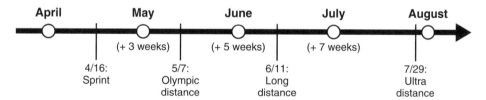

Figure 11.3 Example of race-to-race spacing guidelines for an ultradistance triathlete.

Table 11.4 gives examples of an annual triathlon training plan integrating the concept of periodization and race-to-race spacing guidelines.

Table 11.4 Annual Training Plan Example Including Race-to-Race Spacing Guidelines and Training Focus Based on Periodization

Client:	55-year-old male			
Profile	Six years of triathlon experience up to the intermediate distance. Competing in an ultradistance triathlon in July. Works full-time (1-2 hours available during week) with weekends available for longer training sessions.			
Season goals	1. Qualify for world championships 2. Complete a half-marathon in April as confidence builder 3. Complete a long-distance triathlon in June and practice pacing			
Focus	**Date (week of)**	**Period**	**Events**	**Goals**
Half-marathon (running race)	3/11	Base		Build base + improve strength
	3/18	Base	3/21-3/24: family travel	Easier week (travel)
	3/25	Base		Build base + improve strength
	4/1	Base		Build base + improve strength
	4/8	Peak		Begin taper
	4/15	Taper		Taper
	(4/21)	—	Event day	Race!
Long-distance triathlon	4/22	Transition		Easy
	4/29	Build		Race-specific training
	5/6	Build		Taper
	5/13	Build		Bigger bike week
	5/20	Peak		Peak week
	5/27	Taper		Begin taper
	6/3	Taper		Taper
	(6/9)	—	Event day	Race!

Structuring a Week

Structuring a week for three different sports is challenging because the athlete cannot spend as much time on one sport as a single-sport athlete does; therefore the activities need to be spread out strategically while incorporating recovery.

The principle of specificity of training stipulates that to improve performance in a specific sport or activity, the training must be designed to mimic the specific demands of that activity (9). According to this principle, training requirements for all distance triathlons should include a variation of swim, bike, run, plus back-to-back workouts such as combining bike and run sessions (known as a *brick* workout) in the weeks leading up to the race. The goal of a brick workout is to help the athlete adapt to running immediately after biking in a race.

The athlete should go into a long or interval workout well rested and take at least a day in between these sessions, if possible, which makes it challenging to spread out these types of workouts for three different sports while also including resistance training to improve strength. Also consider that many athletes have full-time jobs and must do long workouts on the weekends. Most seasoned triathletes have a typical weekly routine with a swim, bike, run, and resistance training schedule that provides a good starting point for fine-tuning the training program. Further, athletes can train with other groups such as master's swimming, local running clubs, and strength and yoga classes, which can provide additional coaching and motivation.

Training *consistency* is a concept that involves repeating similarly-structured training sessions, week to week, for a period of time and results in performance improvement. The literature suggests that it takes about 5 to 12 similar sessions for an athlete to make the necessary physiological adaptations that result in fitness gains (14). Based on the number of sessions it takes for the body to adapt to a specific training stimulus and using a 3 to 6 week training cycle or mesocycle, two or three workouts per week per activity (swim, bike, run) is an ideal workout frequency (14).

Following are examples of how to spread out swim, bike, run, and resistance training sessions depending on when athletes can accomplish longer workout sessions, with the goal of achieving two or three workouts per week per activity. Sample training plans that provide specific workouts are detailed later in this chapter. The purpose of the following tables is to break down the planning and show a structured approach to building a training program. By starting with this approach, coaches can ensure that they cover the basics of mapping out weekly swim, bike, and run sessions in a balanced way. While the structure may vary depending on the athlete's time availability, level, and goal races, having a framework in place provides a solid foundation for an effective and tailored training plan.

Table 11.5, which is for the athlete who needs less frequency of training, is an example of how to spread out two workouts per week per activity, with long workouts on the weekend. Table 11.6, which is for the athlete who needs a higher frequency of training, is an example of how to spread out three workouts per week per activity plus a brick, with long workouts on weekends. Table 11.7, which is for the athlete who needs less frequency of training, is an example of how to spread out two workouts per week per activity, with long workouts during the week. Table 11.8, which is for the athlete who needs a higher frequency of training, is an example of how to spread out three workouts per week per activity plus a brick, with long workouts during the week.

Table 11.5 Sample Weekly Workout Structure A (lower frequency and lower volume during the week)

Workout	Mon	Tue	Wed	Thurs	Fri	Sat	Sun
Swim		✓			✓		
Bike			✓			✓ (long)	
Run				✓			✓ (long)
Resistance training			✓				✓

Table 11.6 Sample Weekly Workout Structure B (higher frequency and lower volume during the week)

Workout	Mon	Tue	Wed	Thurs	Fri	Sat	Sun
Swim		✓		✓	✓		
Bike			✓		✓	✓ (long)	
Run		✓ (intervals)		✓		✓ (brick)	✓ (long)
Resistance training	✓		✓				✓

Table 11.7 Sample Weekly Workout Structure C (lower frequency and lower volume during the weekend)

Workout	Mon	Tue	Wed	Thurs	Fri	Sat	Sun
Swim		✓				✓	
Bike			✓ (long)				✓
Run	✓			✓ (long)			
Resistance training				✓			✓

Table 11.8 Sample Weekly Workout Structure D (higher frequency and lower volume during the weekend)

Workout	Mon	Tue	Wed	Thurs	Fri	Sat	Sun
Swim	✓				✓		✓
Bike	✓	✓ (long)				✓	
Run		✓ (brick)	✓ (long)		✓ (intervals)		✓
Resistance training			✓	✓		✓	

Intensity

Training intensity can be measured by a variety of methods including using *rate of perceived effort* (RPE)—that is, how the athlete feels—a heart rate monitor, a certain pace or speed (for the swim and run), or a power meter (bike only).

Using a heart rate monitor in combination with RPE or a power meter for bike workouts and RPE with pacing for swim workouts will provide more feedback.

Training *zones* are given within a workout to differentiate the levels of intensity (effort) that the athlete should be at during each workout. Training at different levels of intensity stimulates different training adaptation responses and can be an effective tool to optimize training time so that training adaptation becomes more specific to the goal while minimizing the risk of overtraining, burnout, and injury (6).

Subjectively Measuring Exercise Intensity

Subjectively measuring exercise intensity using an RPE scale (table 11.9) is a useful tool for athletes who do not have access to heart rate monitors, power meters, or GPS watches or when those tools or equipment malfunction. The scale allows athletes to quantify their intensity by assigning numerical values or ranges to their perceived effort during exercise. Further, it considers an array of different variables that cannot always be measured with a piece of equipment.

Table 11.9 Rating of Perceived Exertion Scale With Definitions

Rating	Description
1	Nothing at all (lying down)
2	Extremely little
3	Very easy
4	Easy (could do this all day)
5	Moderate
6	Somewhat hard (starting to feel it)
7	Hard
8	Very hard (making an effort to keep up)
9	Very, very hard
10	Maximum effort (can't go any further)

Reprinted by permission from M. Martino and N.C. Dabbs, "Aerobic Training Program Design," in *NSCA's Essentials of Personal Training*, 3rd ed., edited for the National Strength and Conditioning Association by B.J. Schoenfeld and R.L. Snarr (Champaign, IL: Human Kinetics, 2022), 432.

A potential pitfall of training by perceived exertion is that it is a subjective measurement—it is the athlete's own self-evaluation (12). Athletes who train only by perceived exertion may not have developed a good feel for their optimal level of effort as compared to their desired level of effort that they can perform at during an event. To become more effective at using perceived exertion, athletes should pay attention to how their body feels when training and racing. Athletes should ask themselves these questions as they exercise:

▶ How hard am I breathing?
▶ How much force am I using to pedal?
▶ How fast are my legs turning over during my run?

- ▶ How do my muscles feel?
- ▶ Do my arms or legs feel heavy?
- ▶ Can I accelerate to pick up speed if needed?
- ▶ How long can I maintain this effort?

With experience, athletes can develop a feel for each intensity level and use RPE as an effective training and racing tool.

Using Tools to Measure Intensity

Besides RPE, several tools are available to measure training intensity and establish training zones, including heart rate, power for cycling, and pace for speed. By using these tools effectively, athletes can optimize their training.

Using Heart Rate   Heart rate is an inexpensive, convenient, and effective method of monitoring intensity because it increases linearly as intensity increases until it reaches a maximum level, making it relatively easy to use to set training zones based on heart rate ranges.

However, heart rate also has its limitations, because factors such as race anxiety, caffeine, fatigue, and hydration levels can influence heart rate up or down. It is important to remember that the heart rate response to changing intensity is not immediate, so using a heart rate monitor in conjunction with perceived exertion can be a powerful tool. Although it can be valuable for athletes to pay attention to their heart rate and see how it reacts in different situations, athletes should not become too reliant on their monitoring device.

Using Power for Cycling   *Power* (usually measured in watts) is a direct measure of the work output that the athlete's legs produce while cycling. Measurement is instantaneous (versus heart rate, which lags effort) and accurate without the subjectivity of perceived effort. The athlete should be sure to calibrate the power meter before using if possible. The athlete can also use a power meter to measure training intensity and set the training zones.

Using Pace or Speed   Pace and speed are measures of how fast the athlete is going. Pace is typically expressed as miles (or kilometers) per hour for biking, minutes per mile (or per kilometer) for running, and time per 100 meters (or yards) for swimming. The athlete can also set the run training zones based on pace ranges.

Keep in mind that pace will vary on uneven terrain while biking and running, and the athlete should expect to go slower uphill and faster downhill at the same level of effort or intensity.

Using Training Zones to Measure Intensity

To simplify specifying training intensity, athletes can use a system of five training zones, ranging from zone 1 (very easy) to zone 5 (very hard), with each zone corresponding to increasing levels of intensity. Within each zone, a " – " or " + " can be used to denote the low or high end of the range, respectively, to provide greater specificity in training intensity (6).

Table 11.10 is an example of how training zones (1 to 5) can be referenced against the RPE scale shown in table 11.9.

Table 11.10 Training Zones Referenced Against an RPE Scale

Zone	RPE (1-10 scale)	Description
—	1	Nothing at all (lying down)
1	2	Extremely little
1+	3	Very easy
2	4	Easy (could do this all day)
2+	5	Moderate
3	6	Somewhat hard (starting to feel it)
3+	7	Hard
4	8	Very hard (making an effort to keep up)
5	9	Very, very hard
5+	10	Maximum effort (can't go any further)

Adapted Friel and Vance (2013); Martino and Dabbs (2022).

Heart rate, power, and pace or speed training zones can be determined by either physiological testing in a lab or by simple field tests for swim, bike, and run.

Determining the Training Zones With Physiological Lab Testing Physiological testing by a qualified exercise physiologist using a metabolic cart to measure $\dot{V}O_2$max or a blood lactate analyzer to measure blood lactate is a controlled means of developing specific, individualized training zones.

Testing may be inconvenient and moderately expensive, but it does provide a greater degree of precision than field tests. If the athlete has easy access to testing, testing with a qualified tester (preferably someone with a college degree in exercise physiology or a related field and with experience testing endurance athletes) is helpful. The following are recommendations regarding lab testing (6):

▶ Perform the tests for the bike and the run separately (and on separate days) because the resulting zones may be different.

▶ Have the athlete go into the test well-rested from training. Any workouts the day before the test should be very light.

▶ Instruct the athlete to avoid eating or consuming caffeine for 3 hours before the test and to show up well hydrated.

Determining the Training Zones With Field Tests Triathletes can conduct field tests to estimate their training zones without the need for specialized equipment or testing facilities. To do a field test, the athlete must perform a specific exercise protocol including a warm-up and maximum sustainable effort for a set period, such as a 20-minute time trial on the bike. The athlete then records the average heart rate or power output for the 20 minutes and uses this value to estimate the lactate threshold heart rate or power output. From there, training zones can be established based on a percentage of this lactate threshold value. Selecting appropriate field test protocols specific to swimming, cycling, and running is crucial to accurately estimating training zones for triathletes. For swimming, an athlete can perform a 1,000-meter (or yard) time trial in a pool and calculate training zones based on a percentage of the athlete's swim pace or speed. For running the athlete can do a 30-minute time trial at maximal effort, with training zones based on a percentage of the athlete's lactate threshold heart rate or running pace (6). Chapter 2 has more information on field and laboratory testing for athletes.

In addition, it is crucial to tailor the tests to an athlete's experience and fitness level by adjusting the length or intensity of the test. For instance, novice athletes can benefit from modifying the test to match their capability by shortening the distance and exerting moderate effort. By projecting longer distances from this modified test, beginners can gauge their progress and gradually increase their stamina. This approach is like performing a 10-repetition maximum (10RM) instead of a 1-repetition maximum (1RM) in resistance training. By consistently adhering to these guidelines and conducting regular field tests, triathletes can precisely establish and fine-tune their training zones, ultimately maximizing their performance potential (6).

TRAINING CONSIDERATIONS

"Nobody is perfect, so don't expect perfection in training. Do your best, don't self-flagellate if you have a bad workout, and most importantly: Have fun."
—Joanna Zeiger, MS, PhD

Carefully planned workouts, implemented into an athlete's weekly workout structure, will help increase the efficiency and effectiveness of their training. It is important for athletes to find the right balance between structure and flexibility in their workout plan, taking into consideration their individual goals, abilities, and needs. A well-designed workout plan can be a valuable tool for improving athletic performance, but it is essential to be adaptable and open to making changes when necessary.

When implementing a workout plan for a triathlete, it is important to consider factors such as injury prevention and the inclusion of resistance training, which was shown in the sample weekly workout structure in tables 11.5 through 11.8, along with swim, bike, run, and brick workouts. Injury prevention should be a top priority, because any setbacks can derail progress and lead to longer recovery times. Incorporating resistance training can improve overall strength and help prevent injuries, making it a valuable addition to any training plan. Missing a day of training can disrupt the carefully crafted plan, so it is crucial to build in flexibility to allow for unexpected events. By considering these factors and designing a detailed workout plan, athletes can achieve their goals and stay on track toward success.

Injury Prevention

Proper recovery and rest are essential for optimal performance and to minimize the chance of overtraining or injury that could end an athlete's race season. Overuse musculoskeletal injuries among triathletes are common especially in the longer distances. Common risk factors for injury during triathlon training include the following:

- ▶ History of high running mileage
- ▶ Previous injury
- ▶ Inadequate warm-up and cooldown regimes
- ▶ Increasing years of experience

It is important to take precautions and consider the individual's history and abilities when developing and increasing the athlete's training loads as mentioned in the training volume guidelines section (2, 10). Athletes and coaches should work with a qualified professional to identify and correct any injuries.

Another coaching consideration related to injury prevention is the *female athlete triad*. In brief, the triad is characterized by three interrelated components: disordered eating, *amenorrhea* (loss of menstrual periods), and *osteoporosis* (loss of bone density). It is important for coaches to be aware of this medical condition and help support the athlete and seek professional help if necessary. An athlete's menstrual cycle can have a significant effect on her workout performance, and tracking how the athlete feels consistently will help establish patterns in energy changes related to hormonal fluctuations so that she can adjust her training accordingly. Changes in intensity can be strategically placed in a triathlon program according to race goals; however, considering the individual and encouraging workout feedback is valuable information for the coach to make training adaptations and help prevent overtraining and injury (11).

Resistance Training

Triathlon training can lead to problems over time, especially as athletes age. Regular resistance training and mobility exercises can help maintain muscular symmetry, improve performance, offset aging declines, and prevent overuse injuries. To target the demands of the triathlon, resistance exercises should simulate swimming, cycling, and running motions. It is important to incorporate resistance training progressively and on nonconsecutive days to avoid interfering with other training sessions for swim, bike, run. Prioritizing resistance training and mobility work is important for injury prevention (3, 4, 15, 16).

It is also important to understand the factors outside of training that will help the athlete. These include sleeping, eating, stretching, massage, and even things such as bike maintenance and laundry. They are all crucially important. Some athletes need more than 9 hours of sleep, while others need only 7 hours. Some athletes need to be conscious of their food and supplements, while others do great by eating what they feel like eating. Athletes and coaches should note (even if just mentally) what works.

Missing a Day of Training

Missing a day of training is common. Coaches should encourage athletes to respect other parts of their lives. On some days, their significant other, kids, work, friends, or social life might get in the way of a workout, and they will not be able to get their planned workouts in. That is completely fine. The athlete should not worry about missing the occasional workout. Consistency is the key, and fitness is gained in the long run. Missing a day here and there will not affect the athlete's performance very much (6).

If the athlete misses a week of sessions in a row (from sickness, travel, etc.) or a few weeks of workouts in a row (from injury), there is no reason for panic. Again, the athlete should resist the temptation to make up for the lost time by adding back in missed workouts, which might make them sick or injured again. Shift the training schedule a week to account for the lost time, and if necessary, adjust race goals or defer the athlete to a different race altogether. In fact, if athletes can consistently get in 70% to 85% of the planned workouts each week, they are doing well.

RACE PREPARATION

Race preparation is a multifaceted process that requires careful attention to detail and a commitment to training. By preparing both physically and mentally, athletes can increase their chances of success and enjoy a positive race experience.

Transitions

Regardless of the distance of the triathlon, the transitions from one discipline to the next are an essential part of every race. Transitions can be considered the fourth sport in triathlon because they require skill and planning and they count toward total race time. The transition from the swim to the bike is typically called *T1*, and the transition from the bike to the run is typically called *T2*. Both transitions are unique and require a different approach for success. Athletes can practice their transitions during training by executing a transition area drill where they set up a transition area in their driveway or indoors and practice doing the transitions while timing themselves.

Transition Area Drill

First the athlete sets up a mock transition area. If the athlete does this outside, a short bike ride and run can be included as part of the practice. To set up the mock transition area, the athlete lays out a small towel with bike shoes and bike helmet toward the back so that they are easily accessible and run shoes in the front. The athlete should include a race belt or visor, if wearing one or both on race day, as well as any nutrition and hydration items.

The athlete starts the drill by doing 10 push-ups, which simulates pumping excess blood into the arms like finishing a swim. Next the athlete stands up and spins around 10 times. The athlete will be dizzy when exiting the water, so spinning helps simulate that experience. After spinning, the athlete runs over to the mock transition area and puts on a bike helmet, sunglasses (if applicable), and bike shoes. Then the athlete runs to the back of the room or about 20 feet (6 m) away from the transition area and back. Finally, the athlete transitions from the bike to the run by removing bike shoes and helmet and putting on run shoes, socks, and visor (the latter two if applicable).

If the athlete is not wearing socks during the bike or the run it is important to practice this beforehand to avoid blisters. A trick an athlete can do beforehand is to use petroleum jelly around the opening of the shoe to avoid rubbing and to put baby powder in the shoe to keep the feet dry. Many athletes use elastic laces in their run shoes, which allows them to slip on the shoes very quickly. It helps to improve speed if the athlete times the drill. Quick transitions offer an opportunity for athletes to surge ahead and create a gap between them and their competition.

Swim

If the athlete is swimming in open water and may need a wetsuit for the race due to cooler water temperatures, it is important to practice sighting in open water and swimming with a wetsuit. (The chapter on swimming discusses drills and techniques for open-water swimming.) To maximize sighting and avoid swimming extra distance, take note of a stationary object beyond the swim finish and locate any turn-around points (usually colored buoys are placed for sighting and to indicate it is time to make a turn). Athletes should practice sighting off the objects in training and implement this during the swim on race day to avoid swimming off course. The course map, race website, and pre-race meeting provide useful information on whether a wetsuit is recommended, where the buoys will be placed, swim entry and exit locations, and water temperature and conditions.

Determining a safe spot for the athlete to start ahead of time will help avoid making a potentially poor decision on race day. A safe position for the athlete is at the back and outside of the pack to avoid getting knocked around by other swimmers, although if the athlete is proficient at open-water swims in large packs, a position near the front and inside the pack is likely preferred. Regardless of their start position, athletes should visualize themselves in their own box and practice relaxed breathing to help avoid potential anxiety from swimming around others. If the athlete has a fear of the water or swimming around others, this can be addressed beforehand by doing group swims and simulating the environment to help avoid panic on race day.

Bike

Most triathlon events are not draft legal. *Drafting* on a bike refers to the practice of riding behind another cyclist to reduce wind resistance and increase speed. The cyclist in front, known as the *drafting leader*, creates a pocket of low-pressure air that the trailing cyclist can ride in, allowing them to expend less energy. This technique is commonly used in road racing, professional-level Olympic-distance triathlons, and group rides, because it allows riders to conserve energy and ride faster as a group.

Although it is helpful to train with groups, the athlete should also ride alone to become comfortable with the effort required when not drafting off other riders. Also, it is helpful for an athlete to become familiar with simple bike maintenance prior to a race and practice things such as changing both front and rear tires and making sure to have a spare tube and CO_2 cartridges or a pump. If the athlete gets a flat on the bike and race support is not available, it could mean the end of the race. Race rules state that an athlete cannot use race support outside of what other athletes have access to as part of the event, and if the athlete gets support from a family member or someone outside of the race, a penalty could be issued.

Run

Learning how to pace on the run after a bike ride is important for the athlete to determine during training, which is why brick workouts help the athlete adapt to the feeling of tired legs when transitioning from the bike to the run. Taking in fluids and calories during the run is a learned skill, and practicing this throughout run workouts will prepare the body to assimilate fluids and digest calories more efficiently at race pace. Additionally, if athletes practice with the tools they want to use on race day (e.g., carrying a bottle or wearing a fuel belt), they can adapt to the extra weight and feeling of wearing or carrying those items.

Nutrition and Hydration

Throughout training and in preparation for race day, it is important to both hydrate and replenish carbohydrate stores. The longer the event, the more vital it becomes for the athlete to have a nutrition plan. The athlete needs to practice drinking and eating during training. It will be helpful for them to get used to what is being offered on the course (or they should plan on bringing their own food and drinks). Athletes should be encouraged to do their best to stick to the nutrition plan and follow recommendations and to resist the temptations from a vendor or fellow athlete to try a new product that could cause stomach distress and may prevent the athlete from finishing the event. The duration and intensity of a particular workout in addition to other factors such as environmental conditions and sweat rate will determine the athlete's caloric and hydration needs.

The athlete's muscle glycogen (carbohydrate) becomes depleted over a period and needs to be replenished; otherwise, the athlete will likely experience a drop in energy and must slow down to maintain activity. Something that works for one athlete may not work for another, which is why it is important for the athlete to practice with what they will be using on race day.

In addition to calories, hydration plays a key role in sustaining energy throughout the event. Successful hydration means replacing both fluids and electrolytes to prevent lack of focus, fatigue, thirst, cramps, body tissue swelling, and dizziness. If the athlete is a salty sweater, experiences cramping, or notices swelling in their hands and feet during and after exercise, the athlete should consider increasing sodium intake. The best sports drinks are formulated to speed absorption of carbohydrates, electrolytes, and fluids into the bloodstream.

As a triathlete, proper nutrition and hydration are crucial for performance and overall health. If the athlete has specific nutrition and hydration concerns and needs, seeking guidance from a registered dietitian who is a board-certified specialist in sports dietetics (CSSD) can help.

It is important to note that nutrition needs vary greatly between individuals and there is no one-size-fits-all approach. Therefore, seeking guidance from a CSSD can help ensure the athlete is meeting their nutritional needs and optimizing their performance.

Mental Practices

Mental preparation comes along with physical preparation. As athletes train their bodies, their minds progressively adapt as well. Many athletes experience race anxiety or get butterflies. In order to decrease anxiety, the athlete can include training practices that can help them relax. For example, some athletes struggle with sleep the night before a race due to race anxiety and it can be helpful to focus on getting more sleep a couple of nights before, especially since most races have early start times. Other practices the athlete can use are controlled breathing and visualization.

Controlled Breathing

Incorporating controlled breathing techniques, such as the *4-7-8 breathing technique*, can have beneficial effects on both mental health and physical performance. The 4-7-8 breathing technique consists of inhaling for a count of 4 seconds, holding the breath for 7 seconds, and exhaling for 8 seconds. This technique has been shown to reduce symptoms of anxiety, improve mood, and improve running economy and performance in triathletes. This suggests that using controlled breathing techniques during training and competition may be a helpful strategy for triathletes looking to enhance their performance and manage their mental state (1, 21).

Visualization

Visualization is a powerful mental practice that can enhance performance for triathletes. Before a workout or race, finding a quiet place to visualize completing the entire event from start to finish can help prepare the mind and improve focus. For example, before getting in the water, an athlete could imagine swimming, exiting the water, entering the first transition, preparing for the bike ride, visualizing riding the entire bike course while taking in fluids and calories according to the plan, entering the second transition, racking the bike, changing into running gear, beginning the run, and crossing the finish line of the race. By doing visualization exercises, the athlete is mentally completing the event before ever actually starting the race—which can be a very powerful practice.

Incorporating visualization techniques into training and competition may prove to be beneficial for triathletes seeking to improve their mental preparation and performance (3, 8).

RACE WEEK

Race week is a culmination of all the hard work athletes have put in. At this point, very little can be done to enhance performance in the few days leading up to the event. Coaches' focus should be on keeping their athletes rested, relaxed, and mentally prepared for the upcoming race. Coaches should trust in the training and let athletes know that they are fully prepared for what is ahead. The primary goals for the days leading up to the race are to rest as much as possible and logistically prepare for the race.

The race is challenging enough, and because many things are out of an athlete's control, planning and practicing will help reduce mishaps. Here are some tips for athletes during race week:

▶ Read through the race information packet as soon as it is available. Longer races tend to be more logistically involved than shorter races. For example, bike check-in at the transition area may occur the day before the race.

▶ Use a watch timer or write the plan on a piece of tape and mount it on the top bike tube to help ensure the race-day plan is carried out as intended.

▶ Plan ahead; here are some questions to help:

• What is the expected water temperature during the swim? Is a wetsuit needed?

• What is the shape of the swim course—rectangle or triangle or something else? Is it a single or double loop? How many buoys are there? Are the turn buoys different shapes than the sighting buoys?

• How do athletes enter and leave the transition area? Is there more than one transition area?

- What is the expected air temperature at the start of the bike? (If it is cold, consider changing into dry clothes after the swim or using arm warmers.)
- What is the bike course like? How are the turns marked?
- What is the run course like? How often will aid stations be available? What foods and drinks will be at the aid stations?

▶ Reduce stress levels and relax as much as possible.

▶ Get more sleep.

▶ Engage in more leisurely activities like reading or watching movies to take the mind off the upcoming race.

▶ On the day before the race, eat in moderation and avoid foods that might upset the stomach on race day.

▶ Become familiar with the course.

▶ Do the practice open-water swims on the race course if available.

▶ Drive the bike course and bike or drive the run course a day or two before the race to become familiar with both.

▶ Avoid doing anything new on race day.

RACE DAY

"Do what you can do in the moment."
—Dave Scott, six-time Ironman world champion

Dave Scott's well-known quote comes from his qualifications as an athlete and is good advice for what to do on race day because it emphasizes the importance of staying present and focused on the task at hand rather than becoming overwhelmed by the magnitude of the overall challenge, which then allows athletes to break the race into manageable chunks and stay motivated until the end.

Before the Race

On race day, athletes should arrive early enough to conduct their preplanned warm-up and complete their transition setup. Most races do not let athletes ride on race morning once they have checked their bikes; bike check-in is typically done the day before the race (plus it can be very crowded).

The athlete starts with setting up the transition area like the practice sessions, making sure everything that will be needed for both T1 and T2 is in position. Additionally, the athlete should double check the bike tires and gears; sometimes tire pressure changes overnight or other athletes accidentally bump into bikes and can cause a bike chain to move out of place. After transition setup is complete the athlete can do a run warm-up if planned and return to the transition area to grab swim gear, leaving enough time for a swim warm-up. Before leaving the transition area, the athlete should take note of where his or her bike is racked and where to enter and exit the transition area to get to it. Some athletes place a bright ribbon around the bike rack or locate stationary landmarks to help them locate their transition spot faster.

Swim

To help them relax, athletes can get in the water prior to the wave start and perform a swim warm-up. When the race begins, athletes should focus on swimming at their own pace, and breathing every stroke can help with stroke rhythm and allow them to access to more oxygen at the beginning of the race. The athlete should keep an eye on the buoy and implement sighting practices about every third or fourth stroke. Buoys and turns can get crowded from other athletes slowing down; the athlete can go wide around each buoy, do breaststroke or a mixture of freestyle and breaststroke, and then recalculate after each turn. Athletes can swim toward one buoy at a time and avoid looking at the finish line too much so that they can focus on their current position and stay on course.

T1

The athlete can start removing the swim cap, goggles, and top portion of the wetsuit (if applicable) immediately after exiting the water. The main thing is to keep moving toward the first transition area and execute what has been rehearsed as part of the race plan. Once athletes reach their spot in T1, they can finish removing their wetsuit, leave removed swim gear in their area, put their bike gear on, and grab anything necessary for the ride before exiting onto the bike course.

Bike

On race day it is important that athletes pace themselves on the bike as planned. Training adaptations have already been made, and deviating by riding faster than planned can sabotage the athletes' race. Because other athletes will be slowing down or stopping at aid stations, those areas can get crowded with people and with litter from used cups and gel wrappers. Athletes must pay careful attention when riding through all aid stations.

Once athletes settle into their pace, they can begin executing their nutrition and hydration plan. It is easier to take in more fluids and calories on the bike as compared to the run since the athlete is seated and non–weight bearing. Also, good hydration and nutrition will set the athlete up for the run segment, and in long-distance events this becomes even more crucial in order for the athlete to sustain energy levels for the duration of the race.

T2

As the athlete approaches T2, it is important to prepare mentally for the transition by visualizing the layout and location of the bike rack, making note of the side the rack is on in flow-through transition areas. Upon reaching the dismount line, the athlete dismounts the bike and heads toward the transition point, using one hand on the seat or stem for control while traveling with the bike. At the bike rack, the athlete carefully places the bike in the designated spot using either the handlebars, seat, or rear tire as specified by the race directions. After racking the bike, the athlete removes the helmet and swaps out cycling shoes for running shoes before beginning the final leg of the triathlon.

Run

After racking the bike, the athlete switches out cycling shoes for running shoes and begins the final leg of the triathlon. Maintaining a steady pace and intensity during the run in a triathlon is crucial for a strong finish. In addition, athletes must adhere to their hydration and nutrition plan to ensure optimal performance.

After the Race

After completing the race, recovery should be a top priority for athletes, which includes immediate hydration and nutrition, cooldown, and massage if possible. It is recommended that athletes take pride in their accomplishment before analyzing their performance in detail. Evaluating performance a couple of hours or days after the race allows athletes to identify areas for improvement and focus on key components during future training sessions.

EXAMPLES OF TRAINING PLANS

A sample week of training is provided in this section, and additional sample training weeks for a sprint, Olympic, and long-distance triathlon can be found at the end of this chapter. See table 11.11 for an explanation of the abbreviations shown in the sample week training plans.

Tables 11.12 through 11.15 provide examples of a base week and 2-week excerpts from the base-build weeks of a 16-week sprint, 18-week Olympic, and 24-week ultradistance triathlon training plan. Coaches and athletes can use the guidelines in the sample plans to help them structure swim, bike, and run workouts for specific distances to create a complete balanced training plan specific to the athlete's needs. A description is provided for each workout, and its duration, distance (swim only), and the level of effort are specified by one or more training zone. Additional program details include the following:

▶ *Workout durations.* Each bike and run workout has a planned duration given in hours and minutes (e.g., 0:30 = 30 min; 1:00 = 1 hour; 1:30 = 1 hour and 30 min). The bike and run workouts are based on time, not distance, because

Table 11.11 Key Terms Used in the Sample Training Plans

Term	Definition
Build	Start out at moderate pace and build to fast pace over the duration of the interval
C/D	Cooldown (easy pace)
Non-free	Swim stroke of choice
Descend	Each successive swim interval gets faster. For example, if workout is 4 × 100 descend, then #4 is faster than #3, which is faster than #2, which is faster than #1.
Easy or EZ	Very little effort, relaxed
Fast	Fast effort, pace to maintain a fast speed for the duration of the interval
Free	Freestyle
M/S	Main set of a workout
Pull	Use a pull buoy between the legs (no kicking during the swim)
r15s, r20s, etc.	Rest period (in seconds) after each interval. For example, "2 × 100 steady, r15s" means swim 100 yards (or meters) at a steady pace then rest for 15 seconds before starting the second 100 interval.
RPM	Revolutions per minute or cadence; i.e., how many times the legs perform one complete rotation on the bike or one complete stride on the run
Single leg drill	Pedal with one leg only
Steady	Moderate effort; somewhat hard
W/U	Warm up (easy pace)
Z1, Z2, Z3, etc.	Zone or training zone is an indicator of how hard the effort is (i.e., intensity)

Adapted from reference 6.

time is easier to consistently measure and follow since only a watch is needed. Each swim workout has a planned duration given in hours and minutes, and some workouts include an estimated distance (which can be in yards or meters). The athlete's goal is to complete the distance, or the time given for each swimming workout. The athlete may take more or less time for the given distance depending on their swimming ability, so do not worry if the planned duration differs from how long the athlete takes to complete the workout. If the athlete normally swims with a master's swim team or other organized swim group, those workouts can be substituted in place of the workouts in the plan. Note that the planned workout time is all inclusive of the given workout. For example, if the workout says, "60 min Z2 with 2 × 3 min Z3 mixed in," the "2 × 3 min Z3 mixed in" is included within the 60-minute workout time. The athlete can use the planned workout time as a target time, not an absolute time. For example, if the athlete completes a workout and is over or under by 5 minutes because of the chosen route, that is close enough. The athlete does not need to spend an extra 5 minutes running around the block, and it is no big deal if the athlete is over by a few minutes. The goal is to finish the workout.

▶ *Rest or "off" days.* Although Monday is the designated off day in the sample, the athlete may swap Saturday or Sunday with Monday in the training plan if there's a desire to have a weekend day be an off day. If the athlete needs an extra rest day, he or she can just take it and does not have to try to make up for the missed workout or workouts. Nothing is gained by doing a workout if the athlete is exhausted. In fact, that is more likely to negatively affect the training especially when overly tired or sore. The athlete must remember that recovery and adaptation happen while resting, not while training.

▶ *Warm-up and cooldown.* Workouts are meant to be started at a light, slow pace for 5 to 10 minutes to warm up the athlete's muscles. Likewise, the athlete should leave the last 5 to 10 minutes as an easier effort to bring the heart rate down slowly. The time devoted to the warm-up and cooldown is included as part of the total workout time.

Sample Base Week Training Plan

Table 11.12 is an example of a weekly plan integrating specific workouts and intensities for a base week of training designed for an amateur triathlete preparing for an Olympic-distance triathlon. The priority is to complete 70% to 90% of the workouts shown.

Table 11.12 Sample of Base Week for an Amateur Triathlete Preparing for an Olympic Triathlon

TOTAL TIME: 5:25	
Day	**Workout type (duration): Description**
Monday	Day off
Tuesday	**Swim** (0:40): W/U: 100 easy 2 × 100 M/S: Pyramid: 100, 200, 300 easy, r15s, 300, 200, 100 steady, r15s C/D: 400 easy with pull buoy
Wednesday	**Long run** (0:50): Start easy Z1 and build into Z2 run on softer surfaces (e.g., dirt, grass) if possible **Resistance training**: Optional
Thursday	**Resistance training**: Optional **Bike drills** (1:00): Z2 of 4 × 30s high-speed spins with moderate resistance and 30s easy in between (quick pedaling as fast as possible without bouncing in the saddle) and 4 × 30s single-leg drill under moderate tension (cadence 60-70 rpm) each leg (alternate legs for total of 8); focus on keeping heels flat and pedaling "circles" (not "squares")
Friday	**Swim** (0:40): W/U: 300 easy practice breathing to both sides, r15s 4 × 25, rest 10s M/S: 200 easy, r30s, 2 × 100 steady, r20s, 200 easy r30s, 2 × 100 steady r20s, 200 steady r30s, 2 × 100 steady r20s C/D: 200 easy with pull buoy
Saturday	**Long bike** (1:40): Z2
Sunday	**Run** (0:35): Easy Z1 **Resistance training**: Optional

Sprint Triathlon Training Plan

Table 11.13 is an example of base-build weeks 3 and 4 excerpted from a 16-week sprint triathlon plan designed for age-group triathletes with full-time jobs and other commitments. The goal of the 16-week structured and periodized plan is to prepare the athlete for a sprint triathlon (typically 750-m swim, 20-km bike, 5-km run). Athletes should be able to complete the following workouts prior to beginning this plan:

- ▶ *Swim.* 50 meters or yards continuously
- ▶ *Bike.* 30 minutes
- ▶ *Run or run/walk.* 20 minutes

The plan includes two swim, bike, and run workouts a week plus one brick run. Workout durations range from 3 to 5 hours across the six to eight sessions per week, with Monday as the designated off day. The weekly breakdown follows:

- ▶ *Swimming.* Average total time: 1:24; longest swim: 1:00
- ▶ *Bike.* Average total time: 2:14; longest ride: 2:00
- ▶ *Run.* Average total time: 1:35; longest run: 1:20

Table 11.13 Sample Base-Build Weeks 3 and 4 From a 16-Week Sprint Triathlon Plan

WEEK 3: TOTAL TIME: 4:55	
Day	**Workout type (duration): Description**
Monday	Day off
Tuesday	**Swim** (0:40): 1,600 total W/U: 100 easy pull, r15s, 2 × 50, r15s M/S: 3 × 400 steady, r30s C/D: 200 easy free
Wednesday	**Bike** (0:45): Z2. Include 3 × 2 min at race pace (Z3/Z4)
Thursday	**Run** (0:30): Z2. Include 3 × 2 min Z4
Friday	**Swim** (0:40): 1,600 total W/U: 200 easy free, r15s, 2 × 50, r15s M/S: 6 × 150 steady, r20s (keep pace consistent), 4 × 50 (25 fast, 25 easy), r15s C/D: 200 easy non-free
Saturday	**Workout #1: Bike** (1:20): Z2 on a course with some hills
	Workout #2: Brick run (0:15): Quickly transition to a steady run after biking
Sunday	**Run** (0:45): Steady Z2

WEEK 4: TOTAL TIME: 5:00	
Day	**Workout type (duration): Description**
Monday	Day off
Tuesday	**Swim** (0:30): 1,400 total W/U: 100 easy free, r15s, 2 × 100, r15s M/S: 2 × 500 steady, r30s C/D: 100 easy any stroke
Wednesday	**Bike** (1:00): Z2 Include 5 × 1 min at race pace (Z3/Z4)
Thursday	**Run** (0:30): Z2. Include 4 × 2 min Z3 with 1 min easy in between
Friday	**Swim** (0:40): 1,700 total W/U: 200 easy pull, r20s, 2 × 50, r15s M/S: 2 × 300 steady, r20s, 6 × 100 (25 steady/50 fast/25 easy), r15s C/D: 200 easy free with long strokes
Saturday	**Workout #1: Bike** (1:30): Steady Z2 on a course with some hills
	Workout #2: Brick run (0:10): Quickly transition to a steady run after biking
Sunday	**Run** (0:40): Steady Z2

Olympic (International) Triathlon Training Plan

Table 11.14 shows weeks 3 and 4 excerpted from an 18-week base-build program for an Olympic-distance triathlon plan designed for experienced triathletes who have completed multiple sprint or Olympic-distance triathlons. The goal of the 18-week training plan is to prepare the athlete for an Olympic-distance triathlon (typically a 1,500-m swim, 40-km bike, 10-km run). Prior to using this plan, athletes should be able to complete the following workouts:

- ▶ *Swim.* 500 meters or yards
- ▶ *Bike.* 60 minutes
- ▶ *Run.* 40 minutes

Starting 18 weeks before the goal race, this plan progresses through two base periods and two build periods (10 hours per week maximum across 8 to 10 workouts each week) prior to peaking and tapering the last 2 weeks. Following the first base period, each week typically contains three swims, three bikes, and three runs plus one brick run and will build up to 3,000 yards (or meters) swimming, 2 hours biking, and 80 minutes running. The long ride is Saturday and the long run is Sunday, with Monday as the off day. The weekly breakdown follows:

- ▶ *Swimming.* Average total time: 2:16; longest swim: 1:00
- ▶ *Bike.* Average total time: 3:05; longest ride: 2:00
- ▶ *Run.* Average total time: 2:12; longest run: 1:20

Table 11.14 Sample Base-Build Weeks 3 and 4 From an 18-Week Olympic Triathlon Plan

WEEK 3: TOTAL TIME: 6:20	
Day	**Workout type (duration): Description**
Monday	Day off
Tuesday	**Swim** (0:40): 1,700 total W/U: 200 easy pull, r15s, 2 × 50, r15s M/S: 3 × 400 steady, r30s C/D: 200 easy free
Wednesday	**Bike** (1:00): Z2. Include 3 × 2 min at race pace (Z3/Z4)
Thursday	**Run** (0:50): Z2. Include 3 × 2 min Z4
Friday	**Swim** (0:40): 2,400 total W/U: 200 easy free, r15s, 2 × 50, r15s M/S: 600 steady, r30s, 6 × 150 steady, r20s (keep pace consistent), 8 × 50 (25 fast, 25 easy), r15s C/D: 200 easy non-free
Saturday	**Workout #1: Bike** (1:40): Z2 on a course with some hills
	Workout #2: Brick run (0:30): Quickly transition to a steady run after biking
Sunday	**Run** (1:00): Steady Z2
WEEK 4: TOTAL TIME: 8:00	
Day	**Workout type (duration): Description**
Monday	Day off
Tuesday	**Swim** (0:30): 2,000 total W/U: 200 easy pull, r20s, 2 × 50, r15s M/S: 4 × 400 steady, r30s C/D: 100 easy any stroke
Wednesday	**Bike** (1:20): Z2. Include 5 × 1 min at race pace (Z3/Z4)
Thursday	**Run** (1:00): Z2. Include 4 × 2 min Z3 with 1 min easy in between
Friday	**Swim** (1:00): 2,500 total W/U: 200 easy pull, r20s, 2 × 50, r15s M/S: 4 × 300 steady, r20s, 8 × 100 (25 steady/50 fast/25 easy), r15s C/D: 200 easy free with long strokes
Saturday	**Workout #1: Bike** (2:00): Z2 on a course with some hills
	Workout #2: Brick run (0:30): Quickly transition to a steady run after biking
Sunday	**Run** (1:20): Steady Z2

Ultradistance Triathlon Training Plan

Table 11.15 shows weeks 3 and 4 excerpted from a 24-week ultradistance triathlon plan designed for experienced triathletes with multiple long-distance triathlon finishes. The goal of the 24-week training plan is to prepare the athlete for an ultradistance triathlon (typically a 2.4-mile swim, 112-mile bike, 26.2-mile run). Prior to using this plan, the athlete should be able to complete the following workouts:

- *Swim.* 300 meters or yards continuously
- *Bike.* 1.5 hours continuously
- *Run.* 45 minutes continuously or a run/walk combination

Starting 24 weeks before the goal race, this plan begins with a 6-week prep period (6-8 hr/week) then progresses through three base periods and one build period (16.5-18 hr/week spanning 6-10 workouts each week) prior to peaking and tapering. Following the prep period, each week typically contains three swims, three bikes, and three runs plus one brick run, and will build up to 3,800 yards (or meters) swimming, 6 hours biking, and 2.5 hours running. The weekly schedule includes optional time allocated for resistance training and a designated off day (Monday). The weekly breakdown follows:

- *Swimming.* Average total time: 2:19; longest swim: 1:40
- *Bike.* Average total time: 4:34; longest ride: 5:00
- *Run.* Average total time: 3:00; longest run: 2:30

Table 11.15 Sample Base-Build Weeks 3 and 4 From a 24-Week Ultradistance Triathlon Plan

WEEK 3: TOTAL TIME: 13:40.	
Day	**Workout type (duration): Description**
Monday	Day off
Tuesday	**Workout #1: Bike** (1:10): Z2 on a hilly course with any hills in Z3
	Workout #2: Swim (1:00): W/U: 300 easy, practice breathing both sides M/S: 4 × 500 start steady and each 400 gets 4-5s faster, r20s C/D: 200 easy
Wednesday	**Workout #1: Run** (1:55): Z2. Run on softer surfaces (e.g., dirt, grass) if possible; practice nutrition and hydration
	Workout #2: Resistance training: Optional
Thursday	**Workout #1: Bike** (1:00): Z1/Z2. Use small chain ring in front and keep cadence >90 rpm
	Workout #2: Swim (1:10): W/U: 300 M/S: 4 × 50 (fast/EZ), r15s, 1 × 1,000 steady, r60s, 1 × 1,000 faster than the first 1 km by 20-30s C/D: 200 non-free
Friday	**Workout #1: Swim** (1:15): W/U: 300 M/S: 75 easy, r15s, 6 × 200 build up to Z3 (fast), r20s, 6 × 100 steady (all at the same pace), r15s, 8 × 50 (25 very fast, 25 EZ), r15s C/D: 200 non-free
	Workout #2: Run (0:45): Z2. Focus on relaxing upper body; include 10 min Z3

(continued)

Table 11.15 Sample Base-Build Weeks 3 and 4 From a 24-Week Ultradistance Triathlon Plan *(continued)*

WEEK 3: TOTAL TIME: 13:40 *(continued)*	
Day	**Workout type (duration): Description**
Saturday	**Workout #1: Bike** (4:00): Z2. Include 2 × 10 min Z3 mixed in; practice nutrition and hydration as if in a race
	Workout #2: Brick run (0:30): Start easy Z1 off the bike (within 5 min of finishing ride) and build up to Z2 to simulate race conditions
Sunday	**Workout #1: Run** (0:55): Z2. Include 4-6 strides of quick accelerations for 20 sec (not all-out efforts)
	Workout #2: Resistance training: Optional
WEEK 4: TOTAL TIME: 16:30	
Day	**Workout type (duration): Description**
Monday	Day off
Tuesday	**Workout #1: Bike** (1:30): Z2 on a hilly course with any hills in Z3
	Workout #2: Swim (1:00): W/U: 300 easy, practice breathing both sides M/S: 5 \x\ 400 start steady, then each one gets 4-5s faster, r20s C/D: 200 easy
Wednesday	**Workout #1: Run** (2:30): Z2. Run on softer surfaces (e.g., dirt, grass) if possible; practice nutrition and hydration
	Workout #2: Resistance training: Optional
Thursday	**Workout #1: Bike** (1:00): Z1/Z2. Use small chain ring in front and keep cadence >90 rpm
	Workout #2: Swim (1:40): W/U: 300 M/S: 1 × 1,000 easy, r30s, 2 × 50 (25 very fast/25 EZ), r20s, 1 × 1,000 start easy and build up to steady, r30s, 2 × 50 (25 very fast, 25 EZ), r20s, 1 × 1,000 steady, r30s C/D: 300 non-free
Friday	**Workout #1: Swim** (1:00): W/U: 300 M/S: Pyramid (use pull buoy on odd intervals, e.g., 100, 300): 100, 200, 300, 400 steady, r15s, 400, 300, 200, 100 steady, r15s C/D: 200 easy
	Workout #2: Run (0:50): Z2. Focus on relaxing upper body; include 3 × 3 min Z3
Saturday	**Workout #1: Bike** (5:00): Z2. Practice nutrition and hydration as if in a race; include 2 × 6 min Z3 mixed in. *Option:* Add 30-60 min to ride if feeling good
	Workout #2: Brick run (0:30): Start easy Z1 off the bike (within 5 min of finishing ride) and build up to Z2 to simulate race conditions
Sunday	**Workout #1: Run** (1:30): Z1/Z1. Relax upper body and glide over the ground
	Workout #2: Resistance training: Optional

CHAPTER 12

Obstacle Course Racing

Roger Earle

The sport of obstacle course racing, typically shortened to *OCR* (which can also stand for obstacle course *race*), is relatively new. The earliest formal event was in 1987 in the United Kingdom and was dubbed the Tough Guy competition. The Muddy Buddy series began in the US in 1999, with OCR events becoming more mainstream in 2010. By 2018 the number of participants in OCRs was over 500,000 annually (3, 5), and in 2020, Spartan Race, the dominant OCR company then and to date, reported over 1.2 million annual participants in more than 250 events in over 40 countries worldwide (6).

Since the sport's inception, many companies have put on OCRs, but most of them have been shuttered, often due to the high cost of liability insurance and building obstacles. Primary companies in existence at the time of this book's publication include BoneFrog, Northman, Nuclear Race, OCR World Championships, Rugged Maniac, Savage Race, Spartan Race, Strong Viking, Tough Mudder, and Toughest. Some of these companies offer a United States, North American, United Kingdom, or European race series, annual championships, or a combination of these.

This chapter provides a brief summary of OCRs, their physiological demands, modes of training, program design guidelines, and sample training plans. Despite that coverage, it is important to point out that the sport's complexity warrants a more comprehensive understanding of additional factors such as mental conditioning, injury prevention strategies, race-day nutrition and apparel recommendations, and obstacle completion tactics, all of which are beyond the scope of this chapter. Further, the sample programs provided are only a glimpse of what complete programs would encompass.

DESCRIPTION OF OCRS

At its roots, an OCR is a running race that commonly takes place on an outdoor trail or multisurface terrain (e.g., grass, field, gravel, sand, dirt, mud) within, for example, a park, nature preserve, ski resort, or off-road track—or very occasionally in an urban area on concrete or asphalt roads, on sidewalks, or within a sport stadium. The distances covered vary and they are interspersed with obstacles that have to be completed or navigated along the way.

OCRs can be categorized (albeit not overtly named as such) as short (3-5 miles [4.8-8.0 km]; e.g., a 5K [3.1 miles]), medium (5-10 miles [8.0-16.1 km]; e.g., a 10K or 15K [6.2 or 9.3 miles]), or long (10-14 miles [16.1-22.5 km]; e.g., a half marathon [13.1 miles; 21.1 km]). Other variations include ultra-length distances (e.g., 50K [30 miles]) or time-based races (e.g., a 12- or 24-hour race that is covered in shorter [e.g., 5-mile or 8K] loops). Despite the distances quoted here, actual race distances are not precise; a race held every year at the same venue is never the same length, and a race type promoted with a certain name by an OCR company can vary in length from venue to venue by a half a mile (0.8 km) up to 2 miles (3.2 km).

The obstacles are deliberately varied in multiple ways, such as

- ▶ type (climbing or crawling up, over, across, or under a structure; traversing monkey bars or a rig with hanging attachments; carrying objects),
- ▶ construction (metal, wood, rope, PVC, chain, cement),
- ▶ use of natural conditions (hills, lakes, streams, hills, sand, gravel, boulders, grass, dry creek beds, fields, forests, bushes, underbrush, sand, dirt, mud),
- ▶ number (10 to over 70, depending on the distance and race type),
- ▶ difficulty (simple or easy completion by all participants, requires one or more attempts to complete but most are successful, or frequently failed by many participants), and
- ▶ spacing in the course (one or more obstacles side-by-side or up to a 3/4-mile [1.2 km] gap between two obstacles).

PHYSIOLOGICAL DEMANDS OF OCRS

Due to the variety in the type of terrain and obstacles that make up an OCR, participants need to possess a range of general fitness qualities to handle the rigor of a race:

- ▶ *Muscular strength:* hoisting or carrying a heavy (40-150-pound [18-68 kg]) weight or pulling the body up and over a 4- to 8-foot (1.2-2.4 m) barrier
- ▶ *Muscular endurance:* performing repeated lower-intensity movements (e.g., crawling on all fours under a span of wires) or holding a sustained isometric contraction (e.g., keeping a sandbag or bucket of rocks held in position on one shoulder while going up a hill)
- ▶ *Muscular power:* jumping up to or onto an obstacle; hopping over and around objects to navigate uncut running paths; or swinging (also called *laché*) to and from ropes, bars, or cargo nets

▶ *Aerobic endurance:* running through a course or (power) walking up a hill

▶ *Anaerobic capacity:* climbing a rope or a tall wooden or cargo net structure; grabbing and moving through a series of handles, bars, ropes; hanging from a rig with the feet off the ground; or completing burpees (a former penalty for failing an obstacle)

Beyond the general fitness qualities, there are OCR-specific abilities that, if acquired, greatly help a participant successfully complete a race:

▶ Ankle and shoulder strength, flexibility, and stability to handle uneven landing surfaces and endure unilateral extremity loading and sheer forces

▶ Grip strength (strength and endurance of the muscles and connective tissue of the forearms, wrists, and hands) for climbing, hanging, holding, and pulling

▶ Obstacle technique skill (execution and efficiency)

▶ *Proprioceptive awareness* (unconscious awareness of body position) and *kinesthetic awareness* (unconscious awareness of body movement); that is, foot-, body-, hand-eye coordination

▶ Repeated effort ability within a single OCR or across multiple races (e.g., a "trifecta" weekend such as completing Spartan Race's three race distances over a 2-day period)

▶ Self-efficacy (the belief in one's ability to be successful despite the highly challenging and unknown aspects of an OCR)

▶ Tolerance of discomfort (often referred to by OCR athletes as "being comfortable with being uncomfortable")

The abilities listed are not in order of importance; rather, the first step of designing an effective training program should be to determine an athlete's current strengths and weaknesses related to OCR performance and prioritize training accordingly. Commonly, those who are new to OCRs typically need to focus on improving overall resilience through multiple-mode physical training, while those who have OCR experience often devote time to gaining obstacle proficiency and learning race-day strategies.

MODES OF OCR TRAINING

Bioenergetically, an OCR is a long-duration aerobic endurance event that contains multiple short, irregularly spaced interruptions (i.e., the obstacles) that require 5 to 10 seconds up to several minutes to complete and that challenge the phosphagen (ATP-PC) and glycolytic energy systems, respectively. Thus, an effective OCR training program should contain workouts consisting of a variety of modalities that tax the full range of metabolic systems: resistance training, plyometric training, running, high-intensity circuit training, obstacle skill training, and multiple-mode (brick) training.

Resistance Training

Among the variables that are manipulated as part of designing a resistance training program, exercise selection is particularly important for OCR training. Because OCR athletes are moving their bodies over, around, and under obstacles, multijoint exercises should be chosen for all phases of training. Minimally, multijoint exercises that are body weight loaded such as the lunge, squat, burpee, pull-up, and push-up should be incorporated into the program because they transfer directly to obstruction hurdling, rope and cargo net climbing, wall scaling, monkey bar traversing, and barbed wire crawling. Over time, it is important to progress the intensity to handling an external load for traditional resistance training exercises (e.g., back or front squat, sumo or standard deadlift, shoulder press, and barbell or dumbbell row) to be able to tolerate the weighted obstacles such as sandbag, bucket (filled with rocks or sand), stone, chain, or log carries (often up a steep hill or in a swamp, sand, or water), or hoists that can exceed 75% of the athlete's body weight. Thus, one primary goal of resistance training for OCRs is to maximize muscular strength, especially in relation to the athlete's body weight, so that it takes less effort to complete an obstacle since the athlete has to carry herself through the obstacle, regardless of any external factor.

As an athlete becomes more resistance trained, further OCR-focused applications of multijoint exercises include the following:

► Total body exercises, such as the power clean and push press (and their derivatives)

► Separate arm or leg exercises, such as the landmine shoulder press or row, Bulgarian squat, and step-up

► Unevenly loaded dumbbell or kettlebell exercises where different weights are used in each hand (e.g., a lunge with a 45-lb or 20-kg dumbbell in one hand and a 12-lb or 6-kg dumbbell in the other hand)

Plyometric Training

Throughout an OCR, an athlete frequently makes quick hops over objects on the trail and across gullies and pockets of water or mud. The ability to tolerate those movements requires a level of power that is gained by plyometric training. Even OCR athletes who are at a beginning level of training can incorporate basic plyometric exercises into their program, such as the squat jump and double-leg hop. It is important to be aware of the physical demand of plyometric training and not overdo it, especially in early stages of training, and to make gradual increases in volume and exercise difficulty (e.g., begin with 1 set of 5 repetitions of double-leg exercises performed in place and steadily progress to multiple sets of 10-15 repetitions of forward, lateral, and diagonal single-leg exercises). An effective way to insert plyometrics to a training program is to perform them after a sufficient warm-up and before a lower body resistance training workout or a run when energy levels are high so maximal effort can be given.

In addition to improvements in power production as an outcome of plyometric training, jumping and hopping exercises may help cramp-proof the calf muscles. Anecdotal evidence shows that cramping due to fatigue caused by repeated (thousands) of small, short jumps throughout a course or running on soft surfaces that result in greater calf and Achilles' tendon stress is one of the most common factors that negatively affect OCR performance. It is not uncommon to see individuals off to the side of a course massaging their spasming calves in obvious pain. While not traditionally categorized as a plyometric exercise, jumping rope is an effective calf training tool to include in an OCR plyometric training program, even if it is part of the warm-up.

Running

At its basic level, an OCR is a running race; observations of this contributor's races revealed that an average of over 92% of total race time was spent running. If penalty loops for failing an obstacle are completed, the ratio of run time versus total time will be even higher. Despite the less than 10% of total race time being taken up by doing obstacles, those intermittently spaced breaks in running creates a variable-intensity, non-continuous event that appears to be unique on how it affects exercise heart rate (1). As a result, the obstacles provide enough of a running break that it is not necessary to work up to a continuous run equal to the total distance of an OCR in training. A minimum threshold of two-thirds of the race distance performed as a continuous run during training is likely sufficient to successfully cover the distance of an OCR; being competitive likely requires greater running volume, however.

The major factors that must be accounted for in a running program for an OCR are the terrain and gradient because they directly affect exercise heart rate (2) and, correspondingly, perceived exertion and carryover to actual race conditions. It is not sufficient to run solely on level, paved streets and running paths. Ideally, at least one running session each week needs to be on a trail—preferably with a rough, uneven surface pockmarked with rocks, sticks, brush, and other debris to mimic an actual race—with elevation changes that challenge the cardiovascular system and lower body musculature. OCR athletes who do not live in areas with outdoor trails or hills need to be creative to remedy that training disadvantage (e.g., by doing incline treadmill running and revolving-step stair machine workouts).

Running workouts should span the gamut of longer, even-paced runs that build an aerobic endurance base, interval-based runs with alternating faster and slower segments that improve anaerobic capacity and recovery ability, and hill-focused runs, ideally as steep as possible because many OCRs take place on ski slopes.

Although running is an OCR athlete's primary mode of aerobic endurance training, *rucking* (walking with a weighted backpack) and *hiking* (power walking on a trail) have training benefits that carry over to an OCR, especially if a ruck or hike is long, such as double or triple the expected time of a targeted OCR, or over particularly hilly terrain.

High-Intensity Circuit Training

The variations in intensity and the variety of movements of an OCR dictates the need to do *high-intensity circuit training* (HICT) consisting of alternated timed intervals of higher-intensity exercise and lower-intensity recovery periods to improve anaerobic capacity and mental resilience (4). The result is an enhanced ability to go from running, completing an obstacle, quickly recovering, and then either resuming running or doing another obstacle in close succession. A wide mixture of upper body, lower body, and total body multijoint exercises that involve similar movement patterns as obstacles should be selected for the work intervals, with an intervening active or absolute rest transition interval that allows the athlete to accumulate more total work than if the work intervals were done consecutively.

One of the advantages of HICT workouts is that they offer many opportunities to increase the overall physiological and mental demand of a given session by

- ▶ changing the complexity or difficulty of the work interval exercise, such as replacing mountain climbers with burpees or increasing the height of the box for the step-up;
- ▶ changing from body-weight-only loading to handling an external load, such as a weight vest, sandbag, one or two dumbbells or kettlebells, barbell, med or slam ball, or heavy rope;
- ▶ changing the order of the work interval exercises so that they intentionally fatigue a certain body area (e.g., change from alternating upper body and lower body exercises to sequencing several upper body and several lower body exercises in a row);
- ▶ increasing the duration of the work interval;
- ▶ adding more circuits (sets); or
- ▶ decreasing the duration of the rest transition interval.

Obstacle Skill Training

Obviously, the aspect of an OCR that differentiates it from a road or trail running race is the inclusion of obstacles. Some only require a low level of skill (e.g., the barbed wire crawl), but others are more complex thereby requiring greater proficiency to be successful (e.g., the rig with hanging attachments such as rings, ropes, T-bars, wheels, horizontal bars). The goal is to maximize proficiency to improve first-attempt success and minimize completion time.

The muscular action of the majority of obstacles involves hanging, grasping, pulling, or a combination of these while in a variety of body positions relative to the obstacle and the ground. The common element of these obstacles is the need for a strong and fatigue-resistant hand grip. For many OCR athletes, simply increasing grip strength and endurance will improve obstacle completion rates. All resistance exercises that focus on the upper back muscles, biceps, and forearms as well as those that involve holding an object that opposes gravity (e.g., the dead hang, farmer's walk, dumbbell or kettlebell lunge and squat) will improve grip strength and endurance due to the need to keep the hand closed for the duration of a set.

Hand-to-hand transfer during a monkey bar or rig crossing requires capable hand-eye timing and coordination that can be practiced. With the popularity of the *American Ninja Warrior* sports entertainment reality show, there are hundreds of facilities in the United States, Australia, Canada, and United Kingdom where OCR athletes can go to receive coaching and rehearse valuable techniques to gain speed and efficiency. Additionally, home gym kits are available that make obstacle practice convenient.

Obstacle proficiency can greatly degrade in a longer OCR and across a multiple-race weekend as a result of accumulated fatigue, both physically and mentally. It is one thing to practice a rig crossing at the gym when fresh, but even the effects of running between obstacles can cause sufficient general fatigue to decrease obstacle success on race day. An effective training tactic to combat this is to do a fatiguing run, HICT session, or resistance training workout immediately before obstacle skill training so that practice occurs under more race-like conditions.

Multiple-Mode (Brick) Training

Obstacle course racing athletes can greatly benefit from *brick* training, a concept borrowed from the sport of triathlon that involves combining two or more modes of training back-to-back with little to no intervening rest within a single session. The objective is to intentionally cause an athlete to have to handle the physical and mental strain of a long training session. For example, a brick session could begin with a lower body plyometric training workout, followed by a lower body resistance training workout, and culminated with a trail run. If an OCR athlete wants to participate in a multiple-race weekend, performing brick workouts must be a training priority. A further application for well-trained athletes is sequential-day brick sessions that simulate the demand of a two- or three-race weekend. For all athletes, it is imperative to allow sufficient recovery from a brick training session because the stress placed on the body is similar to a race or a race weekend.

PROGRAM DESIGN FOR OCRS

For many U.S. and European athletes, the OCR season is commonly mid- to late-spring to late fall or early winter, although there are races in several U.S. areas (e.g., southern California, Arizona, and Florida) and in some African, Central and South American, Asian, European, and Oceanic countries during other times of the year (sometimes on purpose to expose the participants to harsher weather conditions). Often, the national and international championship races are in September, October, and November. In the winter months of the Northern Hemisphere, the OCR-agnostic *general physical preparation* (GPP) phase (i.e., the off-season) generally begins after an active recovery period after the last race of the previous season. Following the GPP phase, a *specific physical preparation* (SPP) build phase (i.e., the preseason) occurs leading up to the competition or race phase (i.e., the in-season).

General Physical Preparation Phase

The first phase of training is designed to create a foundation or base of general readiness that later training phases can expand and progress from. Based on the race schedule and how much postseason recovery is needed, the GPP phase described in this chapter begins in December or January and lasts 2 to 3 months (see table 12.1 for a synopsis of common training priorities).

Table 12.1 OCR General Physical Preparation Phase (Off-Season)

December (or January) through February	2-3 months (8-12 weeks)
Training priorities	• Give special attention to rehabilitating acute or chronic general or OCR-induced injuries from the previous season. • Begin with even-paced, lower-intensity running and progress to include interval running later in the phase. • Perform structural, traditional, bilateral, evenly loaded, general (i.e., not specific to the demands of an OCR) resistance training, and progress from doing more repetitions with lighter loads to fewer repetitions with heavier loads later in the phase (or alternate shorter cycles of each throughout the phase). • Complete single-mode workouts.

Specific Physical Preparation Phase

The SPP phase builds on the GPP phase to focus on OCR-specific training as a precursor to the in-season. Depending on when the first race is scheduled and how training is progressing, preseason training begins in March and can extend past the first several races or race weekends in April or May. For the purposes of this chapter, the SPP phase covers March through May (see table 12.2 for a brief summary of its training priorities).

Table 12.2 OCR-Specific Physical Preparation (Build) Phase (Preseason)

March through April (or May)	2-3 months (8-12 weeks)
Training priorities	• Preferentially select OCR-specific resistance training exercises (e.g., unilateral and unevenly loaded exercises, rowing and pulling movements, forearm- and hand-focused grip exercises); include targeted exercises that focus on muscles and joints that are at a greater risk of injury such as the shoulders, calves, and ankles. • Purposely cause fatigue from an extended training session, back-to-back high-demand training days, or both using multiple-mode (brick) training sessions or days. • Include lower body plyometric training, especially jumping and hopping (increase the intensity gradually and progress to single-leg, multidirectional movements). • Expand the type of running sessions to include hill and trail runs (especially on varying terrain). • Slot in HICT sessions (with exercises that mimic obstacles, the rigor of an OCR, or both). • Learn and practice skills that promote obstacle proficiency.

Competition or Race Phase

The OCR in-season ideally progresses from shorter, sporadic, single-race weekends to longer, more frequent, multiple-race weekends to match the progressive adaptation outcome of an OCR athlete's training program. Often, though, that advantageous progression is not possible due to when OCR companies schedule their races; many factors influence the type and number of races that can be offered and held in a day or during a weekend. Also, the OCR calendar changes each year; although some venues offer one or more races within approximately the same time range, many races may be a month or more sooner (or later) than the previous year. To complicate the calendar further, sometimes popular or high-profile races in different locations are scheduled on the same day or weekend. Therefore, if an OCR athlete wants to do multiple races in various locations throughout a full in-season, it is conceivable that the first (or second or third) race could be a long, difficult event (e.g., a half-marathon-length or longer OCR), part of a multiple-race weekend, or both. As a result, the athlete will have to decide between completing the race at a lower intensity level (just to finish) or focusing on specific aspects of the course for training purposes (e.g., obstacle practice, hill training, mental hardening).

An effective strategy for in-season training is to decide which races are the most important, plan the program around them, and consider the others as an extra-intense training session for a single-race day or 1- or 2-day brick training for a double- or triple-race weekend (see the Multiple-Mode [Brick] Training section for more details). Ideally, the athlete would have one priority race a month to allow for sufficient recovery between them. Depending on the physical demands of an important OCR, it may be necessary to plan a 2- to 7-day taper beforehand and a similar length (or perhaps somewhat longer) recovery period afterward.

By their nature, OCRs have enough unknown race-day factors that, despite how well the training program is developed to account for tapering, racing, and recovering (or training "through" a race), it is important to be flexible enough to allow modifications in the program if a certain race or multiple-race weekend is more challenging than expected due to race conditions (e.g., rain during race week will create muddier conditions that are much harder on the legs), new obstacles, a hillier venue, or a more challenging than usual sequence of obstacles.

Table 12.3 provides a simple overview of the training and race-related priorities of the racing season.

Table 12.3 OCR Competition or Race Phase (In-Season)

May (or June) through October (or November)	6-7 months (24-28 weeks)
Training and race-related priorities	• Choose the primary races and plan the associated tapering and recovery time periods and workouts. • Maximize training progression, especially for OCR-related sessions, during the weeks between primary races. • Modify the training program based on race-induced physical symptoms (i.e., take note of the muscles that are sore after a race as an indication of the muscle groups or body part areas that need more specialized, focused training). • Give ongoing attention to practice self-care (e.g., adequate rest, stress management, quality nutrition) and recovery techniques (e.g., low-intensity active recovery activities, massage). • Do post-race note-taking (e.g., tweaks in obstacle technique, pre-race or race-day food and fluid intake, or apparel). • Decide if the resistance training program will focus on peaking strength via higher-intensity, lower-volume workouts (with a shift to lower-intensity training to reduce fatigue during a taper) or maintaining strength with moderate-intensity and volume training (with manipulations made as needed based on fatigue levels). • Consider setting different resistance training goals for the lower body versus the upper body (e.g., based on race frequency, the legs may not be able to tolerate workouts with heavier loading schemes or higher volumes).

SAMPLE TRAINING PLANS

As previously explained, the training plans in this section are generic examples and, as such, are not directly usable by all athletes. For example, the resistance training exercises listed are common to OCR, but they should be modified to address muscular (and joint, by association) weaknesses and body areas that are at a higher risk of injury based on past injuries or other factors that are specific to the individual.

Also, the intensity and volume assignments and the rate of progression are highly influenced by the athlete's training age, background, and status. For instance, a potential OCR participant might be categorized as fully untrained; other sport or activity trained but OCR untrained (e.g., transitioning from doing running-only races, hybrid sports, or cross-training to OCRs); or beginner-, intermediate-, or elite-level OCR trained, all of which necessitate following a customized training plan. Thus, athletes are encouraged to work with an experienced strength and conditioning professional who has OCR-specific expertise to create a program that is tailored to the individual and the demands of the targeted OCR and to progress that program throughout the sport seasons.

For the purposes of this chapter, the sample off-, pre-, and in-season training plans are for an individual who is moderately trained and has participated in short- to medium-distance OCRs but is looking for a structured, well-rounded program to be more successful in short- to medium-distanced OCRs, graduate to a longer distance OCR, or do more than one race in a weekend. Note the following details:

▶ The first week of the sample off- and preseason's training plans is summarized in tables 12.4 and 12.5, and season-specific details and progression guidelines are described after each table. (*Note*: Day 7 is a full rest day, so only six days of training are shown.) Athletes can align the day numbers with their personal schedule as long as the sequence of the days' workouts is intact (e.g., day 1 is Monday, day 2 is Tuesday, day 3 is Wednesday, and so on, but days 1, 2, 3, etc. could be Sunday, Monday, Tuesday, etc.). The guidelines and recommendations regarding resistance training loads are very simplified; see chapter 6 for a more detailed explanation. The running distances and times in table 12.5 continue from where table 12.4 left off based on the progressions explained in the last row of the table.

▶ An OCR athlete's in-season consists of training, preparing for race day (or a multiple-race weekend), and recovering. Thus, there are two sample in-season training plans; table 12.6 shows a non-race week and table 12.7 shows a week with a Saturday race and a subsequent recovery week. (*Note*: The details and guidelines are isolated to those two circumstances and not progressed from the preceding preseason sample program.)

▶ The sample programs do not show scheduling for recovery weeks (also called *unloading* or *deloading* weeks) that serve to decrease the risk of overtraining and allow the body extra time to adapt to the training stimulus. A common approach is to insert a recovery week after 4 weeks of training throughout off- and preseason training. During the in-season, a recovery week (or half of a week) could be placed midway between two primary races or race weekends. Programming for a recovery week frequently entails workouts of 50% to 75% of an athlete's customary training intensity and volume; see table 12.7 on page 300 for similar guidelines.

Table 12.4 Sample Off-Season OCR Training Plan (8 weeks)

Day 1	Day 2	Day 3	Day 4	Day 5	Day 6
RT: 3 × 12-15[a]	DR: 3.5 mi (5.6 km) or 30 min[b]	RT: 3 × 12-15	DR: 2 mi (3 km) or 17 min	RT: 3 × 12-15[a]	DR: 4 mi (6.4 km) or 35 min[b]

DR = distance running; IR = interval running; RT = resistance training. *Note:* The warm-up procedures for RT are not listed, but they are necessary. [a]Sets × repetitions. [b]There is no intention to imply a certain pace (min/mile or min/km) by providing a distance and time value; simply choose one method or the other of quantifying the workout.

Details about the sample off-season OCR training plan:

▶ RT exercises and order: Leg press, leg (knee) curl, leg (knee) extension, standing calf raise, bench press, lateral raise, lat pulldown (or seated row), triceps extension, biceps curl, machine (or stability ball) back extension, and abdominal crunch. Use loads (if appropriate) that are heavy enough that the last 1 or 2 repetitions in the last set of each exercise are somewhat hard to complete. *Note*: It will likely take 2 or 3 workouts to effectively determine the correct load for each exercise.

▶ DR, days 2 and 6: Run at an even, consistent pace that can be maintained for the full duration of the run (i.e., a full sentence can be spoken in one breath). Warm up first by doing a 5- to 10-minute power walk.

▶ DR, day 4: Run at a varied pace with unstructured fast and slow segments of varying times or distances. Warm up first by doing a 5- to 10-minute power walk, and gradually increase the pace of the fast segments during the run.

▶ Starting in week 5, replace the DR, day 4 session with an IR session: Alternate a 2-minute work interval with a 2-minute recovery interval for 2.5 miles (4 km) or 21 minutes[b] (see the meaning of the [b] superscript under table 12.4). Run at a pace during the work interval that only permits speaking in phrases (not full sentences or only 1-2 words) by the end of the interval, and walk the recovery interval. Fully warm up before the first work interval (e.g., run 5 to 10 minutes, perform several dynamic flexibility exercises, and do 2-3 progressively faster 50-100 yd [or m] warm-up sprints). Run a 5- to 10-minute cooldown after the last interval.

▶ DR and (later) IR: If on the treadmill, use at least a 2% grade.

Guidelines about how to progress the sample off-season OCR training plan:

▸ RT: Weeks 1-4: Perform 3 sets of 12 to 15 repetitions per set. Weeks 5-8: Add weight (5-15 lb [2-7 kg], depending on the exercise) and perform 10 to 12 repetitions per set. Across all weeks, after reaching the maximum number of repetitions in the range and then repeating that success for two RT workouts in a row, add weight for the next workout. For maximum effectiveness, apply this strategy to each set of each exercise independently (and keep track in a workout log).

▸ DR: Add 1/3 mile (0.5 km) or 3 minutes to the total distance or time of each workout each week.

▸ IR: Add 1/2 mile (0.8 km) or 5 minutes to the total distance or time each week (this may result in a final interval of an odd distance or duration). (Another option is to add 30 seconds to each work interval each week while keeping the same recovery interval.)

Table 12.5   Sample Preseason OCR Training Plan (12 weeks)

Day 1	Day 2	Day 3	Day 4	Day 5	Day 6
UB RT: 3 × 12-15[a]	3-part brick: PT: 2 × 5 + LB RT: 3 × 12-15 + IR: 4.5 mi (7.2 km) or 39 min[b]	HICT: 2 circuits of 30-sec work interval, 15-sec transition interval	2-part brick: UB RT: 3 × 12-15 + DR: 6.5 mi (10.4 km) or 56 min[b]	2-part brick: PT: 2 × 5 + LB RT: 3 × 12-15	2-part brick: TR: 5 mi (8 km) or 48 min[b] + OST (>15 min)

DR = distance running; HICT = high-intensity circuit training; IR = interval running; LB = lower body; OST = obstacle skill training; PT = plyometric training; RT = resistance training; TR = trail running; UB = upper body. *Note:* The warm-up procedures for RT are not listed, but they are necessary. [a]Sets × repetitions. [b]There is no intention to imply a certain pace (min/mile or min/km) by providing a distance and time value; simply choose one method or the other of quantifying the workout.

Details about the sample preseason OCR training plan:

▸ UB RT exercises and order: *Alternating single-arm dumbbell bench press, pull-up* (or an alternate version, if needed; e.g., *chin-up* or *band-assisted pull-up*), *single-arm half-kneeling dumbbell shoulder press, alternating hand medicine ball push-up, rope row,* dumbbell shoulder series (front raise, lateral raise, bent-over lateral raise, shoulder shrug), overhead triceps extension, hammer curl, forearms to hands plank, superman back extension, and two grip exercises (choose different exercises each workout: dead hang [holding the bar, a draped towel, or looped rope], plate pinch, farmer's walk or hold, wrist curl, reverse curl, or wrist extension).

▸ LB RT exercises and order: *Squat* (bar or dumbbell), *single-dumbbell lunge, single-dumbbell step-up,* goblet lateral step lunge, single-dumbbell single-leg Romanian deadlift, seated single-leg calf raise, and standing single-leg calf raise. *Note:*

Only use one dumbbell for the load for the three single-dumbbell exercises; begin the exercise holding it in one hand and, during the exercise, transfer the dumbbell to the opposite hand before every full repetition (i.e., each leg does the movement with the dumbbell held in the same hand, and then the dumbbell is moved to the other hand before the next full repetition; this is different than the customary way to handle a single-dumbbell exercise).

▶ RT: Use loads (if appropriate) that are heavy enough that the last 1 or 2 repetitions in every set of each exercise are hard to complete.

▶ Two- (or three-) part brick: Complete the parts of the multiple-mode workout in the order listed with no appreciable rest between each part.

▶ PT: Squat jump, drop freeze (from a 12 in. [30 cm] box), and double-leg hop. Fully warm up before the first exercise (5 to 10 minutes of a mixture of jumping rope, marching, skipping, butt-kickers, etc.).

▶ IR: Alternate a 2-minute work interval with a 2-minute recovery interval. Run at a pace during the work interval that only permits speaking one or two words at a time by the end of the interval, and slowly jog the recovery interval. Fully warm up before the first work interval (e.g., run 5 to 10 minutes, perform several dynamic flexibility exercises, and two or three progressively faster 50- to 100-yard [or m] warm-up sprints). Run a 5- 10-minute cooldown after the last interval.

▶ Starting in week 2, substitute the IR with an HR and alternate the IR and HR parts of the brick workout in subsequent weeks: Find a 100- to 200-yard- (or m) long road or trail hill that is comparable to at least an 8% incline on a treadmill; it should take about 30 to 45 seconds to climb it. Run up the hill at a vigorous pace; be sure the pace is even for the full distance. Recover for three times the duration of the just-completed uphill run by walking or jogging down the hill and then in the nearby area at a slow enough pace to allow for each uphill interval to be at a vigorous pace. Begin with 4 hill repeats. Fully warm up before beginning the hill portion (e.g., run 5 to 10 minutes, perform several dynamic flexibility exercises, and do two or three progressively faster hill segments). Run a 5- 10-minute cooldown after the last hill.

▶ HICT exercises and sequence: Begin with the version of each exercise not in parentheses (i.e., the lower-intensity option): Mountain climber (burpee), incline (flat) push-up, body-weight (goblet) sumo squat, inverted or reverse (rope) row, body-weight squat (squat jump), slam ball drop (slam), single-leg box push-off (floor-to-box jump), hanging knee (leg) raise, and double- (single-) hop jump rope. Set up the stations and program the timer first; warm-up with at least 10 minutes of a general all-body activity then one untimed circuit of 10 to 15 repetitions of each exercise. The goals are to complete the maximum number of repetitions at each station and to reach at least the same number of repetitions at each station in each circuit.

▶ DR: Run at an even, consistent pace that can be maintained for the full duration of the run (i.e., a full sentence can be spoken in one breath). Warm up first by doing a 5- to 10-minute power walk.

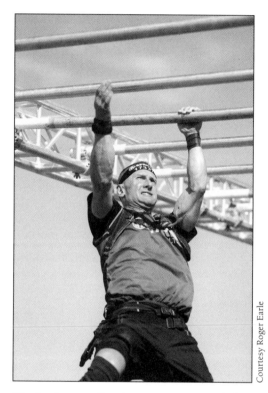

Courtesy Roger Earle

Obstacle practice in preseason training is needed to gain the required skills for monkey bar crossings.

▶ TR: Run (while wearing OCR shoes) on a trail that is comparable to the terrain of an OCR at a pace that only permits speaking in phrases (not full sentences or only one or two words). *Note*: Perceived exertion will be higher during a TR compared to running at the same pace on asphalt or concrete; adjust the TR pace accordingly (e.g., 1 min/mile [37 sec/km] slower). Warm up first by doing a 5- to 10-minute power walk followed by a 5- to 10-minute jog or slower run to lead into the TR pace.

▶ OST: Examples include rope climbing, salmon ladder sequences, wall scaling, swinging, and monkey bar or rig crossing with hanging attachments. Ideally, for safety, learn from and be supervised by a skilled OCR athlete or professional in a controlled environment.

Guidelines about how to progress the sample preseason OCR training plan:

▶ RT: Weeks 1-3: Perform 12 to 15 repetitions per set (for time-based exercises, begin with 15 seconds). Weeks 4-6: Add weight (5-30 lb [2-14 kg], depending on the exercise), increase the difficulty (e.g., remove or change to a thinner band for assisted pull-ups), or add time (aspire to 1 minute or longer) and perform 8 to 10 repetitions per set of the italicized exercises in the list of exercises and 10 to 12 repetitions per set in all others. Weeks 7-9: Reduce the weight (5-15 lb [2-7 kg], depending on the exercise) or decrease the difficulty (e.g., add or change to a thicker band for assisted pull-ups) and perform 12 to 15 repetitions per set in all exercises (keep progressing the time-based exercises as appropriate). Weeks 10-12: Add weight (5-30 lb [2-14 kg], depending on the exercise), increase the difficulty (e.g., remove or change to a thinner band for assisted pull-ups), or add time and perform 8 to 10 repetitions per set of the italicized exercises and 10 to 12 repetitions per set of all others. *Note*: It will likely take one or two UB and one or two LB workouts during weeks 1, 4, 7, and 10 to effectively determine the correct load for each exercise. Across all weeks, after reaching the maximum number of repetitions in the range and then repeating that success for two RT workouts in a row, add weight for the next workout. For maximum effectiveness, apply this strategy to each set of each exercise independently (and keep track in a workout log).

▶ PT: Gradually and cautiously progress to doing more repetitions per set (e.g., add 2 repetitions per set per session); more sets (e.g., add 1 set every 2 to 3 weeks); and greater heights and distances, diagonal and lateral movements, and single-leg versions (e.g., after 6 weeks).

▶ IR: Add 1/2 mi (0.8 km) or 5 minutes to the total distance or time each week (this may result in a final interval of an odd distance or duration). Another option is to add 30 seconds to each work interval each week while keeping the same recovery interval.

▶ HR: Add two hill intervals each session.

▶ HICT: Each week, add 10 seconds per work interval until reaching 60 seconds, then add a circuit (i.e., a set) and lower the work interval back to 30 seconds; keep the transition interval fixed at 15 seconds. Over time, progress to substituting one to three higher-intensity exercise options into the sequence (i.e., those in parentheses): Mountain climber (burpee), incline (flat) push-up, body-weight (goblet) sumo squat, inverted or reverse (rope) row, body-weight squat (squat jump), slam ball drop (slam), single-leg box push-off (floor-to-box jump), hanging knee (leg) raise, and double- (single-) hop jump rope.

▶ DR: Add 1/3 mi (0.5 km) or 3 minutes to the total distance or time each week.

▶ TR: Add 1/2 mi (0.8 km) or 5 minutes to the total distance or time each week.

▶ OST: Progress to more complex combinations and longer practice sessions as obstacle skill and strength improves.

Table 12.6   Sample In-Season OCR Training Plan: Non-Race Week*

Day 1	Day 2	Day 3	Day 4	Day 5	Day 6	Day 7
HICT	3-part brick: PT + IR/HR + LB RT	UB RT	HICT (with running)	3-part brick: Light PT + DR + Light LB RT + UB RT	2-part brick: TR + OST	Rest or recovery walk

*The specifics of the various training modes (e.g., running distance, time, and pace; resistance, plyometric, and HICT exercises, sets, repetitions, interval duration, etc.) depend on how well an OCR athlete adapted to the preseason program. Athletes should not simply follow the sample programs as they are presented; instead, they should consult with an OCR-experienced strength and conditioning professional.

Details about the changes from preseason training to in-season training:

▶ HICT: Add a second weekly session and in that session replace the rest transition interval with a running work interval (outdoors or on a treadmill); begin with 1 to 2 minutes and gradually progress the time, incline (if on a treadmill), speed, or a combination of these. To adjust to this new level of intensity, reduce the length of the work intervals, the number of circuits, or both, and gradually increase them again over time.

▶ PT: Incorporate lateral and diagonal exercises and single-leg versions (e.g., the lateral barrier hop, lateral box push-off, lateral box jump, zig-zap hop, side skip, and single- and double-arm alternate-leg bound).

▶ RT and IR or HR: Running has a higher priority during the in-season, so the order of RT and running workouts are switched from the preseason.

▶ Light PT and light LB RT sessions: Because the TR on day 6 is one of the most important sessions of the week, activities involving the lower body on day 5 are programmed at a lower level of intensity than comparable workouts earlier in the week. Athletes can either reduce training intensity by 50% or reduce training volume by 50%. (The intensity and volume of the UB RT sessions are not reduced.)

▶ Recovery walk: A 20- to 40-minute slower walk (e.g., 20-24 min/mi [12-15 min/km] or 2.5-3 mph [4.0-4.8 kph]) the day after a TR often helps speed recovery.

Table 12.7 Sample In-Season OCR Training Plan: Race Week and Recovery Week[a]

RACE WEEK						
Monday	**Tuesday**	**Wednesday**	**Thursday**	**Friday**	**Saturday**	**Sunday[b]**
TR	HICT	LB/UB RT	DR	Rest	OCR	Rest
I: 25%[c] V: 50%[c]	I: 25% V: 33%	I: 33% V: 33%	I: 50% V: 75%[d]	—	—	
RECOVERY WEEK						
Monday	**Tuesday**	**Wednesday**	**Thursday**	**Friday**	**Saturday**	**Sunday[e]**
Rest	2-part brick: Recovery walk[f] + LB/UB RT	2-part brick: Recovery IR (run/walk) + LB/UB RT	HICT (version with no running work interval)	2-part brick: DR + LB/UB RT	TR	Rest or recovery walk[f]
—	I: 75% V: 66%	IR: I: 50% V: 50% RT: I: 50% V: 33%	I: 50% V: 33%	DR: I: 33% V: 33% RT: I: 25% V: 25%	I: 25% V: 25%	—

[a]The specifics of the various training modes (e.g., running distance, time, and pace; resistance, plyometric, and HICT exercises, sets, repetitions, interval duration, etc.) depend on how well an OCR athlete adapted to the preseason program. Readers should not simply follow the sample programs as they are presented; instead, they should consult with an OCR-experienced strength and conditioning professional. [b]If there is also a race (or two) on Sunday, shift the suggested recovery week training forward by a day. [c]The *percent decrease* in non-race-week intensity ("I") (i.e., load lifted for RT and HICT exercises [as applicable], perceived effort for running) and volume ("V") (i.e., work interval duration and number of HICT circuits, number of RT and PT sets, running distance or time). [d]For example, a 75% decrease in an 8-mile DR results in a 2-mile DR. [e]The Monday that follows begins normal non-race-week training, but if the athlete does not feel sufficiently recovered, complete the training sessions at 100% of non-race-week training volume but at 75% to 90% of non-race-week training intensity until fully recovered. [f]The intensity and volume percentages do not apply to the recovery walk.

CHAPTER 13

Overtraining and Recovery

Michael Naperalsky

Exercise performance is built on the process of training and recovery. The more total load we accumulate and the harder we are able to exercise, the more we adapt for future performance. The stress of training needs a pause in the process; the human body needs time to handle a stress, recover back to a status of *homeostasis* (equilibrium), and adapt to that stress over time. As athletes push the bounds of difficult training, increased attention has been paid to the process of exercise recovery—both the importance of it and how we might positively influence it in order to encourage faster recovery between sessions and achieve improved adaptation over time.

WHAT IS RECOVERY?

Generally speaking, *recovery* is the process by which the body returns to resting levels from a disruption in homeostasis. Exercise causes various disruptions to a baseline resting state, such as elevated heart rate, respiration, and body temperature; increased use of glycogen and fat stores for energy; central and peripheral nervous system fatigue; and psychological stress. Recovery from exercise is dependent on the specific stress involved, how much of the stress was incurred, and the body's previous resilience to the current stress. Because of this, an athlete's return to baseline can be as brief as a few minutes after a single movement or as long as months after a long competition season.

The science of exercise recovery has been studied extensively in many areas, but the broad nature of exercise, training, and sport requires an expansive view of all the confounding factors that can influence recovery. Kellmann and Kallus defined recovery as "an inter- and intra-individual multi-level (e.g., psychological, physiological, social) process in time for the re-establishment of performance abilities" (12). But is recovery to a baseline state really the ultimate goal of training? Or are adaptation, performance, and holistic development the greater goals of physical development? Stone and Stone expanded this traditional view with the idea of *recovery-adaptation* to suggest not simply the return to baseline or refilling of resources, but also the incremental changes that occur as a result of exercise and the repeated cycle of both recovery and adaptation (23). These changes are frequently the original goal that was intended: bike to improve fitness, swim to improve economy, or lift weights to grow stronger. With these intentions in mind, exercise recovery does not simply mean a return to the previous state, but rather an optimization of the adaptation to exercise that might facilitate enhanced training in the future.

STRESS

Exercise training and competitive sport create stress on an athlete. This stress can take various forms, including both physical and psychological, and may come from a variety of sources: physical training, sport practice and competition, social activities, interpersonal relationships, and other areas of daily life. Stress creates a biological and psychological response within the human body, creating periods of acute fatigue, acute response, and long-term adaptation. This cycle of stress, fatigue, recovery, and adaptation is individual, multifactorial, and occurs in repeated cycles. The end result, from an athletic standpoint, is an enhancement of an athlete's level of preparedness for competition (figure 13.1).

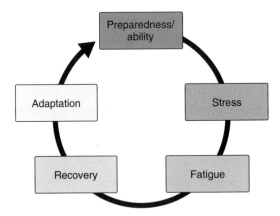

Figure 13.1 The cycle of stress, fatigue, recovery, and adaptation.

Stress occurs in four key areas:

1. *Biomechanical.* Physical stress to muscle, bone, and connective tissue. This can take hours to days to repair.

2. *Metabolic.* The use of substrates for fuel, the accumulation of resulting by-products, and the disruption to the cellular environment. This can take minutes, hours, or even days to restore.

3. *Neural.* Stress that taxes our nervous system, resulting in decreased speed or power, impaired decision making, and decreased reaction time. This can take hours or days to restore.

4. *Psychological.* Mental and emotional stress from a multitude of sources. This can take hours, days, or even weeks to resolve.

It is important to remember that stress and fatigue are the normal results of physical training or sport. Clearly defining and understanding the specific stress involved will help an individual create proactive strategies for hastening recovery and improving adaptation.

RECOVERY MODALITIES

The use of specific recovery modalities can support the body's natural processes for repair and restoration, helping athletes more rapidly return to a state of readiness and improve their abilities over time. Like many products, some modalities are incredibly beneficial, some have mixed results, and some promise more than they deliver. They are categorized as *foundational*, *favorable*, and *uncertain*, respectively.

Foundational Recovery Modalities

As the name implies, these items are not modalities in and of themselves, but are necessary for healthy human life. They are so vital that athletes likely do need to add these to their routines, but instead can optimize the process in their lives and training program.

Rest

The most obvious way to end the stress of exercise is to stop exercising. In the constant pursuit of greater gains and improved performance, athletes often fail to simply take a day off. A scheduled day free of training creates additional time to restore resources, heal tissues, and allow the mind to reset. This simple yet effective technique is all too often overlooked in the competitive world, where the mindset is, "Yesterday went well, so today I should do just a little more." Rest can take a variety of forms but should minimize physical loading and direct one's time away from sport. Suggestions might include additional time with family or friends, meditation or focused breathing exercises, light restorative yoga, or other fun activities that an athlete finds enjoyable. While intentional rest has not been specifically studied outside of research on tapering for competition, it is likely to benefit all four areas of stress.

Sleep

Humans require a period of deliberate rest each day in the form of sleep. Adequate sleep plays a vital role in a variety of cognitive and physiological functions. Sleep allows for memory consolidation and learning, repair of damaged tissues, and optimized growth hormone release, and it supports proper immune function (6, 24).

Strategies to optimize sleep are generally consistent across everyone. Developing good habits around your sleeping environment and behaviors, known as proper *sleep hygiene*, can enhance sleep in your daily routine. These general recommendations include the following (9, 22, 27):

- Most adults need 7 to 9 hours of sleep each night.
- Develop consistent sleep and wake times, rising at the same time and going to bed at the same time each day.
- Create the ideal sleep environment: cool, dark, and quiet. Minimize noise and light interference, aim for a room temperature of 60 °F to 67 °F (16 °C-19 °C), and avoid other activities in bed such as eating or watching television.
- Turn off all screens (TV, computer, phone, tablet) 30 to 60 minutes before bed.
- Avoid caffeine after 3:00 p.m., which may interfere with sleep.
- Late evening exercise may disrupt sleep or make it more difficult to fall asleep.

Athletes can supplement their nightly sleep with daytime naps, especially when following certain guidelines. Naps should last 30 minutes or less or approximately 90 minutes (28). A 30-minute nap allows for a brief psychological reset without falling into deep sleep; a 90-minute nap lasts roughly the length of a single sleep cycle. Naps lasting longer than this may lead to feelings of grogginess or disrupt future sleep–wake patterns. Naps can be placed in the early afternoon and should conclude at least 6 hours before bedtime (29).

Athletes have frequently reported disturbed sleep the night before important competitions, including problems falling asleep, thoughts about competition, and poor sleep quality (11). Because of this, it is important to establish proper sleep hygiene and practice these habits regularly. Restful sleep is likely to benefit all four areas of stress and recovery.

Nutrition

Because endurance exercise frequently involves large fueling demands and extended periods of exercise, adequate and appropriate postexercise nutrition is vital. Endurance exercise relies heavily on stored carbohydrate (glycogen) for fuel, and the time period after immediately after exercise (≤2 hr) is especially optimal for restoring this fuel source (10). Both simple and complex carbohydrates are appropriate sources to help replenish glycogen and glucose. Postexercise snacks and meals should also include protein, which is a vital component for muscle repair, maintenance, and growth, as well as regulating body processes, supporting the immune system, and providing energy.

Athletes can seek out specific help from professionals in the field, especially a registered dietitian (RD). An RD with additional experience in sport may also be a board-certified specialist in sport dietetics (CSSD). If athletes are managing their own nutrition, it is important to understand that nutrition's role in recovery may vary widely depending on the individual and the situation. Important questions athletes might ask themselves include the following:

▶ How long and how intense was the last activity?

▶ How long do I have before my next session?

▶ How long and how intense is my next session?

▶ How does my postexercise recovery snack fit with my regular meal schedule?

▶ Are there any barriers to consuming the food I need (e.g., travel from an event)?

Short recovery windows (e.g., during multiday events or stage races) will likely necessitate prioritizing snacks of carbohydrate plus protein as soon as possible after activity. This is usually followed by a full meal 2 to 3 hours after exercise. Simple carbohydrates (sucrose, glucose) are quickly digested and absorbed, and whey protein is more quickly digested and absorbed than protein sources that are predominantly casein or soy. Athletes can also avoid high-fat or high-fiber foods immediately after exercise, because these will slow overall digestion and absorption. Every athlete will have individual food preferences and even rituals surrounding training and competition, so it is important to experiment with different approaches and find what works best. Appropriate nutrition is likely to benefit all four areas of stress.

Hydration

Proper hydration is important for normal metabolism, thermoregulation, organ function, and strength and power production. Hydration can be especially important during high-intensity activities and exercise in hot, humid conditions or at high altitudes. Body weight loss from dehydration can impair aerobic power output, cognitive tasks and reaction times, and strength production.

It is important to know that hydration can vary from person to person; may depend on environmental conditions; and may change with acclimatization to heat, humidity, or altitude. Important questions athletes might ask themselves include the following:

- ▸ How much did I sweat during my last activity?
- ▸ If possible to measure, how much body weight did I lose?
- ▸ Am I a salty sweater? (Do you find salt deposits on your skin or clothing after exercise?)
- ▸ How long do I have before my next session?
- ▸ What beverages do I prefer?
- ▸ Do I need to include beverages with extra electrolytes or carbohydrate?
- ▸ Are there any barriers to consuming the drinks I need (e.g., availability of cold drinks)?

Rehydration is most important during hot, humid conditions and during short recovery windows (<24 hr). Immediately after exercise, aim to replace fluids of 1.5 times the amount of body weight lost during exercise (e.g., 1.5 L of fluid for every kg of body weight lost) (20). Drinks should include carbohydrate and *electrolytes*, although these additions can be highly variable and individual (19). Electrolytes are minerals such sodium, potassium, magnesium, and calcium that aid in muscle contraction, regulating blood pH, and maintaining proper fluid balance in the body. Athletes are encouraged to add salt to their postexercise beverages, both to encourage thirst and to aid in retaining the fluids consumed. It is also important to sip fluids over an extended period of time as opposed to rapidly drinking or consuming plain water. Rapidly consuming plain water will quickly pass and increase urine production. Cool or cold drinks will aid in thermoregulation and are more likely to be consumed in greater quantities. Hydration should also be taken in the context of an athlete's entire diet, including food intake. Certain snacks or meals such as fruit, vegetables, soups, and salty snacks such as pretzels or pickles can increase overall intake of fluids and electrolytes. In addition to monitoring pre- and postexercise body weight, athletes can monitor their urine color as an approximate gauge of hydration status (consult reference 1 to see a color version of the urine color chart). Clear urine and frequent urination can indicate overhydration, while darker urine is usually a sign of dehydration. Pale or light, yellow-colored urine can indicate adequate hydration levels. Appropriate hydration is likely to benefit all four areas of stress.

Favorable Recovery Modalities

Favorable recovery modalities often have some research backing but may have inconsistent results, lack specific protocols, or lack a specific physiological mechanism by which effectiveness can be assessed. Many of these tools are commonly used, but the precise nature of why they are preferred has not been well established. These same tools often do not appear to elicit any interference effects, so their use is at the discretion of the athlete. Simply put: If you feel it works for you, then have at it. Sometimes we find that a modality is beneficial long before the scientific research can verify why it works.

Compression

Compression often takes one of two primary forms: *static* (using garments or clothing) or *dynamic* (using machines of pulsed air pressure). Compression works by improving venous return, enhancing the removal of waste products, and minimizing inflammation (21). Compression can also decrease pain perception and fatigue, and attenuate strength losses associated with soreness (18).

Compression garments can be worn for 30 minutes to 48 hours after exercise, on areas of heavily involved muscle groups (e.g., pants or tights following cycling) (2, 4). Dynamic compression machines are frequently used for a 20 to 30-minute recovery cycle. Compression socks can also be worn during long-duration travel, especially following strenuous exercise.

Because the human body takes many different sizes and shapes, the specific compression gradient of a garment or machine sleeve may vary greatly from one individual to another. This creates inconsistency across treatment protocols and potential outcomes. Athletes can follow sizing recommendations specific to their apparel manufacturer.

Hydrotherapy

Hydrotherapy—the use of hot, cold, or contrast baths—is suggested to relieve muscle soreness, increase parasympathetic tone (relaxation), and offset the muscle strength and power that can be lost over consecutive days of vigorous efforts (25). Cold water has been shown to be most effective, with some positive results for contrast baths (26). Hot water, frequently a favorite for overall relaxation, has not been shown to help performance or the perception of pain with athletes (26). Hydrotherapy may benefit the biomechanical, neural, and psychological areas of stress.

General recommendations for hydrotherapy are as follows (26):

▶ *Cold:* 50 °F-59 °F (10 °C-15 °C) for 15 to 20 minutes.
▶ *Contrast:* Alternate between 50 °F (10 °C) cold and 102 °F (39 °C) hot for 1 to 2 minutes each, for a total of 12 to 14 minutes.
▶ *Hot:* 100 °F-104 °F (38 °C-40 °C).
▶ Athletes can submerge their lower body (waist-down), entire body (neck-down), or a specific limb or body part.

Emerging research suggests that cryotherapy and the frequent use of cold modalities may blunt inflammation, which can be a key factor in creating physiological change and hypertrophy. A systematic review concluded that cold-water immersion may negatively affect resistance training adaptations, specifically maximal strength and strength endurance (16). At this time, cold-water immersion is not recommended during intense training cycles in the preparatory phase but instead should be prioritized during the competitive season. Additionally, hot-water immersion likely should be avoided if an athlete is looking to minimize swelling following an acute injury (30).

Massage

Human touch and therapeutic massage have been a part of the human condition for millennia. Massage therapy, involving a trained practitioner providing human touch, individualized care, and specific techniques to apply pressure to muscles and skin, has been shown to promote mitochondrial biogenesis and reduce inflammation (3), as well as reduce delayed onset muscle soreness (8).

Hiring a trained professional to help you recover, however, often proves more expensive and more difficult than a device or machine that can accomplish the same task. Such has been the development of self-massage devices over the last century. They come in all shapes and sizes: balls, sticks, rollers, curved hooks for the hard-to-reach places, and percussive-therapy tools, which are all purported to improve soft-tissue tone and pliability, increase range of motion, and ease soreness. Similar to traditional massage therapy, self-massage devices have been shown to briefly improve range of motion, decrease muscle soreness, and minimize power decrements following heavy strength training or eccentric muscle damage (15, 17). Percussive-therapy guns, while newer and less researched, have shown evidence of improving joint range of motion, likely by reducing muscle stiffness (13). It is important to note that while the term *myofascial release* has come into common usage, foam rolling, for example, has been shown to change range of motion without structural changes in the muscle or connective tissue (31). While it does not seem to affect metabolism, self-massage may benefit the biomechanical, neural, and psychological areas of stress.

While self-massage may be used frequently by athletes, there is little agreement in terms of specific protocols or recommendations. Most research studies have involved rolling or self-massaging a target muscle group for 1 to 2 minutes at a time, for 1 or 2 sets, following the guidelines of gentle pressure and only mild discomfort (15, 17). This creates a whole-body routine of 10 to 20 minutes. Various devices have different material densities and shapes, which makes it difficult to say whether one device may offer a specific benefit over another. Athletes should be cautious to avoid self-massage work over injured areas, open wounds, or bony structures.

Uncertain Recovery Modalities

While the foundational recovery components are necessary to support human life, and the favorable modalities are frequently used with positive results, our list of uncertain recovery practices are frequently unsupported by research, lack specific protocols, or lack a physiological explanation for what benefit they provide. In many cases these are not new technologies that are rapidly emerging, but rituals recommended by coaches who learned them from their coaches, and so on. Many of these habits are regularly used by a large population of athletes, but their common use should be questioned without a strong body of evidence or theoretical rationale for their practice.

Static Stretching

Static stretching, the practice of applying a light stretch to a muscle group and holding for a period of time, does not seem to positively affect any of the four key types of stress. No evidence of metabolic benefits exists, because stretching would not increase glycogen synthesis or promote protein synthesis. While static stretching can increase flexibility over time, there is little to no evidence of biomechanical benefits, because stretching does not repair damaged tissue, reduce swelling, or reduce delayed onset muscle soreness (7). While there is not supporting research, one could theorize that the ritual of static stretching might create psychological comfort, where athletes might use such a time for gradual relaxation and a heightened sense of body awareness.

Active Recovery

Active recovery, frequently prescribed as 15- to 30-minute *shakeout sessions*, involves the use of light exercise to increase blood flow, increase range of motion, and encourage physical healing. Active recovery, however, lacks finite physiological mechanisms that might explain its common use. While light exercise has been shown to remove certain metabolic products (e.g., lactate) from the blood more rapidly than passive recovery, lactate specifically has not been shown to negatively affect exercise performance or to increase fatigue or soreness. Active recovery, as with any form of exercise, will elevate metabolism and thus may negatively affect metabolic recovery. Anecdotal evidence suggests that light exercise may decrease muscle soreness following intense exercise but only compared to no activity at all. Athletes may choose to use light exercise sessions as desired but should strongly consider if this additional activity adds to any recovery effects compared to additional rest or relaxation.

PUTTING IT ALL TOGETHER

Direct interventions to promote recovery and adaptation should be individual and based on the specific needs of the athlete at that point in time. An athlete who reports excessive fatigue will likely benefit from a focus on rest, sleep, and adequate nutrition and hydration. An athlete who reports high levels of muscle soreness will likely benefit from massage and cold tub hydrotherapy, and should ensure adequate protein intake.

Recovery modalities should be periodized into the training plan at key times and used within the context of training and competition. Athletes should bear in mind the phrase "recover with a purpose"—in other words, they should understand the nature of the exercise stress, the expected response, and how a proposed intervention will aid in the pursuit of a particular goal. Competition seasons, especially dense periods of repeated maximal efforts, are more appropriate for recovery modalities than an off-season training cycle meant to elicit improvements in strength or fitness.

Physical training, competitive games, and external factors (e.g., life stress) are woven together and often always present. Athletes can approach recovery and adaptation by understanding the long-term plan and manipulating training loads as needed by frequently monitoring themselves and evaluating variable responses to stress. Proper management of stress and adaptation cycles will yield not only improved fitness, but ideally optimal preparedness for peak performance.

OVERTRAINING

Remember that training consists of the continuous cycle of stress, fatigue, recovery, and adaptation. In the short term, the acute phase called *functional overreaching* creates a moderate stress that the body can recover from and adapt to. Without an adequate time frame to synthesize glycogen, repair damaged tissues, recover from neurological fatigue, and restore psychological well-being, the athlete enters the next training session underrecovered. When the process is repeated over and over, the athlete enters a phase of *nonfunctional overreaching*. This is a mismatch between the volume or intensity (or both) of the stress applied and the time used to properly recover from the training stress. If an athlete is unable to recover from one session to the next and stress accumulates without positive adaptation, the clinical presentation of *overtraining syndrome* may apply (5) (figure 13.2). It is important to recognize that overtraining syndrome has a multitude of signs and symptoms, many of which are present with other maladies and illnesses. This can make the overtraining syndrome difficult to specifically identify.

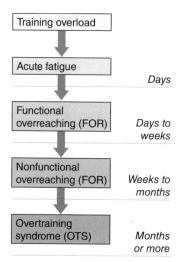

Figure 13.2 The overtraining continuum.

Reprinted by permission from D. French, "Adaptations to Anerobic Training Programs," in *Essentials of Strength Training and Conditioning*, 4th ed., edited by G.G. Haff and N.T. Triplett (Champaign, IL: Human Kinetics, 2015), 108.

The term *overtraining* (also known as *underrecovery*) may be confusing for some. While many athletes recognize that the principle means of improving performance is strenuous and consistent physical training, some coaches and athletes believe that more is always better— that there is no limit beyond which training becomes counterproductive. However, the human body is a biological system with a limit to an athlete's capacity to not only withstand intense training, but also positively adapt to it. Once this threshold is crossed, the athlete fails to progress, and performance or health may decline.

Functionary overreaching is the planned, systematic, and progressive increase in training with the goal of improving performance. A zone of positive training adaptation exists where athletes can reap the benefits of their training. However, this has a scale effect; if an acute overload is too small of a dose (known as *underreaching*), some training adaptations will occur but will only yield small increases in performance. If the athlete maximizes full training adaptations by following a planned program of progressive overload that also includes intentional recovery periods, performance can increase significantly. Nonfunctional overreaching occurs in the long term when an athlete does not allow adequate recovery from the training or intensity. If this situation is not recognized by the athlete or coach, the transient overreaching can become overtraining (14). Athletes need to find the balance between underreaching and overreaching, and they should constantly focus on high-quality training sessions within a recovery-based training model. This will yield consistent improvements in performance without the risk of overtraining. With this concept in mind, it is important for the coach and athlete to objectively quantify training load (external monitoring) and subjectively evaluate the athlete's response to training (internal monitoring). By understanding what training was performed and how the athlete has recovered from that stress, the coach and athlete can properly gauge the next step in the training process.

References

Chapter 1

1. Brooks, GA, Fahey, TD, and Baldwin, KM. *Exercise Physiology: Human Bioenergetics and Its Applications*. New York: McGraw-Hill, 26-29, 59-93, 355-358, 503-505, 2019.

2. Dalley, AF, and Agur, AMR. *Moore's Clinically Oriented Anatomy*. 9th ed. Philadelphia: Lippincott Williams & Wilkins, 28-36, 2022.

3. Haff, GG. Periodization. In *Essentials of Strength Training and Conditioning*. 4th ed. Haff, GG, and Triplett, NT, eds. Champaign, IL: Human Kinetics, 583-604, 2016.

4. Hoffman, J. *Physiological Aspects of Sport Training and Performance*. 2nd ed. Champaign, IL: Human Kinetics, 41-46, 47, 139-143, 155-180, 186-192, 207-218, 219-235, 252-256, 2014.

5. Kenney, WL, Wilmore, JH, and Costill, DL. *Physiology of Sport and Exercise. 8th ed.* Champaign, IL: Human Kinetics, 26-49, 39-42, 58-68, 69, 190-206, 284-309, 2021.

6. Kraemer, W, Fleck, S, and Deschenes, M. *Exercise Physiology: Integrating Theory and Application*. 3rd ed. Philadelphia: Lippincott Williams & Wilkins, 127-130, 427-462, 479-508, 2021.

7. Marieb, EN, and Hoehn, KN. *Human Anatomy and Physiology*. 11th ed. London: Pearson, 279-309, 818-847, 1026-1028, 2018.

8. McArdle, WD, Katch, FI, and Katch, VL. *Exercise Physiology: Nutrition, Energy, and Human Performance*. 9th ed. Philadelphia: Lippincott Williams & Wilkins, 178-184, 185, 294-298, 403-408, 409, 506-507, 507-524, 2022.

9. Mougios, V. *Exercise Biochemistry*. 2nd ed. Champaign, IL: Human Kinetics, 13, 25, 143-160, 171-176, 183-210, 328-336, 416-418, 2020.

10. Reuter, BH, and Dawes, JJ. Program design and technique for aerobic endurance training. In *Essentials of Strength Training and Conditioning*. 4th ed. Haff, GG, and Triplett, NT, eds. Champaign, IL: Human Kinetics, 559-581, 2016.

11. Sharkey, BJ, and Gaskill, SE. *Sport Physiology for Coaches*. Champaign, IL: Human Kinetics, 43-46, 142-148, 2006.

12. Sheppard, JM, and Triplett, NT. Program design for resistance training. In *Essentials of Strength Training and Conditioning*. 4th ed. Haff, GG and Triplett, NT, eds. Champaign, IL: Human Kinetics, 439-469, 2016.

13. Swank, A, and Sharp, C. Adaptations to aerobic endurance training programs. In *Essentials of Strength Training and Conditioning*. 4th ed. Haff, GG, and Triplett, NT, eds. Champaign, IL: Human Kinetics, 115-133, 2016.

Chapter 2

1. Allen, H, Coggan, A, and McGregor, S. *Training and Racing With a Power Meter*. 3rd ed. Boulder, CO: VeloPress, 30-31, 2019.

2. American College of Sports Medicine. *ACSM's Guidelines for Exercise Testing and Prescription*. 11th ed. Philadelphia: Wolters Kluwer, 146-164, 2021.

3. Beaver, WL, Wasserman, K, and Whipp, BJ. Improved detection of lactate threshold during exercise using a log-log transformation. *J Appl Phys* 59:1936-1940, 1985.

4. Beaver, WL, Wasserman, K, and Whipp, BJ. A new method for detecting anaerobic threshold by gas exchange. *J Appl Phys* 60:2020-2027, 1986.

5. Bishop, D, Jenkins, DG, and MacKinnon, LT. The relationship between plasma lactate parameters, Wpeak and 1-h cycling performance in women. *Med Sci Sports Exerc* 30:1270-1275, 1998.

6. Carter, H, Jones, AM, Barstow, TJ, Burnley, M, Williams, C, and Doust, JH. Effect of endurance training on oxygen uptake kinetics during treadmill running. *J Appl Phys* 89:1744-1752, 2000.

7. Cheng, B, Kuipers, H, Snyder, AC, Jeukendrup, A, and Hesselink, M. A new approach for the determination of ventilatory and lactate thresholds. *Int J Sports Med* 13:518-522, 1992.

8. Eigendorf, J, May, M, Friedrich, J, Engeli, S, Maassen, N, Gros, G, and Meissner, JD. High intensity high volume interval training improves endurance performance and induces a nearly complete slow-to-fast fiber transformation on the mRNA level. *Front Physiol* 9, 601, 2018.

9. Gavin, TP, Ruster, RS, Carrithers, JA, Zwetsloot, KA, Kraus, RM, Evans, CA, Knapp, DJ, Drew, JL, McCartney, JS, Garry, JP, and Hickner, RC. No difference in the skeletal muscle angiogenic response to aerobic exercise training between young and aged men. *J Physiol* 585(Pt 1), 231-239, 2007.

10. Gollnick, PD, Armstrong, RB, Saltin, B, Saubert, CW, Sembrowich, WL, and Shepherd, RE. Effect of training on enzyme activity and fiber composition of human skeletal muscle. *J Appl Physiol* 34, 107-111, 1973.

11. Hazell, TJ, Macpherson, RE, Gravelle, BM, and Lemon, PW. 10 or 30-s sprint interval training bouts enhance both aerobic and anaerobic performance. *Eur J Appl Physiol* 110, 153-160, 2010.

12. Hill, DW. The critical power concept. *Sport Med* 16, 237-254, 1993.

13. Ingjer, F. Effects of endurance training on muscle fibre ATP-ase activity, capillary supply and mito-chondrial content in man. *J Physiol* 294, 419-432, 1979.

14. Janssen, P. *Lactate Threshold Training.* Champaign, IL: Human Kinetics, 2001.

15. Jenkins, DG, and Quigley, BM. The influence of high-intensity exercise training on the Wlim-Tlim relationship. *Med Sci Sports Exerc* 25, 275-282, 1993.

16. Jenkins, DG, Palmer, J and Spillman, D. The influence of dietary carbohydrate on performance of supramaximal intermittent exercise. *Eur J Appl Physiol Occup Physiol* 67, 309-314, 1993.

17. Jensen, L, Bangsbo, J, and Hellsten, Y. Effect of high intensity training on capillarization and presence of angiogenic factors in human skeletal muscle. *J Physiol* 557(Pt 2), 571-582, 2004.

18. Jeukendrup, AE, Craig, NP, and Hawley, JA. The bioenergetics of world class cycling. *J Sci Med Sport* 3, 414-433, 2000.

19. Jones, AM, and Vanhatalo, A. The "critical power" concept: Applications to sports performance with a focus on intermittent high-intensity exercise. *Sports Med* 47(Suppl 1), 65-78, 2017.

20. Karsten, B, Petrigna, L, Klose, A, Blanco, A, Townsend, N, and Triska, C. Relationship between the critical power test and a 20-min functional threshold power test in cycling. *Front Physiol* 11, 613151, 2012.

21. Klitzke Borszcz, K, Tramontin, AF, and Costa, VP. Reliability of the functional threshold power in competitive cyclists. *Int J Sports Med* 41(3), 175-181, 2020.

22. Lamberts, RP. *The Development of an Evidence-Based Submaximal Cycle Test Designed to Monitor and Predict Cycling Performance.* Ensdhede, Netherlands: Ipskamp Drukkers, 2009.

23. Lamberts, RP, Rietjens, GJ, Tijdkink, HH, Noakes, TD, and Lambert, MI. 2010. Measuring submax-imal performance parameters to monitor fatigue and predict cycling performance: A case study of a world-class cyclo-cross cyclist. *Eur J Appl Physiol* 108, 183-190, 2010.

24. Lamberts, RP, Swart, J, Noakes, TD, and Lambert, MI. 2010. A novel submaximal cycle test to monitor fatigue and predict cycling performance. *Br J Sports Med* 45, 797-804, 2010.

25. Lamberts, RP. Predicting cycling performance in trained to elite male and female cyclists. *Int J Sports Physiol Perform* 9, 610-614, 2014.

26. Leo, P, Spragg, J, Podlogar, T, Lawley, JS, and Mujika, I. Power profiling and the power-duration relationship in cycling: A narrative review. *Eur J Appl Physiol* 122, 301-316, 2022.

27. Little, JP, Safdar, A, Wilkin, GP, Tarnopolsky, MA, and Gibala, MJ. A practical model of low-volume high-intensity interval training induces mitochondrial biogenesis in human skeletal muscle: Potential mechanisms. *J Physiol* 588(Pt 6), 1011-1022, 2010.

28. Martino, M, and Dabbs, NC. Aerobic training program design. In *NSCA's Essentials of Personal Training.* 3rd ed. Schoenfeld, BJ, and Snarr, RL eds. Champaign, IL: Human Kinetics, 423, 2022.

29. Macpherson, TW, and Weston, M. The effect of low-volume sprint interval training on the devel-opment and subsequent maintenance of aerobic fitness in soccer players. *Int J Sports Physiol Perform* 10, 332-338, 2015.

30. McGrath, E, Mahony, N, Fleming, N, and Donne, B. Is the FTP test a reliable, reproducible and functional assessment tool in highly-trained athletes? *Int J Exerc Sci* 12(4), 1334-1345, 2019.

31. McGuigan, M. Administration, scoring, and interpretation of selected tests. *Essentials of Strength and Conditioning.* 4th ed. Haff, GG, and Triplett, NT, eds. Champaign, IL: Human Kinetics, 277-279, 2018.

32. Pettitt, RW. Applying the critical speed concept to racing strategy and interval training prescription. *Int J Sports Physiol Perform* 11, 842-847, 2016.

33. Skelly, LE, Gillen, JB, Frankish, BP, MacInnis, MJ, Godkin, FE, Tarnopolsky, MA, Murphy, RM, and Gibala, MJ. Human skeletal muscle fiber type-specific responses to sprint interval and moderate-intensity continuous exercise: Acute and training-induced changes. *J Appl Physiol* 130, 1001-1014, 2021.
34. Skiba, PF, Jackman, S, Clarke, D, Vanhatalo, A, and Jones, AM. Effect of work and recovery durations on W\p\ reconstitution during intermittent exercise. *Med Sci Sports Exerc* 46, 1433-1440, 2014.
35. Skiba, PF. *Scientific Training for Endurance Athletes.* Tinton Farms, NJ: PhysFarm Training Systems, 80-81, 2021.
36. Smith, DL, Plowman, SA, and Ormsbee, MJ. Aerobic metabolism during exercise. In *Exercise Physiology for Health, Fitness, and Performance.* 6th ed. Smith, DL, Plowman, SA, and Ormsbee, MJ eds. Philadelphia: Wolters Kluwer, 109, 2023.
37. Vanhatalo, A, Doust, JH, and Burnley, M. 2008. A 3-min all-out cycling test is sensitive to a change in critical power. *Med Sci Sports Exerc* 40, 1693-1699, 2008.
38. Van Proeyen, K, Szlufcik, K, Nielens, H, Ramaekers, M, and Hespel, P. Beneficial metabolic adaptations due to endurance exercise training in the fasted state. *J Appl Physiol* 110, 236-245, 2011.
39. Warnier, G, Benoit, N, Naslain, D, Lambrecht, S, Francaux, M, and Deldicque, L. Effects of sprint interval training at different altitudes on cycling performance at sea-level. *Sports (Basel)* 8, 148, 2020.
40. Wasserman, K, Beaver, WL, and Whipp, BJ. Gas exchange theory and the lactic acidosis (anaerobic) threshold. *Circulation* 81(Suppl 1), II14-II30, 1990.
41. Wasserman, K. Breathing during exercise. *New Eng J Med* 278, 780-785, 1978.

Chapter 3

1. Abou Elmagd M. Common sports injuries. *Int J Phys Educ Sports Health* 3:142-148, 2016.
2. Armstrong, LE. *Performing in Extreme Environments.* Champaign, IL: Human Kinetics, 96, 2000.
3. Armstrong, LE, Casa, DJ, Millard-Stafford, M, Moran, DS, Pyne, SW, and Roberts, WO. American College of Sports Medicine position stand: Exertional heat illness during training and competition. *Med Sci Sports Exerc* 39:556-572, 2007.
4. Armstrong, LE, and Stoppani, J. Central nervous system control of heat acclimation adaptations: An emerging paradigm. *Rev Neurosci* 13:271-285, 2002.
5. Buchheit, M, and Laursen, PB. High-intensity interval training, solutions to the programming puzzle: Part I: Cardiopulmonary emphasis. *Sports Med* 43:313-338, 2013.
6. Buchheit, M, and Laursen, PB. High-intensity interval training, solutions to the programming puzzle: Part II: Anaerobic energy, neuromuscular load and practical applications. *Sports Med* 43:927-954, 2013.
7. Burtscher, M, Niedermeier, M, Burtscher, J, Pesta, D, Suchy, J, and Strasser, B. Preparation for endurance competitions at altitude: Physiological, psychological, dietary and coaching aspects. A narrative review. *Front Physiol* 9:1504-1504, 2018.
8. Busso, T. Variable dose-response relationship between exercise training and performance. *Med Sci Sports Exerc* 35:1188-1195, 2003.
9. Casa DJ, DeMartini JK, Bergeron MF, Csillan D, Eichner ER, Lopez RM, Ferrara MS, Miller KC, O'Connor F, Sawka MN, and Yeargin SW. National Athletic Trainers' Association position statement: Exertional heat illnesses. *J Athl Train* 50: 986-1000, 2015.
10. Castellani, JW, Young, AJ, Ducharme, MB, Giesbrecht, GG, Glickman, E, and Sallis, RE. American College of Sports Medicine position stand: Prevention of cold injuries during exercise. *Med Sci Sports Exerc* 38:2012-2029, 2006.
11. Clemente-Suárez, VJ, and Ramos-Campo, DJ. Effectiveness of reverse vs. traditional linear training periodization in triathlon. *Int J Environ Res Public Health* 16, 2019.
12. Cosca, D, and Navazio, F. Common problems in endurance athletes. *Am Fam Physician* 76:237-244, 2007.
13. Fredette, A, Roy, J-S, Perreault, K, Dupuis, F, Napier, C, and Esculier, J-F. The association between running injuries and training parameters: A systematic review. *J Athl Train* 57:650-671, 2022.
14. González-Ravé, JM, González-Mohíno, F, Rodrigo-Carranza, V, and Pyne, DB. Reverse periodization for improving sports performance: A systematic review. *Sports Medicine - Open* 8:56, 2022.
15. González-Ravé, JM, Hermosilla, F, González-Mohíno, F, Casado, A, and Pyne, DB. Training intensity distribution, training volume, and periodization models in elite swimmers: A systematic review. *Int J Sports Physiol Perform* 16:913-926, 2021.
16. Minghelli, B, Jesus, C, Martins, I, and Jesus, J. Triathlon-related musculoskeletal injuries: A study on a Portuguese triathlon championship. *Rev Assoc Med Bras (1992)* 66:1536-1541, 2020.

17. Mujika, I, and Padilla, S. Detraining: Loss of training-induced physiological and performance adaptations: Part I: Short term insufficient training stimulus. *Sports Med* 30:79-87, 2000.

18. Mujika, I, and Padilla, S. Scientific bases for precompetition tapering strategies. *Med Sci Sports Exerc* 35:1182-1187, 2003.

19. Mujika, I, Padilla, S, Pyne, D, and Busso, T. Physiological changes associated with the pre-event taper in athletes. *Sports Med* 34:891-927, 2004.

20. Powers, S, Howley, E, and Quindry, J. *Exercise Physiology: Theory and Application to Fitness and Performance.* New York: McGraw Hill, 294, 2020.

21. Pyne, DB, Mujika, I, and Reilly, T. Peaking for optimal performance: Research limitations and future directions. *J Sports Sci* 27:195-202, 2009.

22. Reuter, BH, and Dawes, JJ. Program design and technique for aerobic endurance training. In *Essentials of Strength Training and Conditioning.* Haff, GG and Triplett, NT, eds. Champaign, IL: Human Kinetics, 559-582, 2016.

23. Rhind, J-H, Dass, D, Barnett, A, and Carmont, M. A systematic review of long-distance triathlon musculoskeletal injuries. *J Hum Kinet* 81:123-134, 2022.

24. Rundell, KW. Effect of air pollution on athlete health and performance. *Br J Sports Med* 46:407, 2012.

25. Sawka, MN, Leon, LR, Montain, SJ, and Sonna, LA. Integrated physiological mechanisms of exercise performance, adaptation, and maladaptation to heat stress. *Compr Physiol* 1:1883-1928, 2011.

26. Scheer, V, and Krabak, BJ. Musculoskeletal injuries in ultra-endurance running: A scoping review. *Front Physiol* 12:664071, 2021.

27. Seiler, S. What is best practice for training intensity and duration distribution in endurance athletes? *Int J Sports Physiol Perform* 5:276-291, 2010.

28. Smith, GB Jr., and Hames, EF. Estimation of tolerance times for cold water immersion. *Aerosp Med* 33:834-840, 1962.

29. Tønnessen, E, Svendsen, I, Rønnestad, B, Hisdal, J, Haugen, T, and Seiler, S. The annual training periodization of 8 world champions in orienteering. *Int J Sports Physiol Perform* 10:29-38, 2015.

30. Trojian, T, and Amoako, A. Tendinopathy not tendonitis: Now is the time for a change. *ACSM's Health Fit* 19:37-42, 2015.

31. Tsegaw, G, and Alemayehu, Y. Principal air pollutants and their effects on athletes' ealth and performance: A critical review. *Sci Res Essays* 17(7):44-52, 2019.

32. Wilber, RL. Practical application of altitude/hypoxic training for Olympic medal performance: The team USA experience. *J Sci Sport Exerc* 4:358-370, 2022.

33. Wyatt, F. Physiological responses to altitude: A brief review. *J Exerc Physiol Online* 17:90-96, 2014.

34. Zaryski, C, and Smith, DJ. Training principles and issues for ultra-endurance athletes. *Curr Sports Med Rep* 4:165-170, 2005.

Chapter 4

1. Bowman, B. Training for utilization vs. capacity by Bob Bowman (2011). American Swim Coaches Association Archives. December 13, 2016. https://legacy.swimmingcoach.org/training-for-capacity-vs-utilization-by-bob-bowman-2011/. Accessed October 29, 2023.

2. Bompa, TO, and Buzzichelli, CA. *Periodization: Theory and Methodology of Training.* 6th ed. Human Kinetics, Champaign, IL: 91, 2019.

3. Galan-Rioja, MA, Gonzalez-Rave, JM, Gonzalez-Mohino, F, and Seiler, S. Training periodization, intensity distribution, and volume in trained cyclists: A systematic review. *Int J Sports Physiol Perform,* 2023. [e-pub ahead of print].

4. House, S, Johnston, S, and Jornet, K. *Training for the Uphill Athlete: A Manual for Mountain Runners and Ski Mountaineers.* Ventura, CA: Patagonia Works, 49-54, 76-78, 2019.

5. Jones, AM, Burnley, M, Black, MI, Poole, DC, and Vanhatalo, A. The maximal metabolic steady state: Redefining the "gold standard." *Physiol Rep* 7(10):e14098, 2019.

6. Kirkland, A. Aerobic vs. anaerobic exercise: It's missing the point. Kirklandcoaching.myportfolio. com. https://kirklandcoaching.myportfolio.com/aerobic-vs-anaerobic-exercise-its-missing-the-point. Accessed October 29, 2023.

7. Kruger, A. Training theory and why Roger Bannister was the first four-minute miler. *Sport Hist* 26(2):305-324, 2006.

8. Magness, S. History of training. ScienceOfRunning.com. August 18, 2016. www.scienceofrunning. com/2010/06/evolution-and-history-of-training.html?v=47e5dceea252. Accessed October 29, 2023.

9. Martino, M, and Dabbs, NC. Aerobic training program design. In *NSCA's Essentials of Personal Training.* 3rd ed. Schoenfeld, BJ, and Snarr, RL, eds. Champaign, IL: Human Kinetics, 432, 2022.

10. Seiler, S. Seiler's hierarchy of endurance training needs. In *European Endurance Conference, European Athletics Coaching Summit Series, Oslo, Norway, 4-5 November, 2016.*

11. Skiba, PF. *Scientific Training for Endurance Athletes.* Tinton Falls, NJ: PhysFarm Training Systems, 28-34, 80-81, 2022.

12. Spragg, J, Leo, P, and Swart, J. The relationship between training characteristics and durability in professional cyclists across a competitive season. *Eur J Sport Sci* 2:1-10, 2022.

13. Stoggl, TL, and Sperlich, B. The training intensity distribution among well-trained and elite endurance athletes. *Front Physiol* 6:295, https://doi.org/10.3389/fphys.2015.002952015.

14. Tucker, R. The anticipatory regulation of performance: The physiological basis for pacing strategies and the development of a perception-based model for exercise performance. *Br J Sports Med* 43:392-400, 2009.

15. van Der Poel, N. How to Skate a 10K . . . and Also Half a 10K. www.howtoskate.se/_files/ugd/e11bfe_b783631375f543248e271f440bcd45c5.pdf, 2022. Accessed October 29, 2023.

Chapter5

1. Caulfield, S, and Berninger, D. Exercise technique for free weight and machine training. In *Essentials of Strength Training and Conditioning.* 4th ed. Haff, GG, and Triplett, NT, eds. Champaign, IL: Human Kinetics, 351-408, 2016.

2. Lorenz, D, and Reiman, M. The role and implementation of eccentric training in athletic rehabilitation: Tendinopathy, hamstring strains, and ACL reconstruction. *Int J Sports Phys Ther* 6:27-44, 2011.

3. Loturco, I, McGuigan, M, Freitas, TT, Nakamura, F, Boullosa, D, Valenzuela, P, Pereira, LA, and Pareja-Blanco, F. Squat and countermovement jump performance across a range of loads: A comparison between Smith machine and free weight execution modes in elite sprinters. *Biol Sport* 39(4):1043-1048, 2022.

4. Morin, JB, Jiménez-Reyes, P, Brughelli, M, and Samozino, P. When jump height is not a good indicator of lower limb maximal power output: Theoretical demonstration, experimental evidence and practical solutions. *Sports Med* 49:999-1006, 2019.

5. NSCA. *Exercise Technique Manual for Resistance Training.* 4th ed. Champaign, IL: Human Kinetics, xii-xiv, 2022.

6. Sheppard, JM, and Triplett, NT. Program design for resistance training. In *Essentials of Strength and Conditioning.* 4th ed. Haff, GG, and Triplett, NT, eds. Champaign, IL: Human Kinetics, 439-470, 2016.

7. Sheppard, JM, Doyle, TL, and Taylor, K. A methodological and performance comparison of free weight and Smith-machine jump squats. *J Aust Strength Cond* 16:5-9, 2018.

8. Soriano, MA, Jiménez-Reyes, P, Rhea, MR, and Marín, PJ. The optimal load for maximal power production during lower-body resistance exercises: A meta-analysis. *Sports Med* 1191-205, 2015.

9. Williams, KJ, Chapman, DW, Phillips, EJ, and Ball, NB. Load-power relationship during a countermovement jump: A joint level analysis. *J Strength Cond Res* 32(4):955-961, 2018.

Chapter 6

1. Baldwin, KM, Badenhorst, CE, Cripps, AJ, Landers, GJ, Merrells, RJ, Bulsara, MK, and Hoyne, GF. Strength training for long-distance triathletes: Theory to practice. *Strength Cond J* 44:1-14, 2022.

2. Bastiaans, JJ, van Diemen, AB, Veneberg, T, and Jeukendrup, AE. The effects of replacing a portion of endurance training by explosive strength training on performance in trained cyclists. *Eur J Appl Physiol* 86:79-84, 2001.

3. Bazyler, CD, Abbott, HA, Bellon, CR, Taber, CB, and Stone, MH. Strength training for endurance athletes: Theory to practice. *Strength Cond J* 37:1-12, 2015.

4. Beattie, K. Strength training for endurance runners. In *Concurrent Aerobic and Strength Training: Scientific Basics and Practical Applications.* Schumann, M and Rønnestad, BR, eds. Cham, Switzerland: Springer, 341-356, 2019.

5. Berger, J, Harre, D, and Ritter, I. Principles of athletic training. In *Principles of Sports Training: Introduction to the Theory and Methods of Training.* Harre, D, ed. Muskegon, MI: Ultimate Athlete Concepts, 113-150, 2012.

6. Berryman, N, Mujika, I, Arvisais, D, Roubeix, M, Binet, C, and Bosquet, L. Strength training for middle- and long-distance performance: A meta-analysis. *Int J Sports Physiol Perform* 13:57, 2018.

7. Berryman, N, Mujika, I, and Bosquet, L. Concurrent training for sports performance: The 2 sides of the medal. *Int J Sports Physiol Perform* 14:279-285, 2019.

8. Bishop, BJ, Bartlett, J, Fyfe, J, and Lee, M. Methodological considerations for concurrent training. In *Concurrent Aerobic and Strength Training: Scientific Basics and Practical Applications.* Schumann, M, and Ronnestad, BR, eds. Cham, Switzerland: Springer, 183-197, 2019.

9. Blagrove, RC, Howatson, G, and Hayes, PR. Effects of strength training on the physiological determinants of middle- and long-distance running performance: A systematic review. *Sports Med* 48:1117-1149, 2018.

10. Bompa, TO, and Haff, GG. *Periodization: Theory and Methodology of Training.* 5th ed. Champaign, IL: Human Kinetics, 2009.

11. Bosquet, L, Montpetit, J, Arvisais, D, and Mujika, I. Effects of tapering on performance: A meta-analysis. *Med Sci Sports Exerc* 39:1358-1365, 2007.

12. Casado, A, González-Mohíno, F, González-Ravé, JM, and Foster, C. Training periodization, methods, intensity distribution, and volume in highly trained and elite distance runners: A systematic review. *Int J Sports Physiol Perform* 17(6):820-833, 2022.

13. Cuthbert, M, Haff, GG, Arent, SM, Ripley, N, McMahon, JJ, Evans, M, and Comfort, P. Effects of variations in resistance training frequency on strength development in well-trained populations and implications for in-season athlete training: A systematic review and meta-analysis. *Sports Med* 51:1697-1982, 2021.

14. de Salles, BF, Simão, R, Miranda, F, da Silva Novaes, J, Lemos, A, and Willardson, JM. Rest interval between sets in strength training. *Sports Med* 39:765-777, 2009.

15. DeWeese, BH, Hornsby, G, Stone, M, and Stone, MH. The training process: Planning for strength–power training in track and field. Part 1: Theoretical aspects. *J Sport Health Sci* 4:308-317, 2015.

16. DeWeese, BH, Hornsby, G, Stone, M, and Stone, MH. The training process: Planning for strength–power training in track and field. Part 2: Practical and applied aspects. *J Sport Health Sci* 4:318-324, 2015.

17. Doma, K, Deakin, GB, Schumann, M, and Bentley, DJ. Training considerations for optimising endurance development: An alternate concurrent training perspective. *Sports Med* 49:669-682, 2019.

18. Eihara, Y, Takao, K, Sugiyama, T, Maeo, S, Terada, M, Kanehisa, H, and Isaka, T. Heavy resistance training versus plyometric training for improving running economy and running time trial performance: A systematic review and meta-analysis. *Sports Med Open* 8:138, 2022.

19. Furrer, R, Hawley, JA, and Handschin, C. The molecular athlete: Exercise physiology from mechanisms to medals. *Physiol Rev* 103:1693-1787, 2023.

20. Fyfe, JJ, Bishop, DJ, and Stepto, NK. Interference between concurrent resistance and endurance exercise: Molecular bases and the role of individual training variables. *Sports Med* 44:743-762, 2014.

21. Goto, K, Sato, K, and Takamatsu, K. A single set of low intensity resistance exercise immediately following high intensity resistance exercise stimulates growth hormone secretion in men. *J Sports Med Phys Fitness* 43:243-249, 2003.

22. Greig, L, Stephens Hemingway, BH, Aspe, RR, Cooper, K, Comfort, P, and Swinton, PA. Autoregulation in resistance training: Addressing the inconsistencies. *Sports Med* 50:1873-1887, 2020.

23. Grgic, J, Schoenfeld, BJ, Skrepnik, M, Davies, TB, and Mikulic, P. Effects of rest interval duration in resistance training on measures of muscular strength: A systematic review. *Sports Med* 48:137-151, 2018.

24. Guppy, SN, and Haff, GG. Long-term programme design (periodisation). In *Advanced Personal Training: Science to Practice.* 2nd ed. Hough, P and Schoenfeld, BJ, eds. Milton Park, UK: Routledge, 118-128, 2022.

25. Hackett, DA, Johnson, NA, Halaki, M, and Chow, CM. A novel scale to assess resistance-exercise effort. *J Sports Sci* 30:1405-1413, 2012.

26. Haff, GG. Quantifying workloads in resistance training: A brief review. *Prof Strength and Cond* 10:31-40, 2010.

27. Haff, GG. Periodization of training. In *Conditioning for Strength and Human Performance.* 2nd ed. Brown, LE, and Chandler, J, eds. Philadelphia: Lippincott Williams & Wilkins, 326-345, 2012.

28. Haff, GG. Periodization strategies for youth development. In *Strength and conditioning for the young athlete: Science and application.* 2nd ed. Lloyd, R, and Oliver, JL, eds. London: Routledge, 281-299, 2019.

29. Haff, GG. The essentials of periodisation. In *Strength and Conditioning for Sports Performance.* 2nd ed. Jeffreys, I, and Moody, J, eds. Abingdon, UK: Routledge, 394-444, 2021.

30. Haff, GG. Peaking. In *High-Performance Training for Sports*. 2nd ed. Joyce, D, and Lewindon, D, eds. Champaign, IL: Human Kinetics, 330-343, 2022.

31. Haff, GG. Periodization and programming of individual sports. In *NSCA's Essentials of Sport Science*. French, D, and Torres Ronda, L, eds. Champaign, IL: Human Kinetics, 27-42, 2022.

32. Haff, GG, Berninger, D, and Caufield, S. Exercise technique for alternative modes and nontraditional implement training. In *Essentials of Strength Training and Conditioning*. 4th ed. Haff, GG, and Triplett, N, eds. Champaign, IL: Human Kinetics, 409-438, 2016.

33. Haff, GG, and Haff, EE. Resistance training program design. In *Essentials of Periodization*. 2nd ed. Malek, MH, and Coburn, JW, eds. Champaign, IL: Human Kinetics, 359-401, 2012.

34. Haff, GG, and Kendall, K. Strength and conditioning. In *Coaching for Sports Performance*. Baghurst, T, ed. Abingdon, UK: Routledge, 310-350, 2019.

35. Haff, GG, Whitley, A, and Potteiger, JA. A brief review: Explosive exercises and sports performance. *Strength Cond J* 23:13-20, 2001.

36. Haugen, T, Sandbakk, O, Seiler, S, and Tønnessen, E. The training characteristics of world-class distance runners: An integration of scientific literature and results-proven practice. *Sports Med Open* 8:46, 2022.

37. Hausswirth, C, Argentin, S, Bieuzen, F, Le Meur, Y, Couturier, A, and Brisswalter, J. Endurance and strength training effects on physiological and muscular parameters during prolonged cycling. *J Electromyogr Kinesiol* 20:330-339, 2010.

38. Hickson, RC, Dvorak, BA, Gorostiaga, EM, Kurowski, TT, and Foster, C. Potential for strength and endurance training to amplify endurance performance. *J Appl Physiol* 65:2285-2290, 1988.

39. Hornsby, W, Gentles, J, Comfort, P, Suchomel, T, Mizuguchi, S, and Stone, M. Resistance training volume load with and without exercise displacement. *Sports* 6:137, 2018.

40. Issurin, VB. New horizons for the methodology and physiology of training periodization. *Sports Med* 40:189-206, 2010.

41. Kataoka, R, Vasenina, E, Loenneke, J, and Buckner, SL. Periodization: Variation in the definition and discrepancies in study design. *Sports Med* 51:625-651, 2021.

42. Küüsmaa, M, Schumann, M, Sedliak, M, Kraemer, WJ, Newton, RU, Malinen, JP, Nyman, K, Häkkinen, A, and Häkkinen, K. Effects of morning versus evening combined strength and endurance training on physical performance, muscle hypertrophy, and serum hormone concentrations. *Appl Physiol Nutr Metab* 41:1285-1294, 2016.

43. Lima, LCR, and Blagrove, R. Strength training-induced adaptations associated with improved running economy: Potential mechanisms and training recommendations. *Br J Sports Med* 54:302-303, 2020.

44. Luckin-Baldwin, KM, Badenhorst, CE, Cripps, AJ, Landers, GJ, Merrells, RJ, Bulsara, MK, and Hoyne, GF. Strength training improves exercise economy in triathletes during a simulated triathlon. *Int J Sports Physiol Perform* 16:663-673, 2021.

45. Luckin, KM, Badenhorst, CE, Cripps, AJ, Landers, GJ, Merrells, RJ, Bulsara, MK, and Hoyne, GF. Strength training in long-distance triathletes: Barriers and characteristics. *J Strength Cond Res* 35:495-502, 2021.

46. Lum, D, and Barbosa, TM. Effects of strength training on Olympic time-based sport performance: A systematic review and meta-analysis of randomized controlled trials. *Int J Sports Physiol Perform* 14:1318-1330, 2019.

47. Lundberg, TR, Fernandez-Gonzalo, R, Gustafsson, T, and Tesch, PA. Aerobic exercise alters skeletal muscle molecular responses to resistance exercise. *Med Sci Sports Exerc* 44:1680-1688, 2012.

48. Mang, ZA, Ducharme, JB, Mermier, C, Kravitz, L, de Castro Magalhaes, F, and Amorim, F. Aerobic adaptations to resistance training: The role of time under tension. *Int J Sports Med* 43:829-839, 2022.

49. McBride, JM, Cormie, P, and Deane, R. Isometric squat force output and muscle activity in stable and unstable conditions. *J Strength Cond Res* 20:915-918, 2006.

50. Mookerjee, S, Welikonich, MJ, and Ratamess, NA. Comparison of energy expenditure during single-set vs. multiple-set resistance exercise. *J Strength Cond Res* 30:1447-1452, 2016.

51. Morán-Navarro, R, Perez, CE, Mora-Rodriguez, R, de la Cruz-Sanchez, E, Gonzalez-Badillo, JJ, Sanchez-Medina, L, and Pallares, JG. Time course of recovery following resistance training leading or not to failure. *Eur J Appl Physiol* 117:2387-2399, 2017.

52. Mujika, I. Olympic preparation of a world-class female triathlete. *Int J Sports Physiol Perform* 9:727-731, 2014.

53. Mujika, I, and Crowley, E. Strength training for endurance runners. In *Concurrent Aerobic and Strength Training: Scientific Basics and Practical Applications.* Schumann, M, and Rønnestad, BR, eds. Cham, Switzerland: Springer, 369-386, 2019.

54. Nuzzo, JL, McCaulley, GO, Cormie, P, Cavill, MJ, and McBride, JM. Trunk muscle activity during stability ball and free weight exercises. *J Strength Cond Res* 22:95-102, 2008.

55. Paavolainen, L, Häkkinen, K, Hamalainen, I, Nummela, A, and Rusko, H. Explosive-strength training improves 5-km running time by improving running economy and muscle power. *J Appl Physiol* 86:1527-1533, 1999.

56. Pelland, JC, Robinson, ZP, Remmert, JF, Cerminaro, RM, Benitez, B, John, TA, Helms, ER, and Zourdos, MC. Methods for controlling and reporting resistance training proximity to failure: Current issues and future directions. *Sports Med* 36:340-345, 2022.

57. Rønnestad, B. Strength training for endurance runners. In *Concurrent Aerobic and Strength Training: Scientific Basics and Practical Applications.* Schumann, M, and Rønnestad, BR, eds. Cham, Switzerland: Springer, 333-340, 2019.

58. Rønnestad, BR, Hansen, EA, and Raastad, T. Effect of heavy strength training on thigh muscle cross-sectional area, performance determinants, and performance in well-trained cyclists. *Eur J Appl Physiol* 108:965-975, 2010.

59. Rønnestad, BR, Hansen, EA, and Raastad, T. Strength training improves 5-min all-out performance following 185 min of cycling. *Scand J Med Sci Sports* 21:250-259, 2011.

60. Rønnestad, BR, and Hansen, J. A scientific approach to improve physiological capacity of an elite cyclist. *Int J Sports Physiol Perform* 13:390-393, 2018.

61. Rønnestad, BR, Hansen, J, Hollan, I, and Ellefsen, S. Strength training improves performance and pedaling characteristics in elite cyclists. *Scand J Med Sci Sports* 25:e89-98, 2015.

62. Rønnestad, BR, and Mujika, I. Optimizing strength training for running and cycling endurance performance: A review. *Scand J Med Sci Sports* 24:603-612, 2014.

63. Schoenfeld, BJ, Pope, ZK, Benik, FM, Hester, GM, Sellers, J, Nooner, JL, Schnaiter, JA, Bond-Williams, KE, Carter, AS, Ross, CL, Just, BL, Henselmans, M, and Krieger, JW. Longer interset rest periods enhance muscle strength and hypertrophy in resistance-trained men. *J Strength Cond Res* 30:1805-1812, 2016.

64. Schoenfeld, BJ, and Snarr, RL. Resistance training program design. In *NSCA's Essentials of Personal Training.* 3rd ed. Schoenfeld, BJ and Snarr, RL, eds. Champaign, IL: Human Kinetics, 393-425, 2021.

65. Schumann, M, and Rønnestad, BR, eds. *Concurrent Aerobic and Strength Training: Scientific Basics and Practical Applications.* Cham, Switzerland: Springer, 2019.

66. Shimano, T, Kraemer, WJ, Spiering, BA, Volek, JS, Hatfield, DL, Silvestre, R, Vingren, JL, Fragala, MS, Maresh, CM, Fleck, SJ, Newton, RU, Spreuwenberg, LP, and Häkkinen, K. Relationship between the number of repetitions and selected percentages of one repetition maximum in free weight exercises in trained and untrained men. *J Strength Cond Res* 20:819-823, 2006.

67. Snarr, RL, and Batrakoulis, A. Resistance exercise technique. In *NSCA's Essentials of Personal Training.* 3rd ed. Schoenfeld, BJ, and Snarr, RL, eds. Champaign, IL: Human Kinetics, 317-376, 2021.

68. Solli, GS, Tønnessen, E and Sandbakk, Ø. The training characteristics of the world's most successful female cross-country skier. *Front Physiol* 8, 2017.

69. Spiering, BA, Mujika, I, Sharp, MA, and Foulis, SA. Maintaining physical performance: The minimal dose of exercise needed to preserve endurance and strength over time. *J Strength Cond Res* 35:1449-1458, 2021.

70. Stanton, R, Reaburn, PR, and Humphries, B. The effect of short-term Swiss ball training on core stability and running economy. *J Strength Cond Res* 18:522-528, 2004.

71. Stone, MH, and Borden, RA. Modes and methods of resistance training. *Strength Cond J* 19:18-23, 1997.

72. Stone, MH, Collins, D, Plisk, S, Haff, G, and Stone, ME. Training principles: Evaluation of modes and methods of resistance training. *Strength Cond J* 22:65, 2000.

73. Stone, MH, Hornsby, WG, Haff, GG, Fry, AC, Suarez, DG, Liu, J, Gonzalez-Rave, JM, and Pierce, KC. Periodization and block periodization in sports: Emphasis on strength-power training—a provocative and challenging narrative. *J Strength Cond Res* 35:2351-2371, 2021.

74. Stone, MH, Stone, ME, and Sands, WA. Introduction, definitions, objectives, tasks, and principles of training. In *Principles and Practice of Resistance Training.* Stone, MH, Stone, ME, and Sands, WA, eds. Champaign, IL: Human Kinetics, 1-12, 2007.

75. Stone, MH, Suchomel, TJ, Hornsby, WG, Wagle, JP, and Cunanan, AJ. General concepts and training principles for athlete development. In *Strength and Conditioning in Sports: From Science to Practice*. New York: Routledge, 221-251, 2023.

76. Stone, MH, Suchomel, TJ, Hornsby, WG, Wagle, JP, and Cunanan, AJ. *Physical and Physiological Responses and Adaptations*. New York: Routledge, 2023.

77. Stone, MH, Suchomel, TJ, Hornsby, WG, Wagle, JP, and Cunanan, AJ. *Strength and Conditioning in Sports: From Science to Practice*. New York: Routledge, 2023.

78. Suc, A, Sarko, P, Plesa, J, and Kozinc, Z. Resistance exercise for improving running economy and running biomechanics and decreasing running-related injury risk: A narrative review. *Sports (Basel)* 10, 2022.

79. Suchomel, TJ, Nimphius, S, Bellon, CR, Hornsby, WG, and Stone, MH. Training for muscular strength: Methods for monitoring and adjusting training intensity. *Sports Med* 51:2051-2066, 2021.

80. Suchomel, TJ, Nimphius, S, Bellon, CR, and Stone, MH. The importance of muscular strength: Training considerations. *Sports Med* 48:765-785, 2018.

81. Sunde, A, Storen, O, Bjerkaas, M, Larsen, MH, Hoff, J, and Helgerud, J. Maximal strength training improves cycling economy in competitive cyclists. *J Strength Cond Res* 24:2157-2165, 2010.

82. Taipale, RS, Mikkola, J, Vesterinen, V, Nummela, A, and Häkkinen, K. Neuromuscular adaptations during combined strength and endurance training in endurance runners: Maximal versus explosive strength training or a mix of both. *Eur J Appl Physiol* 113:325-335, 2013.

83. Thibaudeau, C. Planning intensity. In *The Black Book of Training Secrets*. Quebec, Canada: F. Lepine Publishing, 87-108, 2006.

84. Tønnessen, E, Svendsen, IS, Ronnestad, BR, Hisdal, J, Haugen, TA, and Seiler, S. The annual training periodization of 8 world champions in orienteering. *Int J Sports Physiol Perform* 10:29-38, 2015.

85. Trowell, D, Fox, A, Saunders, N, Vicenzino, B, and Bonacci, J. Effect of concurrent strength and endurance training on run performance and biomechanics: A randomized controlled trial. *Scand J Med Sci Sports* 32:543-558, 2022.

86. Tufano, JJ, Brown, LE, and Haff, GG. Theoretical and practical aspects of different cluster set structures: A systematic review. *J Strength Cond Res* 31:848-867, 2017.

87. Vikmoen, O, Rønnestad, BR, Ellefsen, S, and Raastad, T. Heavy strength training improves running and cycling performance following prolonged submaximal work in well-trained female athletes. *Physiol Rep* 5, 2017.

88. Willardson, JM, and Burkett, LN. The effect of rest interval length on the sustainability of squat and bench press repetitions. *J Strength Cond Res* 20:400-403, 2006.

89. Yamamoto, LM, Klau, JF, Casa, DJ, Kraemer, WJ, Armstrong, LE, and Maresh, CM. The effects of resistance training on road cycling performance among highly trained cyclists: A systematic review. *J Strength Cond Res* 24:560-566, 2010.

90. Yu Kwok, W, So, BCL, Tse, DHT, and Ng, SSM. A systematic review and meta-analysis: Biomechanical evaluation of the effectiveness of strength and conditioning training programs on front crawl swimming performance. *J Sports Sci Med* 20:564-585, 2021.

91. Zourdos, MC, Klemp, A, Dolan, C, Quiles, JM, Schau, KA, Jo, E, Helms, E, Esgro, B, Duncan, S, Garcia Merino, S, and Blanco, R. Novel resistance training-specific rating of perceived exertion scale measuring repetitions in reserve. *J Strength Cond Res* 30:267-275, 2016.

Chapter 7

1. Aguilar, AJ, DiStefano, LJ, Brown, CN, Herman, DC, Guskiewicz, KM, and Padua, DA. A dynamic warm-up model increases quadriceps strength and hamstring flexibility. *J Strength Cond Res* 26(4):1130-41, 2012.

2. Baron, H. Neural inhibition for continual learning and memory. *Curr Opin Neurobiol* 67:85-94, 2021.

3. Behm, D, and Chaouachi, A. A review of the acute effects of static and dynamic stretching on performance. *Eur J Appl Physiol* 111(11):2633-2651, 2011.

4. Behm, DG, Alizadeh, S, Anvar, SH, Mahmoud, MMI, Ramsay, E, Hanlon, C, and Cheatham, S. Foam rolling prescription: A clinical commentary. *J Strength Cond Res* 34(11):3301-3308, 2020.

5. Bishop, D. Warm-up 2: Performance changes following active warm-up and how to structure the warm-up. *Sports Med* 33(7):483-98, 2003.

6. Chaouachi, A, Castagna, C, Chtara, M, Brughelli, M, Turki, O, Galy, O, Chamari, K, and Behm, DG. Effect of warm-ups involving static or dynamic stretching on agility, sprinting, and jumping performance in trained individuals. *J Strength Cond Res* 24(8):2001-2011, 2010.

7. Cheatham, S, Kolber, M, Cain, M, and Lee, M. The effects of self-myofascial release using a foam roll or roller massager on joint range of motion, muscle recovery, and performance: A systematic review. *Int J Sports Phys Ther* 10(6):827-38, 2015.

8. Distefano, LJ, Blackburn, JT, Marshall, SW, and Padua, DA. Gluteal muscle activation during common therapeutic exercises. *J Orthop Sports Phys Ther* 39(7):532-540, 2009.

9. Dupuy, O, Douzi, W, Theurot, D, Bosquet, L, and Dugue, B. An evidence-based approach for choosing post-exercise recovery techniques to reduce markers of muscle damage, soreness, fatigue, and inflammation: A systematic review with meta-analysis. *Front Physiol* 9:403, 2018.

10. Fauris, P, López-de-Celis, C, Canet-Vintró, M, Martin, JC, Llurda-Almuzara, L, Rodriguez-Sanz, J, Labata-Lezaun, N, Simon, M, and Pérez-Bellmunt, A. Does self-myofascial release cause a remote hamstring stretching effect based on myofascial chains? A randomized controlled trial. *Int J Environ Res Public Health* 18(23):1235, 2021.

11. Fredericson, M, and Wolf, C. Iliotibial band syndrome in runners: Innovations in treatment. *Sports Med* 35(5):451-459, 2005.

12. Gergley, JC. Acute effect of passive static stretching on lower-body strength in moderately trained men. *J Strength Cond Res* 27(4):973-977, 2013.

13. Iwata, M, Yamamoto, A, Matsuo, S, Hatano, G, Miyazaki, M, Fukaya, T, Fujiwara, M, Asai, Y, and Suzuki, S. Dynamic stretching has sustained effects on range of motion and passive stiffness of the hamstring muscles. *J Sports Sci Med* 18(1):13-20, 2019.

14. Jeffreys, I. *The Warm-Up.* Champaign, IL: Human Kinetics, 2018.

15. Joshi, DG, Balthillaya, G, and Prabhu, A. Effect of remote myofascial release on hamstring flexibility in asymptomatic individuals—A randomized clinical trial. *J Bodyw Mov Ther* 22(3):832-837, 2018.

16. Junker, D, and Stoggl, T. The training effects of foam rolling on core strength endurance, balance, muscle performance and range of motion: A randomized controlled trial. *J Sports Sci Med* 18(2):229-238, 2019.

17. Kentta, G, and Hassmen, P. Overtraining and recovery: A conceptual model. *Sports Med* 26(1):1-16. 1998.

18. Kirmizigil, B, Ozcaldiran, B, and Colakoglu, M. Effects of three different stretching techniques on vertical jumping performance. *J Strength Cond* 28(5):1263-71, 2014.

19. Kokkonen, J, Nelson, A, Eldredge, C, and Winchester, J. Chronic static stretching improves exercise performance. *Med Sci Sports Exerc* 39(10):1825-1831, 2007.

20. Kuszewski, M, Gnat, R, and Gogola, A. The impact of core muscles training on the range of anterior pelvic tilt in subjects with increased stiffness of the hamstrings. *Hum Mov Sci* 57:32-39, 2018.

21. Macdonald, G, Button, D, Drinkwater, E, and Behm, D. Foam rolling as a recovery tool after an intense bout of physical activity. *Med Sci Sports Exerc* 46(1):131-412, 2014.

22. Mendiguchia, J, Gonzalez De la Flor, A, Mendez-Villanueva, A, Morin, JB, Edouard, P, and Garrues, MA. Training-induced changes in anterior pelvic tilt: Potential implications for hamstring strain injuries management. *J Sports Sci* 39(7):760-767, 2021.

23. Menzies, P, Menzies, C, McIntyre, L, Paterson, P, Wilson, J, and Kemi, O. Blood lactate clearance during active recovery after an intense running bout depends on the intensity of the active recovery. *J Sports Sci* 28(9):975-982. 2010.

24. Nelson, AG, Driscoll, NM, Landin, DK, Young, MA, and Schexnayder, IC. Acute effects of passive muscle stretching on sprint performance. *J Sports Sci* 23(5):449-454, 2005.

25. Opplert, J, and Babault, N. Acute effects of dynamic stretching on muscle flexibility and performance: An analysis of the current literature. *Sports Med* 48(2):299-325, 2018.

26. Renan-Ordine, R, Alburquerque-Sendín, F, Rodrigues de Souza, DP, Cleland, JA, and Fernández-de-Las-Peñas, C. Effectiveness of myofascial trigger point manual therapy combined with a self-stretching protocol for the management of plantar heel pain: A randomized controlled trial. *J Orthop Sports Phys Ther* 41(2):43-50, 2011.

27. Sander, A, Keiner, M, Schlumberger, A, Wirth, K, and Scmidtbleicher, D. Effects of functional exercises in the warm-up on sprint performances. *J Strength Cond Res* 27(4):995-1001, 2013.

28. Seidi, F, Bayattork, M, Minoonejad, H, Anderson, L, and Page, P. Comprehensive corrective exercise program improves alignment, muscle activation and movement pattern of men with upper crossed syndrome: Randomized controlled trial. *Sci Rep* 10(1):20688. 2020.

29. Sharman, M, Cresswell, A, and Riek, S. Proprioceptive neuromuscular facilitation stretching: Mechanisms and clinical implications. *Sports Med* 36(11):929-939, 2006.

30. Simao, R, Freitas de Salles, B, Figueiredo, T, Dias, I, and Willardson, J. Exercise order in resistance training. *Sports Med* 42(3):251-265, 2012.

31. Siriphorn, A, and Eksakulkla, S. Calf stretching and plantar fascia-specific stretching for plantar fasciitis: A systematic review and meta-analysis. *J Bodyw Mov Ther* 24(4):222-232, 2020.

32. Su, H, Chang, NJ, Wu, WL, Guo, LY, and Chu, IH. Acute effects of foam rolling, static stretching, and dynamic stretching during warm-ups on muscular flexibility and strength in young adults. *J Sport Rehabil* 26(6):469-477, 2017.

33. Taylor, K, Sheppard, J, Lee, H, and Plummer, N. Negative effect of static stretching restored when combined with a sport specific warm-up component. *J Sci Med Sport* 12(6):657-61, 2009.

34. Thomas, E, Bianco, A, Paoli, A, and Palma, A. The relation between stretching typology and stretching duration: The effects on range of motion. *Int J Sports Med* 39(4): 43-254, 2018.

35. Wanich, T, Hodgkins, C, Columbier, J, Muraski, E, and Kennedy, J. Cycling injuries of the lower extremity. *J Am Acad Orthop Surg* 15(12):748-756, 2007.

36. Weldon, EJ, and Richardson, AB. Upper extremity overuse injuries in swimming: A discussion of swimmer's shoulder. *Clin J Sports Med* 20(3):423-38, 2001.

37. Wiewelhove, T, Doweling, A, Schneider, C, Hottenrott, L, Meyer, T, Kellman, M, Pfeiffer, M, and Ferrauti, A. A meta-analysis of the effects of foam rolling on performance and recovery. *Front Physiol* 10:376, 2019.

38. Wong, D, Chaouachi, A, Lau, P, and Behm, D. Short durations of static stretching when combined with dynamic stretching do not impair repeated sprints and agility. *J Sports Sci Med* 10(2):408-16, 2011.

39. Woods, K, Bishop, P, and Jones, E. Warm-up and stretching in the prevention of muscular injury. *Sports Med* 37(12):1089-99, 2007.

40. Zmijewski, P, Lipinska, P, Czajkowska, A, Mróz, A, Kapuściński, P, and Mazurek, K. Acute effects of a static vs. a dynamic stretching warm-up on repeated-sprint performance in female handball players. *J Hum Kinet* 72(1):161-172, 2020.

Chapter 8

1. Albracht, K, and Arampatzis, A. Exercise-induced changes in triceps surae tendon stiffness and muscle strength affect running economy in humans. *Eur J Appl Physiol* 113:1605-1615, 2013.

2. Allen, WK, Seals, DR, Hurley, BF, Ehsani, AA, and Hagberg, JM. Lactate threshold and distance-running performance in young and older endurance athletes. *J Appl Physiol* 58:1281-1284, 1985.

3. Andersen, JJ. The state of running 2019. RunRepeat.com. https://runrepeat.com/state-of-running.

4. Anderson, LM, Bonanno, DR, Hart, HF, and Barton, CJ. What are the benefits and risks associated with changing foot strike pattern during running? A systematic review and meta-analysis of injury, running economy, and biomechanics. *Sport Med* 50:885-917, 2020.

5. Barnes, KR, and Kilding, AE. Running economy: Measurement, norms, and determining factors. *Sport Med* 1:8, 2015.

6. Barnes, KR, McGuigan, MR, and Kilding, AE. Lower-body determinants of running economy in male and female distance runners. *J Strength Cond Res* 28:1289-1297, 2014.

7. Baxter, C, McNaughton, LR, Sparks, A, Norton, L, and Bentley, D. Impact of stretching on the performance and injury risk of long-distance runners. *Res Sport Med* 25:78-90, 2017.

8. Becker, J, Nakajima, M, and Wu, WFW. Factors contributing to medial tibial stress syndrome in runners: A prospective study. *Med Sci Sports Exerc* 50:2092-2100, 2018.

9. Bermon, S, Garrandes, F, Szabo, A, Berkovics, I, and Adami, PE. Effect of advanced shoe technology on the evolution of road race times in male and female elite runners. *Front Sport Act Living* 3:653173, 2021.

10. Berthon, P, Fellmann, N, Bedu, M, Beaune, B, Dabonneville, M, Coudert, J, and Chamoux, A. A 5-min running field test as a measurement of maximal aerobic velocity. *Eur J Appl Physiol* 75:233-238, 1997.

11. Blagrove, RC, Howatson, G, and Hayes, PR. Effects of strength training on the physiological determinants of middle- and long-distance running performance: A systematic review. *Sport Med* 48:1117-1149, 2018.

12. Blagrove, RC, Howatson, G, Pedlar, CR, and Hayes, PR. Quantification of aerobic determinants of performance in post-pubertal adolescent middle-distance runners. *Eur J Appl Physiol* 119:1865-1874, 2019.

13. Blagrove, RC, Howe, LP, Cushion, EJ, Spence, A, Howatson, G, Pedlar, CR, and Hayes, PR. Effects of strength training on postpubertal adolescent distance runners. *Med Sci Sports Exerc* 50:1224-1232, 2018.

14. Blagrove, RC, Howe, LP, Howatson, G, and Hayes, PR. Strength and conditioning for adolescent endurance runners. *Strength Cond J* 42:2-11, 2020.

15. Bramble, DM, and Lieberman, DE. Endurance running and the evolution of Homo. *Nature* 432:345-352, 2004.

16. Brewer, BW, Andersen, MB, and Van Raalte, JL. Psychological aspects of sport injury rehabilitation: Toward a biopsychosocial approach. *Med Psychol Asp Sport Exerc* 4:41-54, 2002.

17. Burnley, M, Bearden, SE, and Jones, AM. Polarized training is not optimal for endurance athletes: Response to Foster and colleagues. *Med Sci Sports Exerc* 54:1038-1040, 2022.

18. Burnley, M, and Jones, AM. Power-duration relationship: Physiology, fatigue, and the limits of human performance. *Eur J Sport Sci* 18:1-12, 2018.

19. Burns, GT, Kozloff, KM, and Zernicke, RF. Biomechanics of elite performers: Economy and efficiency of movement. *Kinesiol Rev* 9:21-30, 2020.

20. Chan, ZYS, Zhang, JH, Au, IPH, An, WW, Shum, GLK, Ng, GYF, and Cheung, RTH. Gait retraining for the reduction of injury occurrence in novice distance runners: 1-year follow-up of a randomized controlled trial. *Am J Sports Med* 46:388-395, 2018.

21. Cochrum, RG, Conners, RT, Caputo, JL, Coons, JM, Fuller, DK, Frame, MC, and Morgan, DW. Visual classification of running economy by distance running coaches. *Eur J Sport Sci* 21:1111-1118, 2021.

22. Conley, DL, and Krahenbuhl, GS. Running economy and distance running performance of highly trained athletes. *Med Sci Sport Exerc* 12:357-360, 1980.

23. Cook, JL, and Docking, SI. "Rehabilitation will increase the 'capacity' of your . . . insert musculoskeletal tissue here. . . ." Defining "tissue capacity": A core concept for clinicians. *Br J Sports Med* 49:1484-1485, 2015.

24. Daniels, J. *Daniels' Running Formula.* 4th ed. Champaign, IL: Human Kinetics, 2022.

25. Decroix, L, De Pauw, K, Foster, C, and Meeusen, R. Guidelines to classify female subject groups in sport-science research. *Int J Sports Physiol Perform* 11:204-213, 2016.

26. Denadai, BS, de Aguiar, RA, de Lima, LC, Greco, CC, and Caputo, F. Explosive training and heavy weight training are effective for improving running economy in endurance athletes: A systematic review and meta-analysis. *Sport Med* 47:545-554, 2017.

27. Dotan, R. A critical review of critical power. *Eur J Appl Physiol* 122:1559-1588, 2022.

28. Edouard, P, Navarro, L, Branco, P, Gremeaux, V, Timpka, T, and Junge, A. Injury frequency and characteristics (location, type, cause and severity) differed significantly among athletics ('track and field') disciplines during 14 international championships (2007-2018): Implications for medical service planning. *Br J Sports Med* 54:159-167, 2020.

29. Fletcher, JR, and MacIntosh, BR. Running economy from a muscle energetics perspective. *Front Physiol* 8:433, 2017.

30. Fokkema, T, van Damme, AADN, Fornerod, MWJ, de Vos, R-J, Bierma-Zeinstra, SMA, and van Middelkoop, M. Training for a (half-)marathon: Training volume and longest endurance run related to performance and running injuries. *Scand J Med Sci Sports* 30:1692-1704, 2020.

31. Foster, C, Casado, A, Esteve-Lanao, J, Haugen, T, and Seiler, S. Polarized training is optimal for endurance athletes. *Med Sci Sports Exerc* 54:1028-1031, 2022.

32. Fuller, JT, Bellenger, CR, Thewlis, D, Tsiros, MD, and Buckley, JD. The effect of footwear on running performance and running economy in distance runners. *Sport Med* 45:411-422, 2015.

33. Gastin, PB. Energy system interaction and relative contribution during maximal exercise. *Sport Med* 31:725-741, 2001.

34. Gent, RN van, Siem, D, Middelkoop, M van, Os, AG van, Bierma-Zeinstra, SMA, and Koes, BW. Incidence and determinants of lower extremity running injuries in long distance runners: A systematic review. *Br J Sports Med* 41:469-480, 2007.

35. Gómez-Molina, J, Ogueta-Alday, A, Camara, J, Stickley, C, and García-López, J. Effect of 8 weeks of concurrent plyometric and running training on spatiotemporal and physiological variables of novice runners. *Eur J Sport Sci* 18:162-169, 2018.

36. Gorostiaga, EM, Sánchez-Medina, L, and Garcia-Tabar, I. Over 55 years of critical power: Fact or artifact? *Scand J Med Sci Sport* 32:116-124, 2022.

37. Halvarsson, B, and von Rosen, P. Could a specific exercise programme prevent injury in elite orienteerers? A randomised controlled trial. *Phys Ther Sport* 40:177-183, 2019.

38. Haugen, T, Sandbakk, Ø, Enoksen, E, Seiler, S, and Tønnessen, E. Crossing the golden training divide: The science and practice of training world-class 800-and 1500-m runners. *Sport Med* 51:1835-1854, 2021.

39. Haugen, T, Sandbakk, Ø, Seiler, S, and Tønnessen, E. The training characteristics of world-class distance runners: An integration of scientific literature and results-proven practice. *Sport Med - Open* 8:46, 2022.

40. Hespanhol, LC, van Mechelen, W, and Verhagen, E. Effectiveness of online tailored advice to prevent running-related injuries and promote preventive behaviour in Dutch trail runners: A pragmatic randomised controlled trial. *Br J Sports Med* 52:851-858, 2018.

41. Hodgson, LE, Walter, E, Venn, RM, Galloway, R, Pitsiladis, Y, Sardat, F, and Forni, LG. Acute kidney injury associated with endurance events—is it a cause for concern? A systematic review. *BMJ Open Sport Exerc Med* 3:e000093, 2017.

42. Hoffman, MD, Pasternak, A, Rogers, IR, Khodaee, M, Hill, JC, Townes, DA, Scheer, BV, Krabak, BJ, Basset, P, and Lipman, GS. Medical services at ultra-endurance foot races in remote environments: Medical issues and consensus guidelines. *Sport Med* 44:1055-1069, 2014.

43. Hollman, H, Ezzat, A, Esculier, J-F, Gustafson, P, and Scott, A. Effects of tailored advice on injury prevention knowledge and behaviours in runners: Secondary analysis from a randomised controlled trial. *Phys Ther Sport* 37:164-170, 2019.

44. Hoogkamer, W, Kipp, S, Frank, JH, Farina, EM, Luo, G, and Kram, R. A comparison of the energetic cost of running in marathon racing shoes. *Sport Med* 48:1009-1019, 2018.

45. Hoppel, F, Calabria, E, Pesta, D, Kantner-Rumplmair, W, Gnaiger, E, and Burtscher, M. Physiological and pathophysiological responses to ultramarathon running in non-elite runners. *Front Physiol* 10:1300, 2019.

46. Horman, S, Browne, G, Krause, U, Patel, J, Vertommen, D, Bertrand, L, Lavoinne, A, Hue, L, Proud, C, and Rider, M. Activation of AMP-activated protein kinase leads to the phosphorylation of elongation factor 2 and an inhibition of protein synthesis. *Curr Biol* 12:1419-1423, 2002.

47. Ingham, SA, Whyte, GP, Pedlar, C, Bailey, DM, Dunman, N, and Nevill, AM. Determinants of 800-m and 1500-m running performance using allometric models. *Med Sci Sport Exerc* 40:345-350, 2008.

48. Jacobsson, J, Kowalski, J, Timpka, T, Hansson, P-O, Spreco, A, and Dahlstrom, O. Universal prevention through a digital health platform reduces injury incidence in youth athletics (track and field): A cluster randomised controlled trial. *Br J Sports Med* 57:364-371, 2022.

49. Jeukendrup, AE. Training the gut for athletes. *Sport Med* 47:101-110, 2017.

50. Jones, AM. The physiology of the world record holder for the women's marathon. *Int J Sports Sci Coach* 1:101-116, 2006.

51. Jones, AM, Carter, H, and Doust, JH. A disproportionate increase in VO2 coincident with lactate threshold during treadmill exercise. *Med Sci Sport Exerc* 31:1299-1306, 1999.

52. Joyner, MJ. Modeling: Optimal marathon performance on the basis of physiological factors. *J Appl Physiol* 70:683-687, 1991.

53. Kalkhoven, JT, Watsford, ML, and Impellizzeri, FM. A conceptual model and detailed framework for stress-related, strain-related, and overuse athletic injury. *J Sci Med Sport* 23:726-734, 2020.

54. Kenneally, M, Casado, A, and Santos-Concejero, J. The effect of periodization and training intensity distribution on middle- and long-distance running performance: A systematic review. *Int J Sports Physiol Perform* 13:1114-1121, 2018.

55. Kluitenberg, B, van Middelkoop, M, Diercks, R, and van der Worp, H. What are the differences in injury proportions between different populations of runners? A systematic review and meta-analysis. *Sport Med* 45:1143-1161, 2015.

56. Knechtle, B, and Nikolaidis, PT. Physiology and pathophysiology in ultra-marathon running. *Front Physiol* 9:634, 2018.

57. Kozinc, Ž, and Šarabon, N. Effectiveness of movement therapy interventions and training modifications for preventing running injuries: A meta-analysis of randomized controlled trials. *J Sport Sci Med* 16:421-428, 2017.

58. Krabak, BJ, Tenforde, AS, Davis, IS, Fredericson, M, Harrast, MA, D'Hemecourt, P, Luke, AC, and Roberts, WO. Youth distance running: Strategies for training and injury reduction. *Curr Sports Med Rep* 18:53-59, 2019.

59. Kulmala, J-P, Kosonen, J, Nurminen, J, and Avela, J. Running in highly cushioned shoes increases leg stiffness and amplifies impact loading. *Sci Rep* 8:1-7, 2018.

60. Lauersen, JB, Andersen, TE, and Andersen, LB. Strength training as superior, dose-dependent and safe prevention of acute and overuse sports injuries: A systematic review, qualitative analysis and meta-analysis. *Br J Sports Med* 52:1557-1563, 2018.

61. Lea, JWD, O'Driscoll, JM, Hulbert, S, Scales, J, and Wiles, JD. Convergent validity of ratings of perceived exertion during resistance exercise in healthy participants: A systematic review and meta-analysis. *Sport Med* 8:1-19, 2022.

62. Lopes, TR, Pereira, HM, and Silva, BM. Perceived exertion: Revisiting the history and updating the neurophysiology and the practical applications. *Int J Environ Res Public Health* 19:14439, 2022.

63. Luedke, LE, Heiderscheit, BC, Williams, DS, and Rauh, MJ. Association of isometric strength of hip and knee muscles with injury risk in high school cross country runners. *Int J Sports Phys Ther* 10:868 876, 2015.

64. Mahieu, NN, Witvrouw, E, Stevens, V, Tiggelen, D Van, and Roget, P. Intrinsic risk factors for the development of Achilles tendon overuse injury a prospective study. *Am J Sports Med* 34:226-235, 2006.

65. Malisoux, L, Ramesh, J, Mann, R, Seil, R, Urhausen, A, and Theisen, D. Can parallel use of different running shoes decrease running-related injury risk? *Scand J Med Sci Sports* 25:110-115, 2015.

66. Malliaropoulos, N, Mertyri, D, and Tsaklis, P. Prevalence of injury in ultra trail running. *Hum Mov* 16:55-59, 2015.

67. Martinez, S, Aguilo, A, Rodas, L, Lozano, L, Moreno, C, and Tauler, P. Energy, macronutrient and water intake during a mountain ultramarathon event: The influence of distance. *J Sports Sci* 36:333-339, 2018.

68. McKay, AKA, Stellingwerff, T, Smith, ES, Martin, DT, Mujika, I, Goosey-Tolfrey, VL, Sheppard, J, and Burke, LM. Defining training and performance caliber: A participant classification framework. *Int J Sports Physiol Perform* 17:317-331, 2022.

69. McLaughlin, JE, Howley, ET, Bassett Jr., DR, Thompson, DL, and Fitzhugh, EC. Test of the classic model for predicting endurance running performance. *Med Sci Sport Exerc* 42:991-997, 2010.

70. Meeusen, R, Duclos, M, Foster, C, Fry, A, Gleeson, M, Nieman, D, Raglin, J, Rietjens, G, Steinacker, J, Urhausen, A; European College of Sport Science; and American College of Sports Medicine. Prevention, diagnosis and treatment of the overtraining syndrome: Joint consensus statement of the European College of Sport Science (ECSS) and the American College of Sports Medicine (ACSM). *Eur J Sport Sci* 13:1-24, 2013.

71. Mendez-Rebolledo, G, Figueroa-Ureta, R, Moya-Mura, F, Guzmán-Muñoz, E, Ramirez-Campillo, R, and Lloyd, RS. The protective effect of neuromuscular training on the medial tibial stress syndrome in youth female track-and-field athletes: A clinical trial and cohort study. *J Sport Rehabil* 30:1019-1027, 2021.

72. Millet, GY, Banfi, JC, Kerherve, H, Morin, JB, Vincent, L, Estrade, C, Geyssant, A, and Feasson, L. Physiological and biological factors associated with a 24 h treadmill ultra-marathon performance. *Scand J Med Sci Sports* 21:54-61, 2011.

73. Milligan, A, Mills, C, Corbett, J, and Scurr, J. The influence of breast support on torso, pelvis and arm kinematics during a five kilometer treadmill run. *Hum Mov Sci* 42:246-260, 2015.

74. Moore, IS. Is there an economical running technique? A review of modifiable biomechanical factors affecting running economy. *Sport Med* 46:793-807, 2016.

75. Moore, IS, Goom, T, and Ashford, KJ. Gait retraining for performance and injury risk. In *The Science and Practice of Middle and Long Distance Running*. Blagrove, RC, and Hayes, P, eds. Abingdon, UK: Routledge, 185-206, 2021.

76. Mountjoy, M, Sundgot-Borgen, J, Burke, L, Ackerman, KE, Blauwet, C, Constantini, N, Lebrun, C, Lundy, B, Melin, A, Meyer, N, Sherman, R, Tenforde, AS, Torstveit, MK, and Budgett, R. International Olympic Committee (IOC) consensus statement on relative energy deficiency in sport (RED-S): 2018 update. *Int J Sport Nutr Exerc Metab* 28:316-331, 2018.

77. Neves, MP, da Conceição, CS, Lucareli, PRG, da Silva Barbosa, RS, Vieira, JPBC, de Lima Brasileiro, AJA, da Silva, GF, and Gomes-Neto, M. Effects of foot orthoses on pain and the prevention of lower limb injuries in runners: Systematic review and meta-analysis. *J Sport Rehabil* 31:1067-1074, 2022.

78. Parmar, A, Jones, TW, and Hayes R, P. The dose-response relationship between interval-training and VO2max in well-trained endurance runners: A systematic review. *J Sports Sci* 39:1410-1427, 2021.

79. Peterson, B, Hawke, F, Spink, M, Sadler, S, Hawes, M, Callister, R, and Chuter, V. Biomechanical and musculoskeletal measurements as risk factors for running-related injury in non-elite runners: A systematic review and meta-analysis of prospective studies. *Sport Med* 8:1-26, 2022.

80. Pethick, J, Winter, SL, and Burnley, M. Physiological evidence that the critical torque is a phase transition, not a threshold. *Med Sci Sport Exerc* 52:2390-2401, 2020.

81. Poole, DC, Burnley, M, Vanhatalo, A, Rossiter, HB, and Jones, AM. Critical power: An important fatigue threshold in exercise physiology. *Med Sci Sport Exerc* 48:2320-2334, 2016.

82. Ruiz-Alias, SA, Molina-Molina, A, Soto-Hermoso, VM, and García-Pinillos, F. A systematic review of the effect of running shoes on running economy, performance and biomechanics: Analysis by brand and model. *Sport Biomech* 22(3):388-409, 2023.

83. Salinero, JJ, Soriano, ML, Lara, B, Gallo-Salazar, C, Areces, F, Ruiz-Vicente, D, Abián-Vicén, J, González-Millán, C, and Del Coso, J. Predicting race time in male amateur marathon runners. *J Sports Med Phys Fitness* 57:1169-1177, 2017.

84. Sandford, GN, and Stellingwerff, T. "Question your categories": The misunderstood complexity of middle-distance running profiles with implications for research methods and application. *Front Sport Act Living* 1:28, 2019.

85. Scheer, V. Participation trends of ultra endurance events. *Sports Med Arthrosc* 27:3-7, 2019.

86. Scheer, V, Basset, P, Giovanelli, N, Vernillo, G, Millet, GP, and Costa, RJS. Defining off-road running: A position statement from the Ultra Sports Science Foundation. *Int J Sports Med* 41:275-284, 2020.

87. Scheer, V, and Krabak, BJ. Musculoskeletal injuries in ultra-endurance running: A scoping review. *Front Physiol* 12:664071, 2021.

88. Scheer, V, and Rojas-Valverde, D. Long-term health issues in ultraendurance runners: Should we be concerned? *BMJ Open Sport Exerc Med* 7:e001131, 2021.

89. Scheer, V, Tiller, NB, Doutreleau, S, Khodaee, M, Knechtle, B, Pasternak, A, and Rojas-Valverde D. Potential long-term health problems associated with ultra-endurance running: A narrative review. *Sport Med* 52:725-740, 2022.

90. Seiler, KS, and Kjerland, GØ. Quantifying training intensity distribution in elite endurance athletes: Is there evidence for an "'optimal'" distribution? *Scand J Med Sci Sport* 16:49-56, 2006.

91. Tiller, NB, Roberts, JD, Beasley, L, Chapman, S, Pinto, JM, Smith, L, Wiffin, M, Russell, M, Sparks, SA, Duckworth, L, O'Hara, J, Sutton, L, Antonio, J, Willoughby, DS, Tarpey, MD, Smith-Ryan, AE, Ormsbee, MJ, Astorino, TA, Kreider, RB, McGinnis, GR, Stout, JR, Smith, JW, Arent, SM, Campbell, BI, and Bannock L. International Society of Sports Nutrition Position Stand: Nutritional considerations for single-stage ultra-marathon training and racing. *J Int Soc Sports Nutr* 16:1-23, 2019.

92. Tjelta, LI. Three Norwegian brothers all European 1500 m champions: What is the secret? *Int J Sports Sci Coach* 14:694-700, 2019.

93. Vanhatalo, A, Black, MI, DiMenna, FJ, Blackwell, JR, Schmidt, JF, Thompson, C, Wylie, LJ, Mohr, M, Bangsbo, J, Krustrup, P, and Jones, AM. The mechanistic bases of the power-time relationship: Muscle metabolic responses and relationships to muscle fibre type. *J Physiol* 594:4407-4423, 2016.

94. Vanhatalo, A, Jones, AM, and Burnley, M. Application of critical power in sport. *Int J Sport Physiol Perform* 6:128-136, 2011.

95. Vernillo, G, Savoldelli, A, La Torre, A, Skafidas, S, Bortolan, L, and Schena, F. Injury and illness rates during ultratrail running. *Int J Sports Med* 37:565-569, 2016.

96. Weyand, PG, Lin, JE, and Bundle, MW. Sprint performance-duration relationships are set by the fractional duration of external force application. *Am J Physiol Regul Integr Comp Physiol* 290:R758-65, 2006.

97. Yeung, SS, Yeung, EW, and Gillespie, LD. Interventions for preventing lower limb soft-tissue running injuries. *Cochrane Database Syst Rev* 7:CD001256, 2011.

Chapter 9

1. Lucía, A, Hoyos, J, and Chicharro, JL. Preferred pedaling cadence in professional cycling. *Med Sci Sports Exerc* 33(8):1361-1366, 2001.

2. Allen, H, and A Coggan. *Training and Racing With a Power Meter.* Boulder, CO: VeloPress, 1-275, 2010.

3. Browning, R, and Sleamaker, R. *Serious Training for Endurance Athletes.* 2nd ed. Champaign, IL: Human Kinetics, 55-70, 1996.

4. Fornusek, C, and Davis, G. Maximizing muscle force via low cadence functional electrical stimulation cycling. *J Rehabil Med* 36:1-7, 2004.

5. Friel, J. *The Cyclist's Training Bible.* 3rd ed. Boulder, CO: VeloPress, 33-50, 2003.

6. Martino, M and Dabbs, N. Aerobic training program design. In *NSCA's Essentials of Personal Training.* Schoenfeld, B, and Snarr, R, eds. Champaign, IL: Human Kinetics, 98-120, 2021.

7. Pruitt, A, and Matheny, F. *Andy Pruitt's Complete Medical Guide for Cyclists.* Boulder, CO: VeloPress, 3-44, 2006.

8. Tanaka, H, Monahan, K, and Seals, D. Age-predicted maximal heart rate revisited. *J Amer Coll Cardiol* 37:153-156, 2001.

9. Trombley, A. *Serious Mountain Biking.* Champaign, IL: Human Kinetics, 3-183, 2005.

10. Valenzuela, P, Muriel, X, Van Erp, T, Mateo-March, M, Gandia-Soriano, A, Zabala, M, Lamberts, R, Lucia, A, Barranco-Gil, D, and Pallarés, J. The record power profile of male professional cyclists: Normative values obtained from a large database. *Int J Sports Physiol Perform* 17(5):701-710, 2022.

11. Wenzel, K, and Wenzel, R. *Bike Racing 101.* Champaign, IL: Human Kinetics, 165-203, 2003.

Chapter 10

1. Brooks, M. *Developing Swimmers.* Champaign, IL: Human Kinetics, 76, 2011.

2. Dekerle, J, Sidney, M, Hespel, JM, and Pelayo, P. Validity and reliability of critical speed, critical stroke rate, and anaerobic capacity in relation to front crawl swimming performances. *Int J Sports Med* 23:93-98, 2002.

3. Keys, M, Lyttle, A, Blanksby, B, Cheng, L, and Honda, K. Analyzing strokes using computational fluid dynamics. In *Science of Swimming Faster.* Riewald, S, and Rodeo, S, eds. Champaign, IL: Human Kinetics, 26-28, 30-31, 123-144, 2015.

4. Lynn, A. *Swimming: Technique, Training, Competition Strategy.* Marlborough, UK: Crowood Press, 77-82, 2006.

5. Maglischo, EW. *Swimming Fastest: The Essential Reference on Technique, Training, and Program Design.* Champaign, IL: Human Kinetics, 6, 113, 2003.

6. Newsome, P, and Young, A. *Swim Smooth: The Complete Coaching System for Swimmers and Triathletes.* West Sussex, UK: John Wiley & Sons, 173-181, 2012.

7. Sander, RH, and McCabe, CB. Freestyle technique. In *Science of Swimming Faster.* Riewald, S, and Rodeo, S, eds. Champaign, IL: Human Kinetics, 26-28, 2015.

8. Skiba, PF. *Scientific Training for Endurance Athletes.* Tinton Falls, NJ: PhysFarm Training Systems, 80-81, 2021.

9. Taormina, S. *Swim Speed Strokes.* Boulder, CO: Velo Press, 33, 39, 42, 45, 62-63, 2014.

10. USA Swimming. 2021 membership demographics report. April 2022. https://www.usaswimming.org/docs/default-source/governance/governance-lsc-website/membership-demographics/2021-membership-demographics-report.pdf?sfvrsn=80510b32_10.

11. USA Triathlon. Membership overview. January 2023. https://www.teamusa.org/usa-triathlon/membership-overview.

Chapter 11

1. Borges, NR, Driller, MW, and Overmayer, RG. Effects of rhythmic breathing on sprint and endurance swimming. *J Strength Cond Res* 29(1):39-45, 2015.

2. Burns, J, Keenan, AM, and Redmond, AC. Factors associated with triathlon-related overuse injuries. *J Orthop Sports Phys Ther* 33(4):177-84, 2003.

3. Cumming, J, Olphin, T, Law, M, and Hall, C. Exploring the relationships between mental skills usage and competitive anxiety responses in elite triathletes. *J Appl Sport Psychol* 18(2):108-120, 2006.

4. Fleck, SJ, and Kraemer, WJ. *Designing Resistance Training Programs.* 3rd ed. Champaign, IL: Human Kinetics, 91, 170, 2004.

5. French, D. Adaptations to anaerobic training programs. In *Essentials of Strength Training and Conditioning.* 4th ed. Haff, GG, and Triplett, NT, eds. Champaign, IL: Human Kinetics, 99, 2016.

6. Friel, J, and Vance, JS. *Triathlon Science.* Champaign, IL: Human Kinetics, 1-336, 2013

7. Haff, GG. Periodization. In *Essentials of Strength Training and Conditioning.* 4th ed. Haff, GG, and Triplett, NT, eds. Champaign, IL: Human Kinetics, 584, 2016.

8. Hays, KF, Thomas, O, and Maynard, I. Enhancing mental toughness and performance under pressure in elite young triathletes: A randomized controlled trial of dry-land-based reflective and video-based interventions. *J Imag Res Sport Phys Act* 12(1):1-14, 2017.

9. Herda, TJ, and Cramer, JT. Bioenergetics of exercise and training. In *Essentials of Strength Training and Conditioning.* 4th ed. Haff, GG, and Triplett, NT, eds. Champaign, IL: Human Kinetics, 59, 2016.

10. Kienstra, CM, Asken, TR, Garcia, JD, Lara, V, and Best, TM. Triathlon injuries: Transitioning from prevalence to prediction and prevention. *Curr Sports Med Rep* 16(6):397-403, 2017.

11. Lloyd, RS, and Faigenbaum, AD. Age- and sex-related differences and their implications for resistance exercise. In *Essentials of Strength Training and Conditioning.* 4th ed. Haff, GG, and Triplett, NT, eds. Champaign, IL: Human Kinetics, 146, 2016.

12. Martino, M, and Dabbs, NC. Aerobic training program design. In *NSCA's Essentials of Personal Training.* 3rd ed. Schoenfeld, BJ, and Snarr, RL, eds. Champaign, IL: Human Kinetics, 423, 2022.

13. Olbrecht, J. *The Science of Winning: Planning Periodizing and Optimizing Swim Training*. 2nd ed. Flanders, Belgium: F&G Partners, 6, 169, 173, 181, 186, 2007.

14. Peveler, W. *Triathlon Training Fundamentals: A Beginner's Guide to Essential Gear, Nutrition, and Training Schedules*. Guilford, CT: Lyons Press, 2014.

15. Reuter, BH, and Dawes, JJ. Program design and technique for aerobic endurance training. In *Essentials of Strength Training and Conditioning*. 4th ed. Haff, GG, and Triplett, NT, eds. Champaign, IL: Human Kinetics, 571-572, 2016.

16. Rittweger, J, di Prampero, PE, Maffulli, N, and Narici, MV. Sprint and endurance power and ageing: An analysis of master athletic world records. *Proc Biol Sci* 276(1657):683-689, 2009.

17. Sharp, MA, and Kilding, AE. Periodization for triathletes: Science and practical application. *Int J Sports Physiol Perform* 10(5):553-561, 2015.

18. Team USA triathlon. 2022 United States Olympic and Paralympic Committee. https://www.teamusa.org/USA-Triathlon/About/Multisport/Disciplines/Triathlon. Accessed March 12, 2023.

19. The Ironman story. www.ironman.com/history. Accessed March 12, 2023.

20. World triathlon history. November 2021. https://triathlon.org/about. Accessed March 12, 2023.

21. Zaccaro, A, Piarulli, A, Laurino, M, Garbella, E, Menicucci, D, Neri, B, and Gemignani, A. How breath-control can change your life: A systematic review on psycho-physiological correlates of slow breathing. *Front Hum Neurosci* 12:353, 2018.

Chapter 12

1. Baghurst, T, Prewitt, SL, and Tapps, T. Physiological demands of extreme obstacle course racing: A case study. *Int J Env Res Public Health* 16(16):2879, 2019.

2. Creagh, U, Reilly, T, and Nevill, AM. Heart rate response to "off-road" running events in female athletes. *Brit J Sport Med* 32(1):34-38, 1998.

3. Davis, MB. State of the Obstacle Racing Industry 2019. February 16, 2019. www.obstacleracingmedia.com/ocr-news/state-of-the-obstacle-racing-industry-2019/https://runrepeat.com/state-of-obstacle-course-racing-in-the-usa. Accessed March 2, 2023.

4. Laursen, P, and Buchheit, M. *Science and Application of High-Intensity Interval Training*. Champaign, IL: Human Kinetics, 2019.

5. Nikolova, V. Fun in the Mud—Trends in Obstacle Course Racing. August 6, 2021. https://runrepeat.com/state-of-obstacle-course-racing-in-the-usa. Accessed March 2, 2023.

6. World Obstacle. World OCR and Spartan Seek 1 M Participants for Virtual Race. May 26, 2020. www.worldobstacle.org/blog/world-ocr-and-spartan-seek-1-m-participants-for-virtual-racehttps://runrepeat.com/state-of-obstacle-course-racing-in-the-usa. Accessed March 2, 2023.

Chapter 13

1. Armstrong, LE. *Performing in Extreme Environments*. Champaign, IL: Human Kinetics, 2000.

2. Brown, F, Jeffries, O, Gissane, C, Howatson, G, van Someren, K, Pedlar, C, Myers, T, and Hill, JA. Custom-fitted compression garments enhance recovery from muscle damage in rugby players. *J Strength Cond Res* 36:212-219, 2022.

3. Crane, JD, Ogborn, DI, Cupido, C, Melov, S, Hubbard, A, Bourgeois, JM, and Tarnopolsky, MA. Massage therapy attenuates inflammatory signaling after exercise-induced muscle damage. *Sci Transl Med* 4:1-8, 2012.

4. de Glanville, KM, and Hamlin, MJ. Positive effect of lower body compression garments on subsequent 40-km cycling time trial performance. *J Strength Cond Res* 26:480-486, 2012.

5. French, D. Adaptations to anerobic training programs. In *Essentials of Strength Training and Conditioning*. 4th ed. Haff, GG, and Triplett, NT, eds. Champaign, IL: Human Kinetics, 108, 2015.

6. Gleeson, M. Immune function in sport and exercise. *J Appl Physiol* 103:693-699, 2007.

7. Herbert, RD, and Gabriel, M. Effects of stretching before and after exercising on muscle soreness and risk of injury: Systematic review. *Br Med J* 325:468-472, 2002.

8. Hilbert, JE, Sforzo, GA, and Swensen, T. The effects of massage on delayed onset muscle soreness. *Br J Sports Med* 37:72-75, 2003.

9. Hirshkowitz, M, Whiton, K, Albert, SM, Alessi, C, Bruni, O, DonCarlos, L, Hazen, N, Herman, J, Adams Hillard, PJ, Katz, ES, Kheirandish-Gozal, L, Neubauer, DN, O'Donnell, AE, Ohayon, M, Peever, J, Rawding, R, Sachdeva, RC, Setters, B, Vitiello, MV, and Ware, JC. National Sleep Foundation's updated sleep duration recommendations. *Sleep Health* 1:233-243, 2015.

10. Ivy, JL, Katz, AL, Cutler, CL, Sherman, WM, and Coyle, EF. Muscle glycogen synthesis after exercise: Effect of time of carbohydrate ingestion. *J Appl Physiol* 64:1480-1485, 1988.

11. Juliff, LE, Halson, SL, and Peiffer, JJ. Understanding sleep disturbance in athletes prior to important competitions. *J Sci Med Sport* 18:13-18, 2015.

12. Kellmann, M, and Kallus, KW. *Recovery-Stress Questionnaire for Athletes: User Manual.* Champaign, IL: Human Kinetics, 8, 2001.

13. Konrad, A, Glashüttner, C, Reiner, MM, Bernsteiner, D, and Tilp, M. The acute effects of a percussive massage treatment with a Hypervolt device on plantar flexor muscles' range of motion and performance. *J Sports Sci Med* 19:690-694, 2020.

14. Kreher, JB, and Schwartz, JB. Overtraining syndrome: A practical guide. *Sports Health* 4:128-138, 2012.

15. Macdonald, GZ, Button, DC, Drinkwater, EJ, and Behm, DG. Foam rolling as a recovery tool after an intense bout of physical activity. *Med Sci Sports Exerc* 46:131-142, 2014.

16. Malta, ES, Dutra, YM, Broatch, JR, Bishop, DJ, and Zagatto, AM. The effects of regular cold-water immersion use on training-induced changes in strength and endurance performance: A systematic review with meta-analysis. *Sports Med* 51:161-174, 2021.

17. Pearcey, GE, Bradbury-Squires, DJ, Kawamoto, JE, Drinkwater, EJ, Behm, DG, and Button, DC. Foam rolling for delayed-onset muscle soreness and recovery of dynamic performance measures. *J Athl Train* 50:5-13, 2015.

18. Sands, WA, McNeal, JR, Murray, SR, and Stone, MH. Dynamic compression enhances pressure-to-pain threshold in elite athlete recovery: Exploratory study. *J Strength Cond Res* 29:1263-1272, 2015.

19. Shirreffs, SM, and Sawka, MN. Fluid and electrolyte needs for training, competition, and recovery. *J Sports Sci* 29:S39-S46, 2011.

20. Shirreffs, SM, Taylor, AJ, Leiper, JB, and Maughan, RJ. Post-exercise rehydration in man: Effects of volume consumed and sodium content of ingested fluids. *Med Sci Sports Exerc* 28:1260-1271, 1996.

21. Sigel, B, Edelstein, AL, Savitch, L, Hasty, JH, and Felix, WR. Type of compression for reducing venous stasis: A study of lower extremities during inactive recumbency. *Arch Surg* 110:171-175, 1975.

22. Stepanski, EJ, and Wyatt, JK. Use of sleep hygiene in the treatment of insomnia. *Sleep Med Rev* 7:215-225, 2003.

23. Stone, MH, and Stone, ME. Recovery-adaptation: Strength and power sports. *Olympic Coach* 15:12-15, 2003.

24. Takahashi, Y, Kipnis, DM, and Daughaday, WH. Growth hormone secretion during sleep. *J Clin Invest* 47:2079-2090, 1968.

25. Vaile, J, Halson, S, Gill, N, and Dawson, B. Effect of hydrotherapy on recovery from fatigue. *Int J Sports Med* 29:539-544, 2008a.

26. Vaile, J, Halson, S, Gill, N, and Dawson, B. Effect of hydrotherapy on the signs and symptoms of delayed onset muscle soreness. *Eur J Appl Physiol* 102:447-455, 2008b.

27. Venter, RE. Perceptions of team athletes on the importance of recovery modalities. *Eur J Sport Sci* 14:S69-S76, 2014.

28. Waterhouse, J, Atkinson, G, Edwards, B, and Reilly, T. The role of a short post-lunch nap in improving cognitive, motor, and sprint performance in participants with partial sleep deprivation. *J Sports Sci* 25:1557-1566, 2007.

29. Werth, E, Dijk, DJ, Achermann, P, and Borbely, AA. Dynamics of the sleep EEG after an early evening nap: Experimental data and simulations. *Am J Physiol Regul Integr Comp Physiol* 271:R501-R510, 1996.

30. Wilcock, IM, Cronin, JB, and Hing, WA. Physiological response to water immersion: A method for sport recovery? *Sports Med* 36:747-765, 2006.

31. Yoshimura, A, Inami, T, Schleip, R, Mineta, S, Shudo, K, and Hirose, N. Effects of self-myofascial release using a foam roller on range of motion and morphological changes in muscle: A crossover study. *J Strength Cond Res* 35: 2444-2450, 2021.

Index

Note: The italicized *f* and *t* following page numbers refer to figures and tables, respectively.

About the NSCA

The **National Strength and Conditioning Association (NSCA)** is the world's leading organization in the field of sport conditioning. Drawing on the resources and expertise of the most recognized professionals in strength training and conditioning, sport science, performance research, education, and sports medicine, the NSCA is the world's trusted source of knowledge and training guidelines for coaches and athletes. The NSCA provides the crucial link between the lab and the field.

About the Editor

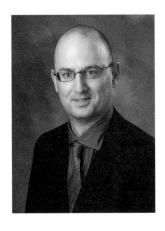

Ben Reuter, PhD, CSCS,*D, ATC, is an associate professor in the department of exercise, health, and sport science at PennWest University–California. He earned his doctorate in exercise physiology from Auburn University and his master's degree, with an emphasis on athletic training, from Old Dominion University. He has been a member of the NSCA since 1988 and was the 2020 NSCA Sports Medicine and Rehabilitation Professional of the Year.

Reuter is an associate editor for the *Strength and Conditioning Journal*, a journal of the NSCA. His research interests include injury prevention and performance enhancement for age-group endurance athletes. He has authored or coauthored chapters in several NSCA Essentials textbooks, and he also served as editor for the first edition of *Developing Endurance*.

About the Contributors

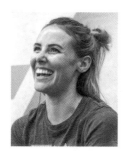

Kate Baldwin, PhD, is a sport scientist and physiotherapist with over 10 years of experience working with endurance athletes. She is the owner of Valere Endurance and Endurance Movement, both of which promote and encourage strength training in endurance athletes. She has worked with multiple professional triathletes and runners and is also a lecturer at the University of Notre Dame in Australia. Her PhD dissertation examined the effects of strength training on performance in long-distance triathletes.

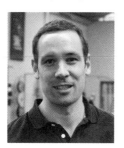

Richard C. Blagrove, PhD, ASCC, CSCS, is a senior lecturer in physiology and the leader of the master's strength and conditioning program at Loughborough University. Richard is accredited by the United Kingdom Strength and Conditioning Association (UKSCA) as a strength and conditioning coach and is certified by the NSCA as a strength and conditioning specialist. He has provided coaching support for 15 years to endurance runners, including Olympians and athletes who have won medals at major international championships. Blagrove's current research investigates issues relating to performance and health in endurance runners, including physiological determinants of performance, the use of strength-based exercise, prevention of injury, and recovery from relative energy deficiency in sport syndrome.

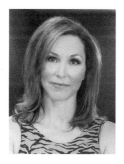

Rachel Cosgrove, CSCS, co-owns and operates Results Fitness, a fitness center in Southern California that was voted one of the top 10 gyms in the United States by *Men's Health* magazine. Cosgrove earned her bachelor's degree in physiology from the University of California–Santa Barbara and holds the Certified Strength and Conditioning Specialist credential from the NSCA. In 2012 Cosgrove was named IDEA Personal Trainer of the Year. An athlete herself, Cosgrove is an Ironman triathlete and obstacle course racer. Extremely goal-oriented, she is always looking for a new physical challenge, and she draws on these experiences to make her a better coach.

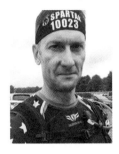

Roger Earle, MA, CSCS,*D, NSCA-CPT,*D, RSCC*D, has over 35 years of experience as a sport performance coach and behavior modification facilitator for all ages and fitness levels. He is a coauthor, coeditor, or contributor for 10 fitness and resistance training books, including *Essentials of Strength Training and Conditioning, Weight Training: Steps to Success,* and *Fitness Weight Training.* Earle competes in obstacle course racing and has over 40 top-five placings in his open age group in Spartan races. He began racing in 2013 and has qualified for the OCR World Championships each year since 2015. Earle is a brand ambassador for MudGear and Honey Stinger.

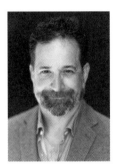

G. Gregory Haff, PhD, CSCS,*D, ASCC, ASCA L2, FNSCA, is a professor of strength and conditioning at Edith Cowan University. He is the author of the *Scientific Foundations and Practical Applications of Periodization* and the coeditor of *Essentials of Strength Training and Conditioning.* He is a past president of the NSCA, holds the Certified Strength and Conditioning Specialist With Distinction credential from NSCA, is accredited by the United Kingdom Strength and Conditioning Association (UKSCA) as a strength and conditioning coach, and is accredited by the Australian Strength and Conditioning Association (ASCA) as a Level 2 Strength and Conditioning Coach. He is a Level 3 Weightlifting Coach in both Australia and the United States. Haff was awarded the NSCA's Impact Award in 2021 in recognition of the impact of his research, teaching, and service to the strength and conditioning profession. In 2014, the UKSCA recognized him as the Strength and Conditioning Coach of the Year for Education and Research for the impact of his work. He was the 2011 winner of NSCA's William J. Kraemer Outstanding Sport Scientist Award.

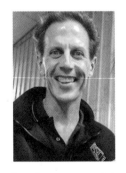

Dave Joensen, MA, MS, ASCA, is a swim coach with over 38 years of swim coaching experience. He is certified by the Australian Strength and Conditioning Association (ASCA) as a Level 4 Coach. He has coached multiple junior national, national, and Olympic Trial qualifiers. He has had swimmers invited to USA Swimming's National Select Camp and their National Diversity Camp. Joensen has been on the coaching staff of the USA Swimming Central Zone Select Camp and the USA Swimming National Select Camp. He has been named Iowa Coach of the Year on three occasions. Joensen has degrees in food science and nutrition, exercise science, and coaching. He has also been the coauthor of several research articles.

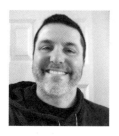

Will Kirousis, MS, CSCS, has coached endurance athletes for over 25 years. Kirousis has also written for various popular press sources and professional organizations, and he has presented on coach education and athlete development for USA Triathlon, NSCA, USA Cycling, and other organizations. Kirousis has been fortunate to help athletes achieve various goals, from finishing their first race to winning age-group world championships or professional national championships. Kirousis can be reached at will@tri-hard.com or @willkirousis.

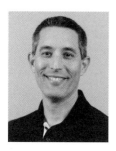

Joshua Miller, DHSc, CSCS, ACSM-EP, ISAK-2, is the director of undergraduate studies at the University of Illinois at Chicago and is a clinical associate professor in the department of kinesiology and nutrition. He is currently teaching undergraduate and graduate students in the area of exercise physiology. Additionally, Miller has worked in various areas of the exercise physiology field, including working with elite endurance athletes and active duty military personnel. Miller has coauthored more than 20 peer-reviewed journal articles, has coauthored book chapters, and recently coauthored a book on strength and conditioning.

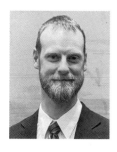

Michael Naperalsky, MS, MSCC, RSCC*D, has over 15 years of experience in athletic development and performance management. Currently an assistant director of sport performance at the University of Louisville, Michael oversees three teams and teaches graduate courses in the department of health and sport sciences. He previously worked as a senior strength and conditioning coach with the U.S. Ski and Snowboard Association, where he helped athletes win 3 Olympic medals, 6 World Championship medals, 16 X Games medals, and 93 World Cup podiums. Michael earned a master's degree in health and human performance, and he holds certifications from NSCA, Collegiate Strength and Conditioning Coaches Association (CSCCa), USA Weightlifting (USAW), and American College of Sports Medicine (ACSM).

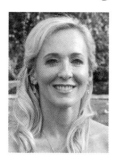

Krista Schultz, MEd, CSCS, CPT, is a former elite triathlete with over two decades of experience in the health and fitness industry. Her athletic journey began as a Division I track and cross country runner at the University of New Orleans before transitioning to triathlon, where she competed in events such as the Ironman Triathlon World Championship in Kona, Hawaii. Schultz's athletic background serves as the foundation for her role as a health and fitness consultant, leveraging her expertise to optimize sport performance and holistic well-being for her clients. With a diverse professional background that includes roles in physical therapy, strength and conditioning coaching, and medical product education management, Schultz is uniquely positioned to deliver personalized fitness training to clients of all levels. She holds a master of education degree in athletic administration and a bachelor of science degree in exercise physiology. She holds the Certified Strength and Conditioning Specialist credential from the NSCA. Krista is passionate about empowering individuals to achieve their health and fitness goals, drawing inspiration from her upbringing and family background in medicine.

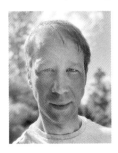

Mike Schultz, CSCS, NSCA-CPT, is the head coach and founder of Highland Training, and he has more than 20 years of racing, coaching, and training experience from endurance and ultraendurance events. Schultz has coached and provided consulting services to more than 400 athletes over the years, and he currently works with a wide range of cyclists. Schultz has a passion for cycling and gaining strength on the bike. He chased ultraendurance mountain bike 24-hour solo podiums throughout the 2000s, followed by 100-mile off-road races and multiple-day bike pack events over the past 12 years.

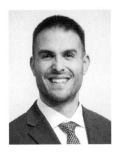

Antonio Squillante, PhD, CSCS,*D, RSCC*D, SENr, is the head of sport performance and training at USA Cycling's Track Sprint Program. He graduated summa cum laude with a bachelor's degree in physical education from the Università San Raffaele in Rome, Italy. Antonio earned a master of science degree in sport performance and orthopedic rehabilitation from A.T. Still University and a master of science degree in biokinesiology from the University of Southern California. He is currently conducting research at the Clinical Exercise Research Center in the department of biokinesiology and physical therapy at University of Southern California in Los Angeles. Squillante is a faculty member at California State University at Long Beach and is a member of the NSCA board of directors. Squillante holds the Registered Sport and Exercise Nutritionist credential.

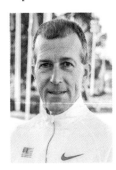

Randy Wilber, PhD, FACSM, is a senior sport physiologist for the United States Olympic and Paralympic Committee (USOPC). In that position, he works closely with Team USA athletes and coaches in the areas of altitude training, heat and humidity acclimatization, blood chemistry analysis, overtraining, international air travel and jet lag, and environment-induced asthma. Wilber has been a member of the official delegation of Team USA at six Summer Olympics (Athens 2004, Beijing 2008, London 2012, Rio de Janeiro 2016, Tokyo 2020, and Paris 2024), six Winter Olympics (Salt Lake City 2002, Torino 2006, Vancouver 2010, Sochi 2014, PyeongChang 2018, and Beijing 2022), two Pan American Games (Santo Domingo 2003 and Rio de Janeiro 2007), and multiple world championships.

Contributors to the Previous Edition

Stephanie Burgess, BS

Denny DePriest, RSCC

Jason Gootman, MS, CSCS

G. Gregory Haff, PhD, CSCS,*D, ASCC, ASCA L2, FNSCA

Neal Henderson, MS, CSCS

Will Kirousis, CSCS

Peter Melanson, MS, CSCS,*D, RSCC*D

Bob Seebohar, MS, RD, CSSD, CSCS

Suzie Snyder, MS, CSCS

Randy Wilber, PhD, FACSM

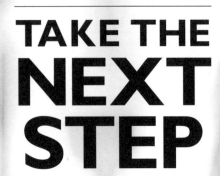